Immunological Aspects of Oral Diseases

IMMUNOLOGY AND MEDICINE SERIES

IMMUNOLOGY
· SERIES · SERIES · SERIES · SERIES **AND** SERIES · SERIES · SERIES · SERIES ·
MEDICINE

Immunological Aspects of Oral Diseases

Edited by
L. Ivanyi
Department of Clinical Pathology and Immunology,
Institute of Dental Surgery,
Eastman Dental Hospital, London

Series Editor: Professor W. G. Reeves

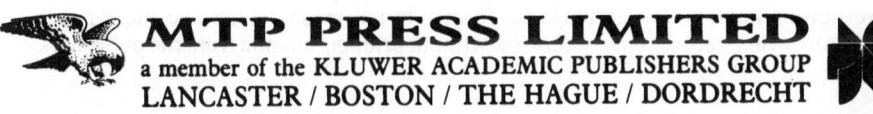

MTP PRESS LIMITED
a member of the KLUWER ACADEMIC PUBLISHERS GROUP
LANCASTER / BOSTON / THE HAGUE / DORDRECHT

Published in the UK and Europe by
MTP Press Limited
Falcon House
Lancaster, England

British Library Cataloguing in Publication Data

Immunological aspects of oral disease. —
    (Immunology and medicine series)
    1. Mouth — Diseases — Immunological aspects
    I. Ivanyi, L.   II. Series
    616.3'1079   RC815

ISBN-13: 978-94-010-8350-8   e-ISBN-13: 978-94-009-4167-0
DOI: 10.1007/978-94-009-4167-0

Published in the USA by
MTP Press
A division of Kluwer Academic Publishers
101 Philip Drive
Norwell, MA 02061, USA

Library of Congress Cataloging-in-Publication Data

Immunological aspects of oral diseases.

    (Immunology and medicine series)
    Includes bibliographies and index.
    1. Mouth — Diseases — Immunological aspects
I. Ivanyi, L. (Ludmila), 1936–   . II. Series.
[DNLM: 1. Mouth Diseases — immunology. 2. Oral
Manifestations — immunology. 3. Tooth Diseases —
immunology. WU 140 I33]
RC815.I46   1986   616.3'1079   86-18536

Typeset in Times and Helvetica by David John (Services) Ltd, Maidenhead, UK

Contents

Foreword

Progress in medical sciences over the past two decades has witnessed great advances in immunology. The demonstration of immunoglobulin structure, complement cascade and monoclonal antibodies are only some of the milestones in humoral immunity. The cellular basis of immune responses, with phenotypic and functional definition of subsets of immunoregulatory T cells, B cells and accessory cells, have generated a wealth of new concepts in the pathogenesis of many diseases. The discovery that the major histocompatibility antigens are esssential in genetic restriction and in antigen presentation has placed immunogenetics in the centre of investigations of a great number of diseases. Molecular immunology has been the most recent advance which almost solved one of the greatest dilemmas in immunology, namely the nature of the T cell receptor. Diagnostic medicine has also benefited greatly from the specificity and sensitivity of antibody dependent assays such as radioimmunoassay.

Oral diseases are no exception to the benefits bestowed by immunology. Indeed, the subject is now taught both at the undergraduate and postgraduate levels. This new book brings together experts in oral immunology and presents concepts and knowledge in this specialized area. The remarkable point is that immunology has taken the centre stage in our understanding not only of two of the most common dental diseases, periodontal disease and caries, but also of mucosal conditions, such as recurrent oral ulceration.

The demand for information in oral immunology is considerable and this volume should fulfil the objectives of presenting the subject to those who wish to improve their understanding of the aetiology, pathogenesis, treatment and prophylaxis of a large number of oral diseases.

T. Lehner MD, MB, BDS, FDS, FRCPath
Professor of Oral Immunology
Head of Department of Immunology
United Medical and Dental Schools of Guy's
and St Thomas (Guy's Campus), London

Series Editor's Note

The modern clinician is expected to be the fount of all wisdom concerning conventional diagnosis and management relevant to his sphere of practice. In addition, he or she has the daunting task of comprehending and keeping pace with advances in basic science relevant to the pathogenesis of disease and ways in which these processes can be regulated or prevented. Immunology has grown from the era of anti-toxins and serum sickness to a state where the study of many diverse cells and molecules has become integrated into a coherent scientific discipline with major implications for many common and crippling diseases prevalent throughout the world.

Many of today's practitioners received little or no specific training in immunology and what was taught is very likely to have been overtaken by subsequent developments. This series of titles on IMMUNOLOGY AND MEDICINE is designed to rectify this deficiency in the form of distilled packages of information which the busy clinician, pathologist or other health care professional will be able to open and enjoy.

Professor W. G. Reeves, FRCP, FRCPath
Department of Immunology
University Hospital, Queen's Medical Centre
Nottingham

List of Contributors

S.J. CHALLACOMBE
Department of Oral Immunology
and Microbiology
United Medical and Dental
Schools
Guy's Hospital
London SE1 9RT
UK

A.E. DOLBY
Department of Peridontology
University of Wales
College of Medicine
Heath Park
Cardiff CF4 4XN
UK

M.M. FERGUSON
Department of Oral Medicine
and Oral Surgery
School of Dentistry
University of Otago
PO Box 647
Dunedin
NEW ZEALAND

J.J.H. GILKES
Department of Oral Medicine
Institute of Dental Surgery
University of London
Eastman Dental Hospital
256 Gray's Inn Road
London WC1X 8LD
UK

L. IVANYI
Department of Clinical Pathology
and Immunology
Institute of Dental Surgery
Eastman Dental Hospital
256 Gray's Inn Road
London WC1 8LD
UK

P.-J. LAMEY
Department of Oral Medicine
and Pathology
Glasgow Dental Hospital and
School
378 Sauchiehall Street
Glasgow G2 3JZ
UK

K.W. LEE
Department of Oral Pathology
Institute of Dental Surgery
Eastman Dental hospital
Gray's Inn Road
London WC1 8LD
UK

E.E. MACFADYEN
Department of Oral Medicine
and Pathology
Dental Hospital and School
378 Sauchiehall Street
Glasgow G2 3JZ
UK

P.D. MARSH
Bacterial Metabolism Research
Laboratory
PHLS Centre for Applied
Microbiology and Research
Porton Down, Salisbury SP4 1JG
UK

F.F. NALLY
Department of Oral Medicine
Institute of Dental Surgery
University of London
Eastman Dental hospital
256 Gray's Inn Road
London WC1X 8LD
UK

H. NEWMAN
Department of Periodontology
Institute of Dental Surgery
Eastman Dental Hospital
256 Gray's Inn Road
London WC1X 8LD
UK

S.R. PORTER
University Department of Oral
  Medicine and Oral Surgery
Bristol Dental Hospital and School
Lower Maudlin Street
Bristol BS1 2LY
UK

W.D. ROBERTSON
Department of Oral Medicine and
  Oral Pathology
University of Edinburgh
Old Surgeons Hall
High School Yards
Edinburgh EH1 1NR
UK

C. SCULLY
University Department of Oral
  Medicine and Oral Surgery
Bristol Dental Hospital and School
Lower Maudlin Street
Bristol BS1 2LY
UK

J.C. SOUTHAM
Department of Oral Medicine
  and Oral Pathology
University of Edinburgh
Old Surgeons Hall
High School Yards
Edinburgh EH1 1NR
UK

D.M. WALKER
Department of Oral Medicine
  and Oral Pathology
Dental School, University of Wales
College of Medicine
Heath Park
Cardiff, CF4 4XY
UK

D.M. WILLIAMS
Department of Oral Pathology
London Hospital Medical College
Turner Street
London E1 2AD
UK

D. WRAY
Department of Oral Medicine
  and Oral Pathology
School of Dental Surgery
Chambers Street
Edinburgh EH1 1JA
UK

1
The Host Defence System of the Mouth

A. E. DOLBY

THE BARRIERS OF THE ORAL MUCOSA

The most effective way of isolating the host from potentially harmful agents would be by the establishment of a completely impermeable barrier. In the case of the mouth this problem is in fact dealt with in a number of ways; partly through the creation of a series of physicochemical barriers and partly through specific and non-specific humoral and cellular barriers within and on the mucosa. In addition, the resident flora afford some protection to the host; they may prevent colonization by pathogens through the phenomenon of 'bacterial interference'. How this mechanism works is not clear, but it may involve competition for sites on the host cells, for nutrients or mutual inhibition by toxic products. The first of the barriers provided by the host is saliva (see Figure 1.1).

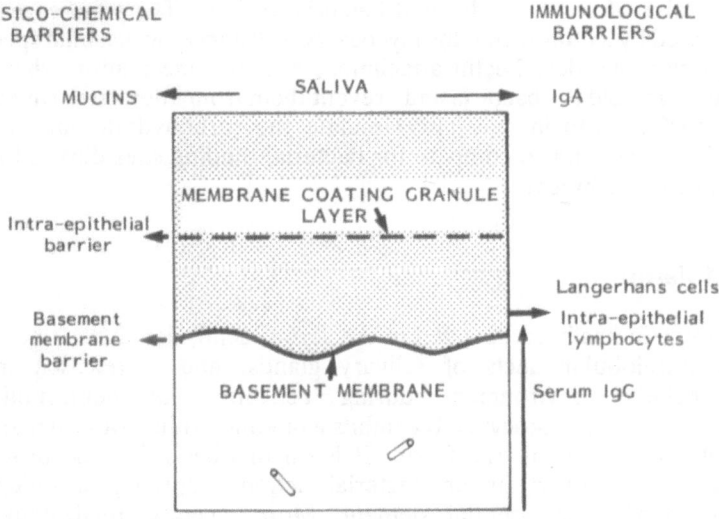

Figure 1.1

1

THE PHYSICOCHEMICAL BARRIERS

Saliva as a protective barrier

The mouth is bathed in saliva, secreted by both major and minor salivary glands, and organisms trapped within the saliva are transported to the hostile environment of the stomach. Attachment and colonization of the mouth by organisms occurs nonetheless. Several constituents of saliva are non-specifically protective: mucin, lactoferrin, lysozyme and lacto-peroxidase.

Antibacterial role of mucin

Other, protective constituents of saliva also rely to some extent upon mucin for their action. For example, lysozyme, which is a basic protein, is strongly associated with the sialic acid portion of mucin and is therefore presented to bacteria entrapped by the mucin. Secretory immunoglobulin A (IgA) appears to interact with mucin. Human IgA contains a large number of oligosaccharides linked to the protein core in the 'hinge' region of the molecule where the Fc (non-antigen-binding) portion is linked to the Fab (antigen-binding) portions. This and other structural peculiarities of IgA have led to the suggestion that IgA and mucins form a complex with the antibody combining site of the Ig protruding from the surface. In this way bacteria are made 'mucophilic' and retained within the mucus layer through antigen–antibody interaction. Non-immune mechanisms of bacterial clearance by mucin appear to depend upon the presence of the oligosaccharide side-chains as well as the protein core. Bacteria possess an interlacing polysaccharide coat or glycocalyx, and can adhere to the glycocalyx of another cell, be it bacterial or host. The adherence is often mediated by lectins within the glycocalyx, substances which bind specifically to polysaccharides. Lectin attachment is also a mechanism whereby the mucin can hold the bacteria and prevent them from interacting with the host cell surface. Mucin may also simulate the carbohydrate surface of the epithelial cell and so compete for bacterial binding sites directed towards host cell attachment.

Lactoferrin

Lactoferrin has been detected in the serous acini, demilunes, intercalated and intralobular ducts of salivary glands, and is released into the extracellular environment during activation of neutrophil poly-morphonuclear leukocytes. It exhibits a binding avidity for iron many times greater than that of transferrin. It is on this basis that the protein was presumed to exert its antibacterial action, depriving iron-dependent bacteria of their essential element. More recently, realization of the importance of the superoxide species in bacterial killing by phagocytic cells, and the fact that the production of the hydroxyl radical (OH·) could be catalysed by iron, led to the suggestion that lactoferrin acted as an iron-bearing catalyst in the modified Haber–Weiss reaction where hydrogen peroxide is reduced by reduced molecular oxygen (O_2^-). However, since lactoferrin is not fully saturated, it would function best at sites of infection. Levels of lactoferrin are raised where there is inflammation in the gut and the gingival sulcus is one example of a site where this occurs.

Mucus is subject to oxidative degradation, a reaction in which iron or copper can serve as a catalyst. Thus lactoferrin probably acts also as an inhibitor of this degradation, helping to maintain the rheological properties of saliva.

Lysozyme

Lysozyme is a cationic protein with the enzymic potential (muramidase) of hydrolysing bacterial cell wall peptidoglycan. Its origin is primarily from the salivary glands where it is present, in soluble and free form, in the acinar and intralobular ducts. It is found also in macrophages and neutrophils; since these cells are also present in gingival sulcus fluid they will contribute to the salivary lysozyme via this route.

In its muramidase capacity the enzyme may play a role in combating *Streptococcus mutans*, either by lysis of the bacterial cell wall or by disaggregation of the chains of streptococci with subsequent reduction in growth potential.

In addition lysozyme, since it is a cationic protein, can act as an aggregating agent and again lead to autolysis of bacteria. In this role lysozyme is not inactivated by competitive inhibitors of the enzyme muramidase, and Gram-negative organisms have been lysed in *in vitro* studies.

Lactoperoxidase

The lactoperoxidase of saliva oxidizes thiocyanate ions, in the presence of hydrogen peroxide, to intermediate toxic products such as hypothiocyanate. Gram-negative bacteria seem to be more susceptible; they may actually be killed while Gram-positive organisms are only slowed in their growth. The presence or absence of catalase ($2H_2O_2 \rightleftharpoons H_2O_2 + O_2$) in bacteria is important, since the H_2O_2 is a rate-limiting factor in the production of the toxic oxidized thiocyanates.

The two physicochemical barriers of the oral epithelium

Studies of oral mucosal permeability have included the buccal absorption test, in which materials are applied which may elicit a response in the underlying tissue; *in vitro* systems with mucosal epithelium suspended in a diffusion cell; and tracer studies involving lanthanum (electrodense for electron microscopy) or horseradish peroxidase (demonstrable by histochemistry). Passage of materials from below appears to be hindered at a level which at the first, intra-epithelial barrier, corresponds to the site of discharge of the membrane coating granules into the extracellular space during maturation of the epithelial cells. Membrane coating granules, in keratinizing oral epithelium, are membrane-bound, elongated structures containing a series of parallel lamellae. They are composed mainly of phospholipid and appear to play a role in the formation of a water barrier. Non-keratinizing oral epithelial membrane coating granules are circular with a dense non-lamellar central core. Both types of granules appear to fuse with the cell membrane and discharge their contents into the extracellular space. Membrane coating granules are not present in the epithelium of the gingival attachment.

The second barrier is that of the basement membrane; here large molecules are impeded, for example antigen–antibody complexes will not pass through. In inflammation the efficiency is reduced and larger molecules can pass through.

THE CELLULAR BARRIER

Inter-epithelial lymphocytes

These occur singly and in clusters; they are capable of migrating into and out of epithelium. Even germ-free animals possess these inter-epithelial lymphocytes which do not increase in number on antigen challenge. Some of the cells possess the cell surface markers of helper and suppressor/cytotoxic T cells; others are presumably B cells since they are not completely absent even in the athymic nude mouse oral mucosa. These cells may have a variety of roles: in the intestine inter-epithelial lymphocytes have been shown to function as natural killer cells, to participate in antibody-dependent cell mediated cytotoxicity and to proliferate in response to non-specific mitogens and alloantigens. However, inter-epithelial lymphocytes in the intestine increase in number with inflammation; for example in coeliac disease the inter-epithelial lymphocytes may outnumber the enterocytes. Unlike oral mucosa, the conversion of a germ-free animal to normal does lead to an increase in the number of intestinal inter-epithelial lymphocytes. The intestine therefore appears to behave like a secondary lymphoid organ, whereas the oral mucosa lymphoid cells constitute a primary lymphoid organ. One other possible role of the inter-epithelial lymphocytes is that of the control of the Langerhans cells.

Langerhans cells

These are dendritic inter-epithelial cells which possess adenosine triphosphate, cell surface glycoproteins which have been linked to the

4

immune response (Ia antigens) and receptors for the functional non-antigen combining portion of immunoglobulin (Fc receptors) and for the third component of complement (C3). They therefore have several features of macrophages and are thought to fill this role, processing antigen at an intra-epithelial site. Unlike inter-epithelial lymphocytes Langerhans cells do increase in number with inflammation; in human gingival epithelium when oral hygiene is withdrawn and in the oral mucosa of germ-free animals exposed to conventional surroundings. As with inter-epithelial lymphocytes, Langerhans cells are found in normal uninflamed mucosa. Presumably they process antigen which is transported to the lymph nodes to evoke a response in resting lymphocytes. The Langerhans cells, like the other macrophages, produce variable amounts of interleukin-I, a non-antigen-specific factor that augments lymphocyte reactions by activating T helper cells. Keratinocytes can also produce interleukin-I, the summation of the two soluble mediators from Langerhans cells and keratinocytes has been termed epidermal cell-derived thymocyte-activating factor or ETAF, which has been detected in gingival sulcus fluid. The thymocytes referred to in the acronym are mouse thymocytes which are used in assays of interleukin-I.

Antigen processing and major histocompatibility antigens

Antigen is apparently presented to the lymphocyte as a package composed also of the Class II major histocompatibility (MHC) antigens of the Langerhans cell – the Ia (or immune response associated) antigens referred to above. Experiments *in vitro* have shown that antigens which require T cell cooperation for antibody production are processed most effectively when there is matching of the Class II MHC antigens of the macrophage and the lymphocyte. The importance of this rather complex restriction in antigen presentation probably lies in the resistance to autoimmunity it induces, since only cells with Class II MHC antigens can effectively present antigen to the lymphocytes. Interestingly, other cells which do not normally display Class II MHC antigens can be persuaded to do so, by, for example, γ interferon. Even keratinocytes can display Class II MHC antigens under the influence of interferon, so that the potential for autoimmune responses is then increased.

The Langerhans cell is also required in the processing of cell surface associated antigens, for example *in vitro* studies using unmatched epidermal cells have revealed that Langerhans cells are necessary for the generation of cell-mediated cytotoxic reactions occurring against such epidermal cells.

Distribution of Langerhans cells

The Langerhans cells are distributed unevenly throughout the mouth. Keratinized oral mucosa has fewer Langerhans cells than skin; the number within the oral mucosa appears to vary inversely with the degree of keratinization. Thus in the hard palate and dorsal tongue there are areas

5

with no Langerhans cells. This uneven distribution may give a clue to the role of the oral mucosa in sensitization of the host as there is a parallel between the absence of Langerhans cells from some sites of the oral mucosa and from rodent tail skin. Tolerance, rather than hypersensitivity, to the sensitizer dinitrofluorobenzene is induced by painting the Langerhans cell devoid tail skin of the rodent.

Langerhans cells in skin can be reduced by adhesive tape stripping, ultraviolet irradiation and topical corticosteroid therapy. Although ultraviolet irradiation is limited, orally, to the lips, topical corticosteroid application does have relevance to oral mucosa. It should be remembered that topical corticosteroid therapy influences this afferent limb of the immune response in addition to other anti-inflammatory effects.

The cells of the gingival sulcus

Gingival crevice fluid contains desquamating epithelial cells from the oral sulcular epithelium and leukocytes. The gingival sulcus is in fact the major route for the passage of leukocytes into the oral cavity. Of these leukocytes 95–97% are neutrophils, 1–2% lymphocytes and 2–3% monocytes and of the lymphocytes, the ratio of T cells to B cells is 1 : 2.7. Studies of labelled leukocytes show that they migrate from blood into the gingival sulcular fluid. The number of leukocytes entering the mouth from the gingival sulcus is often thought to be very large. In the presence of gingival or periodontal disease this is indeed the case, but in health the number of leukocytes entering the mouth by this route is remarkably small. Examination by *in vitro* methods, of the functional capacity of the cells, reveals that the neutrophils retain their phagocytic function, albeit at a lower level than those of peripheral blood.

Phagocytosis by the gingival sulcus leukocytes

When a foreign particle is deposited in the gingival sulcus, it may be coated with specific host protein such as immunoglobulin (Ig) or complement. These proteins, defined as opsonins, facilitate ingestion of the particle by the phagocytic cell through binding to specific receptors on the phagocytic cell surface (Fc receptor, complement receptor). The engulfed particles are internalized within cytoplasmic vacuoles which, with the fusion of enzyme-rich lysosomal granules, forms the phagolysosome. The process of fusion is known as degranulation. These lysosomal enzymes may also be released to the exterior under certain circumstances and B glucuronidase and elastase, for example, have been detected in gingival sulcus fluid.

The oxidase system of phagocytosis

Initiation of the phagocytosis is accompanied by a cellular 'respiratory burst' characterized by an increase in oxygen consumption (2–20-fold background) and generation of reactive oxygen derived radicals (superoxide anion O_2^-, HO_2). These may also be released into the gingival sulcus. Other materials such as Ig or immune complex may initiate the respiratory burst. Two molecules of O_2^- react to form H_2O_2, a reaction catalysed by superoxide dismutase. The highly reactive oxygen-derived metabolites which are produced include hydroxyl radical, singlet oxygen and hypochlorous acid. Singlet oxygen is very unstable and will readily interact with other molecules. This return to the more stable form of molecular oxygen is accompanied by the release of energy leading to light emission which may be measured, and is interpreted as a measure of phagocytic activation.

The role of the leukocyte myeloperoxidase

Both neutrophil and macrophage myeloperoxidase will react with hydrogen peroxide in the presence of a halide (the chloride ion is abundant in tissue fluid and transudates) to form highly reactive toxic substances such as hypochlorous acid. Individuals lacking the myeloperoxidase system are not unusually susceptible to recurrent infections, whereas subjects with a deficient oxidase system (chronic granulomatous disease) do experience severe and recurrent infections including oral mucosal ulcerations.

Damage to the host by the leukocyte defence mechanisms

During the phagocytic process, and in other methods of neutrophil activation, the antibacterial substances released are capable of damaging host cells. The host is protected from the action of the lysosomal enzymes released by phagocytic cells by enzyme inhibitors such as the α_2-macroglobulin and α_1-antitrypsin of gingival sulcus fluid. The oxidase system is counterbalanced by superoxide dismutase which converts the superoxide anion to hydrogen peroxide, and catalase which deals with the hydrogen peroxide. The selenium-dependent enzyme glutathione peroxidase works at lower concentrations of H_2O_2 and may therefore be more important than catalase. Finally, and perhaps not unexpectedly, some bacteria found in the gingival sulcus also provide superoxide dismutase.

THE BARRIER PROVIDED BY IMMUNOGLOBULIN

The immunological barrier of oral mucosa: immunoglobulin in the epithelium

Immunoglobulin (Ig) may be present in the oral mucosal epithelium in a free or bound form. Free Ig represents the Ig of serum and tissue fluid and can be removed by prolonged washing of the tissue prior to histological examination. Bound Ig is that which cannot be removed by such washing; in reaction with antigen it may form insoluble complexes that are trapped

7

within the tissue, probably also bound, by the Fc portion (the non-antigen binding part) of the antibody to Fc receptors on the surface of phagocytic cells.

Normal oral mucosa contains free Ig, which can be detected within the intercellular spaces of the lower two-thirds of the mucosal epithelium. IgG and IgA are found most commonly and are most pronounced at the junction of the outer one-third and inner two-thirds of the epithelium. This is the area where the physicochemical permeability barrier is also sited. In inflamed oral mucosa inter-epithelial IgM and fibrinogen are also detectable, an indication of the loss of the molecular sieving effect of the normal basement membrane. Pooling of Ig within the epithelium may explain the eosinophilic bodies which are observed there. Thus a protective barrier of Ig lies within the epithelium: IgA which should lead to 'quiet' elimination of the antigen or IgG which would lead to an inflammatory response.

Immunoglobulins of the oral cavity: gingival sulcus fluid

IgG, IgM and IgA are all present in gingival sulcus fluid but at levels lower than those found in serum. The third component of complement is also found and may explain the presence of ghosts of bacterial cells found at the apical border of dental plaque. This functional role of immunoglobulin and complement in the gingival sulcus appears to be limited by the fact that only approximately 20% of the total IgG and IgA in dental plaque is specific for bacterial antigen found within the plaque. Activation of the classical complement pathway appears to occur to a small extent in the normal gingival sulcus; both the classical and alternate pathways are activated in disease and some complement components (C3 and C4) are then produced in the gingiva itself.

Immunoglobulins of the oral cavity: saliva

Saliva contains immunoglobulin which is derived from several sources. In addition to the secretory IgA which is produced by plasma cells closely associated with the major and minor salivary glands, it contains variable amounts of IgG which is derived from the gingival sulcus and from transudate of oral mucosa. The amount of IgG is raised with increased gingival inflammation partly because there is an increased gingival sulcus flow of serum IgG and partly because inflamed gingiva acquires additional IgG-producing plasma cells. Other immunoglobulins, IgE and IgD, may be found in saliva; they also will be of gingival sulcus fluid origin having come originally from serum. It is for this reason also that IgM is low in saliva; it is at a diffusion disadvantage compared with IgG in passing from serum into the gingival sulcus or pocket. The IgA which is found in saliva arises from two sources: that of the common mucosal defence system described below and that which may be locally induced.

Secretory IgA

Secretory IgA (SIgA) is the predominant Ig in saliva and is synthesized by plasma cells associated with the major and minor salivary glands. Minor salivary gland secretions contain much higher concentrations of SIgA than do parotid secretions or mixed saliva. Most minor salivary glands have short ducts and are probably exposed to antigens; lymphoid cells are often associated with these ducts. Further characterization of the lymphoid cells associated with the minor salivary glands into the T and B variety of cells suggests that a separate mucosal Ig system may exist in the mouth, dependent partly on the circulating large lymphocyte pool but capable also of local stimulation and modulation of the response via accompanying T cells. That local stimulation may occur is supported by the finding of cells with the characteristics of antigen presenting cells in association with the minor salivary glands of experimental animals. Thus in addition to mucosal IgA arising from the common mucosal immune defence system described below, a proportion would appear to be induced locally.

Secretory IgA has the advantage in terms of mucosal protection that it is neither complement activating nor opsonizing. Unlike complement activating immunoglobulins, there is no cell lysis with release of enzymes into the tissues or ingress of polymorphs to further enhance the local damage. IgA is in this sense a 'quiet' defender of mucosal surfaces.

The value of IgA to the newborn is shown by the concentration of IgA in colostrum, more than 20 times that of whole saliva.

Secretory component

SIgA is conveyed to the mucosal surfaces as a dimer joined to a glycoprotein termed secretory component, which is synthesized by epithelial cells of the salivary glands. The dimeric SIgA is linked by a J chain; this and the secretory component are complexed and extruded from the epithelial cells as a product highly resistant to proteolytic attack. However, certain pathogenic organisms such as *Streptococcus pneumoniae* and *Haemophilus influenzae* secrete a protease capable of selectively cleaving the IgA1 subclass in humans. The IgA2 subclass is resistant to this enzyme; since IgA1 and IgA2 are often present in approximately equal amounts in secretions the fact has importance in terms of attempts to stimulate immunity.

Stimulation of the mucosal immunoglobulin system

In a simplistic explanation immunoglobulin produced by plasma cells which have been stimulated by an antigen should be presented to the same site. In some instances this is true, a large proportion of the immunoglobulin produced in a granuloma relates to antigens present there and local mucosal responses are as much as 30 times higher at the site of antigen presentation compared with elsewhere. However, in the case of the mucosal immune

9

system, other factors prevail which result often in immunoglobulin appearing at sites remote from the stimulatory site. The primary site of antigen processing in the gut is the Peyers patches. After population of the Peyers patches before birth, B cells are apparently sensitized by antigen of gut origin, then divide and migrate to other sites within the body. Essentially, small lymphocytes migrate to the peripheral lymph nodes and spleen, whereas large lymphocytes migrate to the lamina propria of the gut. Those cells committed to IgA production seem to have a predilection for the lamina propria of the gut and the exocrine tissues such as salivary and mammary glands. This route of induction of cells capable of producing IgA, followed by production of the IgA at other distant mucosal sites, has been termed the common mucosal immune defence system; the mechanism underlying the phenomenon is not known. What determines the homing of the IgA cell to specific sites is also not clear, although there is some evidence that the presence of antigen increases the homing rate and that hormones play a role, at least, in the mammary gland and uterine cervix. It does mean, however, that circulating cells may settle at a site where they produce IgA which is irrelevant to that situation.

Modulation of the mucosal IgA response

Stimulation of the mucosal immune response within the gut is of considerable interest since it has been realized that protection by IgA is one of the major sources of protection against such intestinal diseases as cholera or shigellosis. In the mouth the major interest has been with the enhancement of a mucosal response to the organisms associated with dental caries or, hopefully, specific periodontal disease-associated organisms.

The route of presentation of the antigen is of importance in the stimulation of the mucosal response. For example, B-lactoglobulin (a constituent of cows' milk) stimulates tonsillar lymphocytes *in vitro* to produce IgA, whereas tetanus toxoid stimulation leads to the production of IgG. Parenteral antigens appear to lead to an IgG response whereas those antigens priming the mucosa-associated lymphoid system stimulate mainly IgA-producing cells. Mucosal IgA responses are stimulated most effectively by repeated or prolonged antigen exposure. Thus an organism replicating continuously in contact with mucosa would act this way. However, the response is transient; the mucosal IgA system has a poor memory. For example, the protective mucosal secretory IgA antibodies which accompany gonorrhoea last for little more than 6 weeks. Periodontal pocket bacteria are thus more likely to evoke a continued mucosal immune response than *Streptococcus mutans*; the latter attaches preferentially to teeth rather than mucosa.

Oral tolerance

Tolerance to an antigen may exist at the mucosal site, systemically or at both sites. Immunization by the oral route may lead to systemic tolerance, but there are no instances of oral immunization leading to mucosal tolerance. Parenteral immunization evokes suppression of mucosal IgA responses by two mechanisms, that of the production of suppressor T cells and of high-avidity IgG serum antibody which interferes with the normal function of the mucosal IgA responses. The factors that determine whether mucosal antigens would evoke systemic tolerance or immunity are not well understood; clearly they are of importance in attempts at combating caries or periodontal disease by enhanced immunity. Circulating antigen–IgA complexes or T-suppressor cells may be responsible for the tolerance.

SUMMARY

The mouth is protected from harmful substances and organisms by a series of barriers. Physicochemical barriers exist within the oral mucosa, but are not absolute. Immunoglobulin pervades the mucosal epithelium and enters the gingival sulcus. Cells within the mucosa process antigen to initiate a response which leads to the immunoglobulin presence or to sensitized cells capable of mounting a cellular immune response. Potentiation of the humoral response presents difficulties.

Enhancement of the immune component of the barrier is short-lived in terms of IgA, damaging in terms of IgG and poorly understood in the cellular sense.

FURTHER READING

Bos, U. R. and Burkhardt, A. (1980). Inter-epithelial cells of the oral mucosa. *J. Oral Pathol.*, **9**, 65–81

Brandtzaeg, P. and Tolo, K. (1977). Immunoglobulin systems of the gingiva. In Lehner, T. (ed.) *The Borderland between Caries and Periodontal Disease*. (New York: Grune & Stratton)

Carlstedt, I. and Sheehan, J. K. (1984). Macromolecular properties and polymeric structure of mucous glycoproteins. In *Mucus and Mucosa*, Ciba Foundation Symposium No. 109, pp. 157–172. (London: Pitman)

Cimasoni, G. (1983). *Crevicular Fluid Updated*. 12. Monographs in Oral Science. (Howard, M. and Myers, S., eds). (Basel: Karger)

Daniels, T. E. (1984). Human mucosal Langerhans cells: post-mortem identification of regional variations in oral mucosa. *J. Invest. Dermatol.*, **82** (1), 21–24

Reibel, J. (1984). Immunohistochemical demonstration of plasma proteins in squamous epithelium of formalin fixed, paraffin embedded oral mucosa. *J. Oral Pathol.*, **13**, 75–84

Roitt, I. M. and Lehner, T. (1980). *Immunology of Oral Diseases*. pp. 297–304. (Oxford: Blackwell Scientific Publications)

Sauder, D. N., Carter, C., Katz, S. I. and Oppenheim, J. J. (1982). Epidermal cell production of thymocyte activating factor (ETAF). *J. Invest. Dermatol.*, **78**, 452–56

Squier, C. A. (1977). Membrane coating granules in non-keratinising oral epithelium. *J. Ultrastruct Res.*, **60**, 212–20

Wilton, J. M. A., Renggli, H. H. and Lehner, T. (1976). The isolation and identification of mononuclear cells from the gingival crevice in man. *J. Periodont. Res.*, **11**, 262–8

11

SUMMARY

FURTHER READING

2
The Microbiology of Dental Plaque in Health and Disease

P. D. MARSH

INTRODUCTION

A unique feature of the ecology of the mouth is the provision of hard, non-shedding surfaces (teeth) for microbial colonization. Elsewhere in the body, bacteria attach to epithelial surfaces, and regular desquamation ensures that the bacterial load at any site is small. Commonly, only around 100 bacteria are found per human buccal epithelial cell and these belong to only a limited number of bacterial genera (e.g. *Streptococcus* and *Haemophilus* spp.). In contrast, relatively thick *films* of micro-organisms are able to accumulate on teeth, particularly at those sites (pits and fissures, approximal surfaces, the gingival crevice) that afford protection from saliva flow and mastication. These films of micro-organisms are embedded in a matrix of polymers of microbial and salivary origin and are termed dental plaque. Although dental plaque is associated with disease it is important to remember that it is also found *naturally* on sound enamel surfaces. Indeed, one of the main problems when attempting to determine the causative organisms of plaque-mediated infections arises from the fact that disease occurs at sites where there is already a normal flora. Bacteriological studies have shown that these diseases are not attributable to any of the common, medical pathogens but appear to result from an imbalance in the commensal flora. Thus, the bacteria that have been implicated with disease (and which will be described later in detail) are also found at healthy sites, although usually less frequently and in lower numbers. Consequently, many microbiological studies of plaque are concerned with:

1. what constitutes a normal, healthy plaque flora;

2. which plaque bacteria can act as opportunistic pathogens and cause disease (and under which conditions);

13

3.   what are the properties of these opportunistic pathogens that contribute to their pathogenicity; and

4.   what are the environmental factors that trigger the transition of the plaque flora from having a commensal to a pathogenic relationship with the host?

The answers to many of these questions will be provided in this chapter, but as a prelude to any study attempting to relate the microbial composition of plaque to the clinical status of the site, methods for the optimum recovery of all the viable bacteria present in a sample have to be developed. These will be described in the following section.

METHODS FOR THE RECOVERY, ENUMERATION AND IDENTIFICATION OF BACTERIA IN DENTAL PLAQUE

The study of the bacterial composition of dental plaque has proved to be one of the most challenging areas of contemporary microbiology. Some of the features of dental plaque that make it so demanding to analyse are shown in Table 2.1 while the main stages in the processing of plaque are shown in Figure 2.1.

Table 2.1 Some properties of dental plaque that contribute to the difficulty in determining its bacterial composition

Property	Comment
High species diversity	Plaque contains a wide range of different bacteria, some of which are present only in low numbers
Cell adhesion and aggregation	Plaque bacteria adhere to one another, and therefore have to be dispersed without causing undue cell damage
Anaerobic	Many plaque bacteria lose their viability if exposed to air
Variability in composition	Plaque flora varies in composition over relatively small areas; therefore small, discrete samples are necessary
Confused taxonomy/difficult identification of plaque bacteria	The classification of some of the bacterial groups (taxa) found in plaque has yet to be resolved; this leads to difficulties in identifying isolates which can be compounded by the lack of simple criteria for speciation

Sampling procedures

An important fact that has to be borne in mind (and which will be developed in more detail later) is that the microbial composition of plaque varies from site to site. Therefore large plaque samples or, indeed, a number of smaller samples from different sites but which are pooled together, are of little value

14

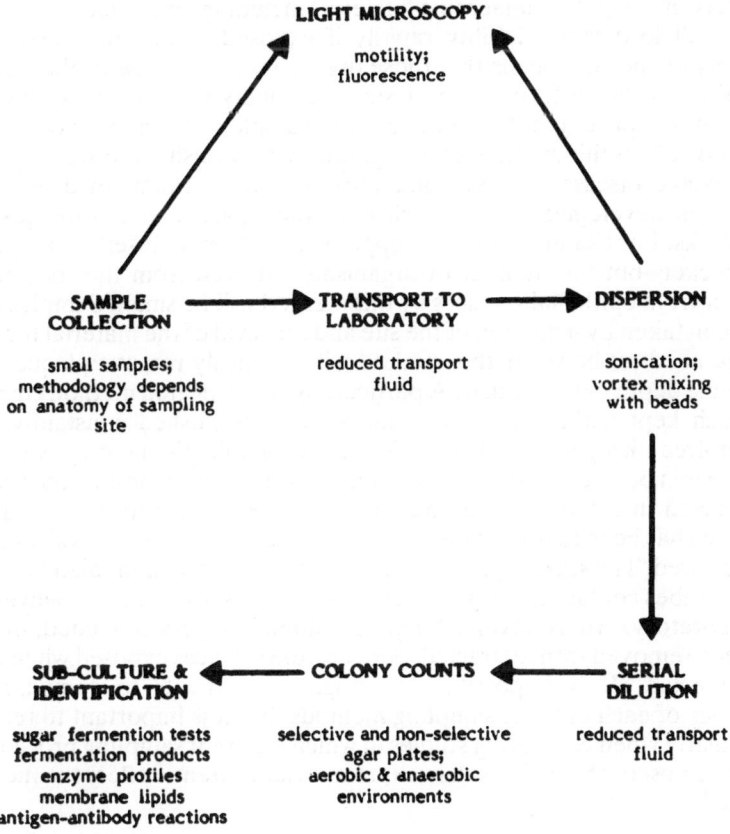

Figure 2.1 Schematic representation of the stages involved in determining the microbial composition of dental plaque

because important site differences will be obscured. The method of sampling plaque will depend on the site under study, but individual research groups often develop their own specific techniques. The accessible smooth surfaces of enamel pose few problems and a range of dental instruments have been used. Care has to be taken to avoid 'contamination' of the specimen with saliva which contains around 10^8 bacteria/ml. It is more difficult to remove plaque from approximal sites although dental probes, scalers, dental floss and abrasive strips have all been used with different degrees of success. Pits and fissures are also difficult to sample and generally the amount of plaque recovered is dependent on the anatomy of the site. Fine probes, pieces of wire and sterile needles have been used, although as an alternative approach some groups used artificial fissures or crowns which can be easily inserted and removed from the mouth for study.

Sub-gingival plaque has proved to be the most difficult to sample because of the anaerobic nature of the site. The flora is now known to comprise high numbers of obligately anaerobic bacteria, including spirochaetes, most of which will lose their viability rapidly if exposed to air. In disease, the anatomy of the site means that those organisms at the base of the pocket, near the advancing front of the lesion, are likely to be of most interest. Again, it is important not to remove with a sample material from other sites in the pocket, as this might obscure significant relationships between specific bacteria and disease. To overcome these problems a number of methods have been developed, all of which have their particular advantages and drawbacks. For example, a simple approach has been to insert paper points into pockets but the number of organisms removed from the root of the tooth or from epithelial surfaces by this method will be small. Samples have also been taken by irrigation of the site and retrieval of the material through syringe needles; however this method will obviously remove plaque from the whole depth of the pocket. A particularly sophisticated method employs a broach kept withdrawn in a cannula which is flushed constantly with oxygen-free nitrogen. The broach is used to sample plaque only when the cannula is in position near the base of the pocket. After sampling, the broach is retracted into the cannula and withdrawn. Perhaps the most frequent approach has been to use a curette or scaler after the supra-gingival area has been cleared. The scaler tips can be detached and placed immediately in gas-flushed tubes containing reduced (anaerobic) transport fluid for delivery to the laboratory. Alternatively, when periodontal surgery is needed, plaque has been removed from extracted teeth or from surfaces exposed when flaps are reflected. It is impossible to design experiments to compare the efficiency of each of these sampling methods, but it is important to realize, particularly when comparing studies in which different sampling procedures have been used, that the results will, to a certain extent, reflect the method adopted.

Transport and dispersion

All samples need to be transported to the laboratory for processing as quickly as possible. Specially designed transport fluids help to reduce the loss of viability of some of the more delicate organisms during delivery to the laboratory. These fluids usually contain reducing agents such as cysteine to maintain a low redox potential, thus helping to preserve the obligate anaerobes.

Plaque by definition is a complex mixture of a range of micro-organisms which are bound tenaciously to one another. These clumps and aggregates of bacteria must be dispersed efficiently (ideally to single cells) if the specimen is to be diluted accurately. It is now accepted that mere vortex mixing of a sample is inadequate. Mild sonication produces the maximum number of particles from a specimen but it exerts a selective effect by specifically damaging spirochaetes and some other Gram-negative bacteria, particularly *Fusobacterium* species. One of the most efficient methods, particularly for sub-gingival plaque, is to vortex samples with small glass beads in a tube filled with carbon dioxide.

Cultivation

Once dispersed, samples are usually serially diluted in transport fluid and aliquots are spread on to a number of freshly prepared, pre-reduced agar plates. These plates are chosen to grow either the maximum number of bacteria (generally, various forms of blood agar are used for this purpose) or, in order to encourage the growth of some of the minor components of plaque, a number of selective media have been devised which permit the growth of only a limited number of species. For example, the addition of vancomycin to blood agar plates will inhibit nearly all Gram-positive bacteria, a high sucrose concentration encourages the growth of oral streptococci, while plates with a low pH favour lactobacilli. It should be stated that these media are selective and not *specific*. The identity of the colonies on these plates must be confirmed; their colonial appearance or growth on a particular medium should not be regarded as diagnostic. Also, some bacteria will not grow unless additional factors are added to the medium. Haemophili were only recovered from plaque when the appropriate co-factors were added to the isolation media. Depending on the bacteria being cultivated, plates have to be incubated for different times and under different atmospheric conditions. For example, to grow some *Bacteroides* species, plates will need at least 7 days incubation at 37 °C in an anaerobic jar or cabinet filled with a gas mix containing $CO_2/H_2/N_2$, while *Neisseria* require only 2 days incubation in air.

Identification

The first stage usually involves colony counting; colonies with a similar appearance are counted and subcultured for further analysis. This assumes that:

1.   cells of the same micro-organism produce colonies with an identical morphology, and

2.   cells of different micro-organisms produce colonies with distinct morphologies.

Generally this assumption holds true, but on occasions it has been shown that different bacteria can produce identical colonies. The first level of discrimination involves the Gram-staining of subcultured colonies; bacteria are then grouped according to whether their cells are Gram-positive or Gram-negative, and are rod- or coccal-shaped. This dictates which tests will be necessary to achieve speciation. Some bacteria can be identified using simple criteria – for example, sugar fermentation tests – while others require a more sophisticated approach such as the application of gas–liquid chromatography to determine their acid end-products of metabolism. The main groups of bacteria found in plaque, together with an outline of the methods employed in their identification, will be described in the next section.

17

Microscopy

An idea of the principal morphological groups of bacteria found in plaque can be obtained using light microscopy. Dark-field illumination techniques have been used to quantify the numbers of motile bacteria in 'unprocessed' plaque, including spirochaetes, which are extremely difficult to cultivate by conventional means. As the numbers of spirochaetes and motile organisms have been related to the severity of some periodontal diseases, and because microscopy is relatively cheap and gives results quickly, it has been hoped that these techniques could be used in the clinic to monitor the progress of patients undergoing treatment. However, a major disadvantage of dark-field microscopy is that most of the putative pathogens in plaque-mediated diseases cannot be recognized by morphology alone. To overcome this problem, some groups are raising antisera (monoclonal or specific polyclonal) against a limited number of bacteria that are believed to be implicated in disease. These antisera can be either conjugated with a fluorescent dye (direct fluorescence) or used in conjunction with commercially prepared, conjugated anti-rabbit IgG (indirect fluorescence) to quantify rapidly the approximate numbers of selected key bacteria in plaque. This methodology would obviate the need for many of the lengthy and labour-intensive steps described above (Figure 2.1), but to date only a limited number of specific antisera have been described and close correlations between results obtained by these serological approaches and conventional bacteriology on the same material have not always been found. Electron microscopy has proved useful in studying plaque formation, and it has also been used to show that bacteria invade gingival tissues in aggressive forms of periodontal disease: immunocytological techniques have enabled some of the observed bacteria to be identified.

TYPES AND PROPERTIES OF THE PRINCIPAL BACTERIA FOUND IN DENTAL PLAQUE

The normal flora of dental plaque is complex, comprising a wide range of bacterial species; yeasts such as *Candida* spp. can also be found. The microbial composition of plaque is not constant but varies from site to site, both between and within mouths, and with time. Before these variations can be discussed, the main bacterial types commonly recovered from plaque will be described briefly; these are listed in Table 2.2. Emphasis is placed on the taxonomy of plaque bacteria because, without valid subdivision and accurate identification of isolates, any possible association of particular species with disease will not be made.

Gram-positive cocci

Streptococci comprise on average around 30% of the total cultivable flora of plaque. The majority are α-haemolytic on blood agar and consequently were

Table 2.2 Some of the commonly isolated bacteria from dental plaque

Gram-positive cocci	**Gram-negative cocci**
Streptococcus mutans	*Branhamella* spp.
sobrinus	*Neisseria* spp.
sanguis	*Veillonella alkalescens*
'mitior'	
milleri	
salivarius	
Peptostreptococcus spp.*	
Gram-positive rods	**Gram-negative rods**
Actinomyces israelii	*Actinobacillus actinomycetemcomitans*
naeslundii	*Bacteroides* spp.
viscosus	*Campylobacter concisus*
odontolyticus	*Capnocytophaga sputigena*
Arachnia propionica	*gingivalis*
Bacterionema matruchotii	*ochracea*
Bifidobacterium spp.	*Eikenella corrodens*
Eubacterium spp.	*Fusobacterium* spp.
Lactobacillus acidophilus	*Haemophilus* spp.
casei	*Leptotrichia buccalis*
spp.	*Selenomonas sputigena*
Propionibacterium spp.	*Treponema* spp.
Rothia dentocariosa	*Wolinella recta*

*The term spp. is used where there is confusion or controversy as to the number and nomenclature of species in a genus

originally grouped together as viridans streptococci or as *Streptococcus viridans*. More recent taxonomic studies have shown that these can be divided into a number of well-defined species with distinct properties, often with a different potential to act as opportunistic pathogens. Most work has been published on *Streptococcus mutans*, mainly because of its primary role in the aetiology of dental caries. In particular its antigenic make-up has received considerable attention because of the possibility of:

1.   immunizing humans with *S. mutans*, or specific antigens of *S. mutans*, as a protective measure against caries; and

2.   using serological techniques for the rapid identification of clinical isolates, for example, for use in epidemiological surveys.

So far, at least eight serotypes of *S. mutans* have been recognized (a–h) on the basis of carbohydrate antigens which are covalently linked to the peptidoglycan of the cell wall (Table 2.3). Although they are serotype-specific they can also be responsible for cross-reactions among some of the other serotypes. For example, there is cross-reactivity among serotypes c, e and f, probably because of a common poly-rhamnose backbone to the antigen. More recent studies have suggested the differences between some of these serotypes are so great that they should be regarded as separate

19

species (Table 2.3). This proposal has been slow to gain widespread acceptance but, in future, it is likely that the specific epithet *S. mutans* will be limited to the c, e, f serogroups only.

Table 2.3 Proposed nomenclature and cell wall carbohydrates of the '*S. mutans*' group

Present serotype	Cell wall carbohydrate	Proposed species name
c, e, f	Glucose, rhamnose	S. mutans
d, g, h	Glucose, galactose, rhamnose	S. sobrinus
a	Glucose, galactose, rhamnose	S. cricetus
b	Galactose, rhamnose	S. rattus

Note: Another "mutans-like" species, *S. ferus*, which reacts with antisera raised against *S. mutans* (serotype *c*), has been isolated from wild rats.

Other components of the outer surfaces of the '*S. mutans* group' of bacteria have been found to be antigenic (Figure 2.2). Lipoteichoic acids are negatively charged amphipathic molecules, composed of sugar phosphates (e.g. glycerol phosphate), that are attached to the cell membrane but which protrude through the cell wall and are secreted in high concentrations into the environment. The function of lipoteichoic acids (LTA) is not known, but they are responsible for wide serological cross-reactions among oral streptococci. These molecules do have biological activity; they are involved in bacterial adherence and can cause bone resorption in periodontal disease. A great deal of attention has been focused in recent years on the protein antigens of *S. mutans*. A number have been isolated and purified and shown to have a range of molecular weights; they are probably covalently linked to the cell wall although they are also released into the environment, and

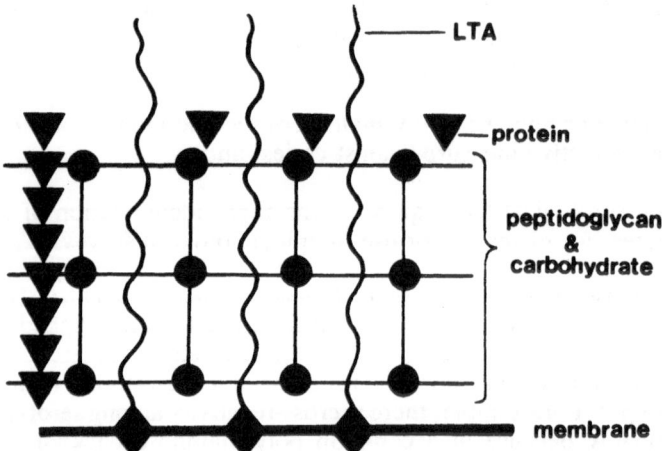

Figure 2.2 Schematic representation of the outer layers of a streptococcal cell

growth conditions can effect their secretion. In many cases the function of these proteins is not clear, although some have been found to have enzyme activity, particularly with respect to sucrose metabolism (e.g. glucosyltransferase, fructosyltransferase, or invertase activity) or to act as receptors (glucan-binding proteins, salivary protein-binding proteins). The main interest in these proteins has been due to the fact that some have been used with success as immunogens in an anti-caries vaccine, reducing both caries and the numbers of *S. mutans* in plaque in monkeys.

In plaque overlying sound enamel, *S. mutans* is found spasmodically and often only in low numbers. In caries the numbers of this group of bacteria increase, although the factors responsible for this shift are not yet clear. A notable feature of these bacteria is that they can proliferate under low pH conditions (i.e. they are aciduric) whereas most other plaque bacteria, with the exception of lactobacilli, would be inhibited. *S. mutans* is also highly acidogenic, and these bacteria can also synthesize from sucrose several water-soluble and water-insoluble polysaccharides using glycosyl-transferases. There are several enzymes involved; in simple terms, glucosyltransferase-I synthesizes the insoluble glucan while glucosyl-transferase-S produces the soluble glucans. Together they synthesize a highly branched, water-insoluble poly-glucan rich in $\alpha,1-3$ linkages, termed 'mutan'. This polysaccharide plays an important role in the consolidation of attachment of cells in plaque, and may localize acidic fermentation products producing environments with a low local pH, thus encouraging demineralization of enamel. *S. mutans* also produces a fructosyltransferase that synthesizes an unusual fructan with an inulin ($\beta,2-1$)-like structure.

Other streptococci are associated more with sound enamel and unfortunately, because of this, have received much less attention. *Streptococcus sanguis* is an early colonizer of the tooth surface and also produces glucosyltransferases. The product has fewer $\alpha,1-3$ linkages than the polymer made by *S. mutans*. Generally, *S. sanguis* is regarded as not producing a fructosyltransferase although, under certain growth conditions, one strain has been shown to make a poly-fructan from sucrose. Some strains produce neuraminidase, which removes the terminal sialic acid residues on the side-chains of salivary glycoproteins, while others have IgA_1 protease activity. This may affect how the particular organism competes with the host and colonizes certain sites. *S. sanguis* also possesses carbohydrate, lipoteichoic acid and protein antigens but they have received little detailed attention. '*S. mitior*' and *S. milleri* are also commonly isolated from dental plaque; some strains of '*S. mitior*' also make insoluble glucans from sucrose while *S. milleri* makes no polymers at all. These bacteria are potential opportunistic pathogens, particularly if they gain entry to the blood stream. '*S. mitior*' is the most common isolate from cases of infective endocarditis while *S. sanguis* and *S. mutans* are also recovered regularly. In contrast, *S. milleri* is rarely associated with infective endocarditis but it has been isolated from abscesses (particularly of the brain and liver), appendicitis and peritonitis. Despite its name, *S. salivarius*, is also found regularly in plaque. A characteristic of this species is the production from sucrose of a fructan with a levan-like ($\beta,2-6$) structure. This molecule is

21

highly labile and can be metabolized by a number of plaque bacteria. Some strains of *S. salivarius* have also been shown to produce glucans from sucrose. Other streptococci are recovered less frequently from plaque. Obligately anaerobic streptococci (e.g. *Peptostreptococcus* spp.) have been found in periodontal pockets, and in infected root canals and abscesses. Occasionally, enterococci such as *S. faecalis* have been isolated from plaque and also infected root canals. In contrast to the skin and nose, staphylococci and micrococci are not considered to be regular members of the plaque flora although they have been found in fissures. Generally, simple physiological tests can be used to identify oral streptococci and there are a number of commercially produced galleries of tests now available for this purpose.

Gram-positive rods

This is one of the predominant groups of bacteria in healthy plaque and includes a wide range of species. Indeed, certain genera such as *Actinomyces*, *Bacterionema* and *Rothia* appear to have the mouth as their sole natural habitat. However, many species can act as opportunistic pathogens, e.g. *Actinomyces israelii*, *A. viscosus* and *A. naeslundii* are commonly isolated from cases of actinomycosis and, more recently, have also been recovered from infections associated with inter-uterine devices. *Actinomyces* spp. have both carbohydrate and protein antigens, some of which are associated with specific types of fimbriae on the cell surface, and an amphipathic molecule distinct from LTA has also been identified. *A. viscosus* produces an extracellular slime which is a heteropolysaccharide, and a fructan (levan) from sucrose. The numbers of *Actinomyces* in plaque increase at the onset of gingivitis, and they have also been implicated in root surface caries.

Lactobacilli are another group of bacteria that have received a great deal of attention in the past, mainly because it was believed that they were the causative organisms of dental caries. They are now believed to play more of a role in the progression of incipient lesions and in dentinal caries rather than with initiation *per se*. Both homo- and heterofermentative strains are present in plaque; commonly isolated species include *L. casei*, *L. acidophilus*, *L. fermentum* and *L. plantarum*. Their numbers are very low at healthy sites but they are probably the most acid-tolerant species of bacteria in dental plaque and thrive at sites with a low pH. Lactobacilli are generally more resistant to fluoride and chlorhexidine than other plaque bacteria. A number of the Gram-positive rods in plaque are obligately anaerobic, including *A. israelii*, *Arachnia propionica*, *Bifidobacterium* spp., *Eubacterium* spp. and *Propionibacterium* spp. Therefore, appropriate precautions have to be taken when attempting to isolate these organisms from plaque. The use of gas–liquid chromatography to identify the acid end-products of carbohydrate metabolism is necessary to differentiate between these diverse groups of bacteria, although the analysis of cell wall carbohydrates by thin-layer chromatography is also useful. Simple physiological tests or serology may be needed to speciate isolates once the genus has been determined by the above-mentioned chemotaxonomic methods.

Gram-negative cocci

Branhamella spp. and *Neisseria* spp. are early colonizers of the enamel surface. *Branhamella* can be distinguished from *Neisseria* by their inability to make acid from carbohydrates. Oral isolates of both of these genera are poorly described but can be differentiated from *Veillonella* spp. by being facultatively anaerobic (i.e. strains can grow in the presence or absence of air). In contrast, *V. alkalescens* is an obligate anaerobe that cannot metabolize sugars but does utilize intermediary metabolites such as lactate. Thus they can form food chains with lactate-producing bacteria and they have recently been shown to be highly acid-tolerant, growing in the laboratory in mixed cultures at pH 4.1. Large numbers of this species may reflect sites where there are high concentrations of lactic acid.

Gram-negative rods

This is probably the most diverse and taxonomically confused group of bacteria found in plaque. The majority of aerobic or facultatively anaerobic Gram-negative rods belong to the genus *Haemophilus*, many of which cannot be cultivated unless their growth medium is supplemented with haemin (X-factor) or nicotinamide adenine dinucleotide (V-factor) or both. The species isolated from plaque include *H. parainfluenzae, H. segnis* and *H. aphrophilus*. Other facultatively anaerobic Gram-negative rods have been identified as *Eikenella corrodens*, the colonies of which characteristically pit the surface of agar plates. These facultatively anaerobic bacteria can be opportunistic pathogens and have been isolated from infections of the jaw and from cases of infective endocarditis. A group of bacteria that have come into prominence more recently are micro-aerophilic, CO_2-requiring strains that have been classified as *Capnocytophaga* spp. and *Actinobacillus actinomycetemcomitans*. The latter strain has also been isolated from cases of infective endocarditis, and it is strongly implicated in the aetiology of juvenile periodontitis. At present its taxonomic position is being reassessed and it has been proposed that it should be reclassified as *Haemophilus actinomycetemcomitans*. Strains of *Capnocytophaga* have also been isolated in high numbers from pockets in subjects with juvenile periodontitis.

The obligately anaerobic Gram-negative rods are currently undergoing considerable taxonomic reorganization. Problems have arisen because some strains are asaccharolytic and therefore simple physiological tests, such as sugar fermentation tests, cannot be used in their identification. The application of gas–liquid chromatography to determine the pattern of metabolic products from glucose or peptide catabolism is usually necessary in order to place isolates into their appropriate genus. However, a problem can arise because some strains are slow-growing and it can be difficult to distinguish between such bacteria and those that are genuinely asaccharolytic. As an alternative approach some research groups have applied more sophisticated methods to classify and identify these difficult isolates. These methods include:

1. enzyme profiles, particularly aminopeptidases (commercially prepared galleries containing a range of substrates are available for these studies);

2. enzyme mobilities;

3. analysis of the chemical composition of cell walls;

4. analysis of the lipid components of the cell membranes.

The obligately anaerobic genera include *Leptotrichia*, *Fusobacterium*, *Campylobacter* (*C. concisus* is a new species recently isolated from periodontal pockets), *Bacteroides*, *Selenomonas* (*S. sputigena* has a tuft of flagella), and *Wolinella* (*W. recta* is also motile due to a single polar flagellum). These bacteria are found in the highest numbers in the gingival crevice and the periodontal pocket; indeed, many of these Gram-negative rods are strongly implicated in the aetiology of different periodontal diseases.

One group of fastidious, obligately anaerobic bacteria that can be easily recognized are those *Bacteroides* that produce colonies with a characteristic black pigment when grown on blood agar plates. These black-pigmenting *Bacteroides* were originally named *B. melaninogenicus*, although the pigment is now known not to be melanin but to be derived from haemin, an essential growth factor for these bacteria. Recent studies have shown that there are a number of distinct black-pigmenting species including *B. melaninogenicus*, *B. intermedius*, *B. gingivalis*, *B. loescheii*, *B. denticola* and *B. endodontalis*. These black-pigmenting *Bacteroides* are found in high numbers in cases of chronic periodontitis, although the predominant species may vary with the depth of the pocket. The classification of the non-pigmenting *Bacteroides* is undergoing a reformation; it would be inappropriate and, indeed, impossible in this chapter to attempt to describe the taxonomy of this diverse and nutritionally demanding group of bacteria.

A number of spirochaetes of different sizes have been recognized in plaque using dark-field microscopy. They have proved difficult to cultivate in the laboratory although species such as *Treponema denticola*, *T. orale*, and *T. macrodentium* have been described based on differences in their metabolic activities in simple physiological tests, their fermentation products, and on the number and arrangement of their axial filaments. Mycoplasmas have also been recovered from dental plaque and some believe that they may play a role in periodontal diseases; however, little is known of their pathogenic properties as yet.

DEVELOPMENT OF DENTAL PLAQUE

Three approaches have been adopted in the study of the development of plaque on a clean tooth surface. Microscopy, and particularly scanning electron microscopy, has been valuable in following the appearance of the different morphological types of microbe during colonization and plaque build-up, while conventional bacteriological techniques have been used to identify and enumerate the attached micro-organisms. The attachment of these organisms to surfaces (for example, hydroxyapatite beads) and to other plaque bacteria, in the presence and absence of saliva, has been quantified in the laboratory and a number of specific molecular interactions have been described. The combined results' of these studies suggest that plaque does not develop in a random manner but rather that bacteria colonize in a relatively specific sequence. Four distinct (but arbitrary) stages in plaque development can be recognized:

1.   a reversible phase, whereby cells are adsorbed to a surface primarily by electrostatic forces; this is followed by:

2.   an irreversible phase involving specific molecular interactions between the cell and saliva-coated enamel surfaces;

3.   a repeat of phases (1) and (2), but in which salivary bacteria attach to organisms that are already adhering (this stage is termed co-aggregation); and finally

4.   the division of the attached micro-organisms until growth is confluent and a film is formed.

Each of these stages will now be described in more detail, but it should be remembered that these divisions are artificial. Plaque formation is a dynamic process; the adsorption, growth, removal and reattachment of bacteria is a continuous process and so the structure of plaque will undergo regular reorganization.

Bacteria rarely come into contact with clean enamel. Within seconds of a tooth surface being cleaned, certain salivary polymers are selectively adsorbed, forming the 'acquired pellicle'. This pellicle is less than 1 μm thick and consists of various proteins (including proline-, tyrosine-, and histidine-rich proteins), glycoproteins, lysozyme, amylase, immunoglobulins (particularly IgA), and blood group reactive proteins. It is the outcome of the interaction between these molecules and those on the bacterial surface that determines whether an organism will attach. Bacteria also become coated with polymers from saliva to increase still further the possible number of interactions. However, the first stage in adherence is believed to involve electrochemical forces. All surfaces in nature have an electrical charge. Therefore as a bacterium approaches a surface it experiences both a weak van der Waals attractive force and an electrostatic repulsive force. The summation of these forces produces a theoretical area (known as the

25

'secondary minimum') where a cell will experience a weak attraction towards the surface. Depending on the ionic strength of saliva, this secondary minimum will lie approximately 5–10 nm from the tooth surface. While bacteria are held (reversibly) in this secondary minimum, the outer layers of bacteria are able to (1) adsorb either non-specifically to the pellicle or (2) interact specifically with receptors or polymers present in the pellicle. This polymer bridging increases the probability of irreversible attachment and it has been proposed that these molecules may span the distances over which electrochemical forces apply, particularly if they are located on surface appendages of bacteria such as fimbriae. Some of the specific polymer interactions that have been recognized include:

> lipoteichoic acid
> or glucosyltransferase – blood group reactive proteins
> antigen – antibody (particularly IgA)
> protein receptor – lysozyme
> glucosyltransferase – dextran/glucan

Only a few bacterial types are able to colonize a clean tooth surface. These pioneer species are generally coccal-shaped and the majority are *Neisseria* spp. or streptococci, and in particular *S. sanguis*. The synthesis of neuraminidase IgA$_1$ protease by the latter may aid its early colonization of enamel. The surface never becomes saturated with adsorbed bacteria (Figure 2.3a). Those that are present grow, forming microcolonies which will eventually merge (Figure 2.3b). Salivary polymers will continue to be adsorbed on to the bacteria already attached to the pellicle, and therefore several of the adhesive mechanisms described above will continue to operate. An important mechanism that aids plaque build-up and encourages species diversity is the recently described phenomenon of coaggregation between oral bacteria. Coaggregation can occur between:

1. Gram-positive species,

    e.g. *S. sanguis or*   and   *Actinomyces* spp., or
         S. mitis   *Bacterionema matruchotii*
                                                         Propionibacterium acnes

2. Gram-negative species,

    e.g. *Bacteroides melaninogenicus*   and   *Fusobacterium nucleatum*

3. *Gram-positive* and *Gram-negative* species,

    e.g. *Streptococcus* spp. or   and   *Bacteroides* spp.
         Actinomyces spp.   *Capnocytophaga* spp.
                                          F. nucleatum
                                          Eikenella corrodens
                                          Veillonella sp.

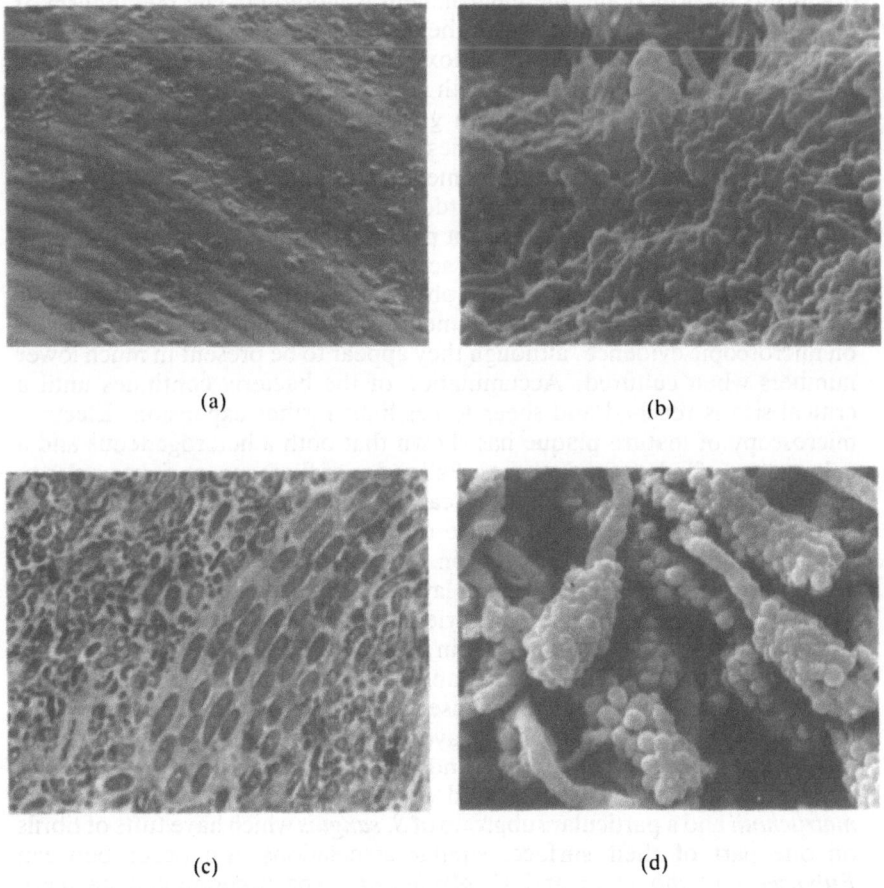

(a)

(b)

(c)

(d)

Figure 2.3 Scanning electron micrographs of developing plaque showing (a) microcolony formation during colonization, (b) the complexity of plaque when growth is confluent and a complete microbial film is formed, (c) a section of plaque showing a microcolony type of substructure, and (d) 'corn-cob' formation. These photographs were kindly provided by Alan Saxton (Unilever Research)

Coaggregation involves lectins; lectins are carbohydrate-binding proteins that interact with the complementary carbohydrate-containing receptor on another cell. Thus the lectin-mediated interaction between streptococci and actinomyces can be blocked by adding galactose or lactose or by treating the receptor with a protease. Another important factor in plaque development is the synthesis of extracellular polysaccharides by streptococci. The water-insoluble glucans, and in particular mutan, make an important contribution to the structural integrity of plaque. Also, they are believed to localize acidic fermentation products which may encourage demineralization. As the microcolonies of attached bacteria grow and merge, a film of micro-

27

organisms is formed and the environment is modified. The metabolism of the early colonizers, together with the development of gradients in plaque, creates conditions with a lower redox potential which are therefore more suited to obligate anaerobes. Growth rates of bacteria are faster during the early stages of colonization; mean generation times of approximately 2 hours have been measured in studies of animals. As the coverage of the surface becomes confluent, so the mean generation times become longer, and in established plaque bacterial doubling times of 24 hours have been recorded. During the early stages of plaque development, few rod-shaped bacteria are seen, although *Rothia*, actinomyces and lactobacilli have been isolated. After several days, anaerobes including *Veillonella* spp. appear more frequently and eventually filamentous bacteria become predominant on microscopic evidence, although they appear to be present in much lower numbers when cultured. Accumulation of the bacteria continues until a critical size is reached and sheer forces limit further expansion. Electron microscopy of mature plaque has shown that both a heterogeneous and a colony type of substructure exists. Pallisades of filaments at right angles to the enamel surface can be seen, as can microcolonies of apparently single species (Figure 2.3c). The structure of plaque varies from site to site. A vertical stratification can be seen on smooth surfaces: the early stages of colonization result in a condensed layer of a limited number of bacterial types, while a bulk layer shows less orientation but a higher species diversity. Impacted food particles can be seen in fissures; there is also little evidence of pallisading. In the gingival crevice and periodontal pocket a loose layer is found over the surface of a condensed layer. Many bacterial associations have been observed in these 'loose layers', of which the most common is the attachment of coccal cells to one end of a filamentous cell (Figure 2.3d). These associations have been termed 'corn-cobs' and the components are *B. matruchotii* and a particular subgroup of *S. sanguis* which have tufts of fibrils on one part of their surface; similar associations also occur between *Eubacterium sabbuream* and *V. alkalescens*. The predominant bacterial types found on sound enamel at different sites on the tooth surface will now be described in detail.

BACTERIAL COMPOSITION OF PLAQUE AT DIFFERENT SITES OF THE TOOTH SURFACE

The main factors affecting the distribution of bacteria on the tooth surface are:

1. The affinity of an organism for a site. Certain streptococci have a predilection for saliva-coated enamel because of the specific molecular interactions described previously.

2. The redox potential of a site. Obligately anaerobic bacteria will be limited to those sites with a low Eh. Such conditions exist in the deeper layers of plaque, particularly in the gingival crevice and at approximal surfaces.

3. The provision of essential nutrients. Many of the more fastidious oral bacteria are dependent on the provision of nutrients (particularly peptides and amino acids) and growth factors (vitamins and haemin) by crevicular fluid. The gingival crevice is therefore able to satisfy the nutritional demands of certain bacteria that could not survive elsewhere in the mouth.

From the above, it is not surprising that the predominant cultivable flora from fissures, approximal surfaces and the gingival crevice are different, or that variations occur in the flora at a particular site in different individuals. The microbiology of fissure plaque has been determined using either 'artificial fissures' implanted in occlusal surfaces of pre-existing restorations, or by sampling 'natural' fissures. The flora is mainly Gram-positive and is dominated by streptococci, and extracellular-polysaccharide producing streptococci in particular. In one study no obligately-anaerobic Gram-negative rods were found, although other anaerobes including *Veillonella, Arachnia* and *Propionibacterium* were isolated in low numbers (Table 2.4). Other studies have found *Neisseria* spp. and *Haemophilus parainfluenzae* on occasions. A striking feature of the flora is the wide range of numbers and types of bacteria in the different fissures. This suggests that the ecology of each fissure might be different. The factors that determine the final composition of the flora in fissures are not known, but the influence of saliva at this site must be of great significance. The simpler community found in fissures compared to other enamel surfaces probably reflects a more severe environment, perhaps with a limited range of nutrients.

Table 2.4 The predominant cultivable flora of 10 occlusal fissures in adults

Bacterium	Median percentage of total cultivable flora	Range	Percentage isolation frequency
Streptococcus	44.9	7.9–86.3	100
Staphylococcus	8.5	0–23.0	80
Actinomyces	18.2	0–45.9	80
Arachnia	1.6	0–20.8	60
Propionibacterium	0.9	0– 7.5	50
Eubacterium	0	0–27.1	10
Lactobacillus	0	0–28.6	20
Veillonella	3.3	0–44.4	60
Individual species:			
S. mutans	24.7	0–86.3	70
S. sanguis	0.8	0–14.9	50
'*S. mitior*'	0	0–13.0	30
S. milleri	0	0– 3.2	10
A. naeslundii	3.3	0–44.3	70
A. viscosus	3.3	0–17.0	80
L. casei	0	0– 9.8	10
L. plantarum	0	0–28.6	10

The main organisms isolated from 58 samples of approximal plaque taken from 10 subjects are shown in Table 2.5. Although streptococci are present in high numbers, these sites are frequently dominated by Gram-positive rods, particularly *Actinomyces* spp. The more reduced nature of this site compared to that of fissures can be gauged from the higher recovery of obligately anaerobic organisms. Again, the range and percentage isolation frequency of most bacteria is high, suggesting that each site represents a distinct ecological niche which should be looked at in isolation with regard to the relationship between the resident flora and the clinical state of the enamel.

Table 2.5 The predominant cultivable flora of approximal plaque

Bacterium	Mean percentage of total cultivable flora	Range	Percentage isolation frequency
Streptococcus	22.9	0.4–70.0	100
Gram-positive rods (predominantly *Actinomyces*)	42.1	4.0–81.0	100
Gram-negative rods (predominantly *Bacteroides*)	7.8	0–66.0	93
Neisseria	1.5	0–44.0	76
Veillonella	13.1	0–59.0	93
Fusobacterium	0.4	0– 5.4	55
Lactobacillus	0.5	0– 1.9	24
Rothia	0.4	0– 5.7	36
Individual species:			
S. mutans	2.2	0–23.0	66
S. sanguis	5.9	0–64.0	86
S. salivarius	0.7	0– 7.0	54
S. milleri	0.5	0–33.0	45
A. israelii	16.5	0–78.0	72
A. viscosus/naeslundii	19.1	0–74.0	97

Viable counts were derived from 58 samples of approximal plaque from 10 schoolchildren

The variability of plaque has again been highlighted in a recent study in which several small samples have been taken from different sites around the contact area of teeth extracted for orthodontic purposes. An example is shown in Table 2.6; at each approximal site the total numbers, as well as the range and types, of bacteria vary, again emphasizing the need for accurate sampling of discrete sites when attempting to correlate the composition of plaque with disease.

An obviously distinct ecological climate is found in the gingival crevice. This is reflected in the high species diversity of the bacterial community at this site. Obligately anaerobic bacteria form a major part of the crevice flora and spirochaetes are isolated almost exclusively from this region. In contrast to the flora of fissures and approximal surfaces, the predominant bacteria in the gingival crevice are obligately anaerobic and many are Gram-negative

Table 2.6 The cultivable flora from three sites on the approximal surface of an extracted tooth from a schoolchild

Bacterium	Viable count (colony-forming units)		
	Site 1	2	3
Total count	1.7×10^4	6.8×10^2	7.9×10^5
Streptococcus	0	0	6.1×10^5
Actinomyces	5.8×10^2	0	1.8×10^5
Neisseria	25	25	1.5×10^4
Veillonella	0	0	6.5×10^4
Capnocytophaga	0	0	1.3×10^2
Haemophilus	1.7×10^4	6.0×10^2	0
Individual species:			
S. mutans	0	0	3.7×10^4
S. sanguis	0	0	1.1×10^5
S. mitior	0	0	1.0×10^4
S. salivarius	0	0	1.8×10^4
A. viscosus	5.8×10^2	0	1.8×10^5
A. naeslundii	0	0	$6..5 \times 10^3$
Gram-negative 'spreading' bacillus	0	+	0

Table 2.7 The predominant cultivable flora of the healthy gingival crevice of seven adults

Bacterium*	Mean percentage of total cultivable flora	Range	Percentage isolation frequency
Gram-positive facultatively anaerobic cocci (predominantly *Streptococcus*)	39.6	2.4–73.2	100
Gram-positive obligately anaerobic cocci (predominantly *Peptostreptococcus*)	0.8	0– 5.6	14
Gram-positive facultatively anaerobic rods (predominantly *Actinomyces*)	35.1	9.8–62.5	100
Gram-positive obligately anaerobic rods	9.5	0–36.6	86
Gram-negative facultatively anaerobic cocci (predominantly *Neisseria*)	0.3	0– 1.8	14
Gram-negative obligately anaerobic cocci (*Veillonella*)	2.0	0– 4.9	57
Gram-negative facultatively anaerobic rods	Not detected		0
Gram-negative obligately anaerobic rods	12.7	7.5–20.4	100

*Spirochaetes were not looked for in this study, but they have been found at this site using dark-field microscopy techniques in other investigations

(Table 2.7). In disease, the gingival crevice becomes a periodontal pocket; the flora from these pockets is also complex and is predominantly Gram-negative and will be described in detail in the following section. The complexity of the flora from these sites is not only due to the low redox potential (Eh) and the provision of essential nutrients by crevicular fluid, but also because many of the indigenous bacteria are able to form food chains. Thus, the products of metabolism of one organism become primary sources of nutrients for another. Examples include the production of isobutyrate and putrescine or spermine by *Fusobacterium* spp., and succinate by Gram-positive rods, which are utilized by some spirochaetes. Similarly, *Fusobacterium* and *Bacteroides* spp. provide hydrogen and formate for the growth of vibrio-like organisms, while the metabolism of black-pigmented *Bacteroides* is dependent on the synthesis of vitamin K by other bacteria. Lactate, produced by a number of oral bacteria, can be utilized by *Veillonella* sp. and *Treponema oralis*. The high pH (the pH of deep pockets is pH 8.5) of the site will also favour certain bacteria including *B. gingivalis* which have alkali-stable enzymes. The majority of asaccharolytic bacteria found in the mouth are recovered from the gingival crevice and periodontal pocket.

DENTAL PLAQUE AND DISEASE

Impetus for much of the work on oral microbiology has stemmed from the finding of a relationship between the numbers and metabolism of certain bacteria in plaque and the most prevalent diseases affecting industrialized societies – namely, caries and periodontal diseases. As stated earlier, this area of study has proved to be one of the most challenging in contemporary microbiology, primarily because of the presence of a complex, *normal* flora at sites of infection. The bacterial aetiology of these diseases will be described in detail shortly, but it should be remembered that many plaque bacteria can also act as opportunistic pathogens, particularly if they gain entry to the blood stream. Bacteria can then be disemminated to other parts of the body causing abscesses at a number of sites (including the brain, liver and abdomen) and infective endocarditis in 'at-risk' subjects with damaged or prosthetic heart valves. Most of the bacteria isolated from these infections are sensitive to the antibiotics used in routine clinical practice. However, low numbers of resistant bacteria (particularly penicillin-resistant streptococci and *Bacteroides* spp.) are carried by many people, and therefore the response of patients to antibiotic treatment should be carefully monitored.

DENTAL CARIES

Dental caries has been defined as the localized destruction of the tissues of the tooth by bacterial action. Cavities begin as small demineralized areas in the enamel but commonly progress into the dentine or pulp, and it is now believed that the bacterial flora changes as the lesion progresses through these tissues. Evidence for dental caries as an infectious disease will be presented in the next chapter. In brief, studies using germ-free animals have shown that caries only develops when animals fed on a cariogenic (high sucrose) diet are infected with certain bacterial species. In these studies, *S. mutans* has been shown to be the most cariogenic species, causing caries of smooth surfaces as well as in pits and fissures in hamsters, gerbils, rats and monkeys. Immunization of rodents and monkeys with whole cells or specific antigens of *S. mutans* can lead to a reduction in the numbers of the organism in plaque and a decrease in the number of carious lesions that develop compared with sham-immunized animals. Other bacterial species can cause caries when mono-infected in germ-free animals including *S. sanguis*, '*S. mitior*', *S. milleri*, *S. salivarius*, enterococci, *Lactobacillus* spp., *A. viscosus* and *A. naeslundii*, although the cavities are usually restricted to fissures.

In humans the evidence for the involvement of bacteria in caries is obviously indirect. Patients on long-term antibiotic therapy usually exhibit a reduced caries experience, while the bacterial flora of a carious lesion is usually different from that found on sound enamel. The difference that has attracted most attention has been the finding that *S. mutans* is isolated more commonly and in higher numbers from carious lesions. Thus a large number of cross-sectional epidemiological studies around the world, on a number of sites and surfaces, have demonstrated a positive correlation between the presence of a carious lesion and an increase in the isolation frequency and percentage viable count of *S. mutans* in the overlying plaque compared with control sites on sound enamel. For example, in one particularly interesting study several small samples of plaque were taken from a number of individual incipient ('white spot') lesions and the percentage viable counts of *S. mutans* were compared with those in a similar number of samples taken from neighbouring, clinically sound enamel on the same tooth. The proportions of *S. mutans* from carious areas were considerably higher than those from the adjacent sound surface areas although, except at one site, the percentage counts of *S. mutans* were low (Table 2.8). The bacteria making up the remainder of the flora were not identified but would undoubtedly include other streptococci and actinomyces which can make significant concentrations of acid from carbohydrates. In studies of carious fissures, higher levels of *S. mutans* have been recovered from carious sites. For example, in one study, 71% of carious fissures had viable counts of *S. mutans* of 10% or more of the total cultivable flora, whereas 70% of the fissures that were caries-free at the time of sampling had no detectable *S. mutans*. The collective evidence from this type of cross-sectional study has been taken as proof by many that *S. mutans* is the *sole* pathogen in human caries. However, cross-sectional studies do *not* allow cause-and-effect relationships to be determined. It is possible that *S. mutans* may increase in numbers in plaque only once a carious lesion has been initiated, perhaps in response to a change in environmental conditions. *Streptococcus mutans* grows well at low pH and the pH of a carious lesion is generally below pH 4.0 and can be as low as pH 3.2. Furthermore, the development of a carious lesion is favoured by a high and regular intake of sucrose, and this has been shown to lead to an increase in the proportions of *S. mutans* at a site while other bacteria (e.g. *S. sanguis*) that are less tolerant of excess carbohydrate and low pH values, are inhibited. Longitudinal epidemiological studies, in which initially sound, but caries-susceptible, surfaces are monitored both clinically and microbiologically for a fixed length of time, are the only way that true cause-and-effect relationships between bacteria and disease can be established. Several longitudinal surveys of fissures have demonstrated a strong relationship between the presence of high levels of *S. mutans* (>20% of the total cultivable flora) and the initiation of dental caries, while no correlation between *S. sanguis* and caries was found. In one study, *S. mutans* was only a minor component (0.1%) of plaque from five fissures that became carious; however, counts of lactobacilli (bacteria also able to tolerate low pH) were higher in these samples and it was concluded that these were the causative organisms in these fissures. There was also a group that remained caries-free during the study, but who had previously a high caries experience; *S. mutans* comprised, on average, nearly 10% of the total cultivable flora of these fissures over a 12-month period. Thus, although a strong correlation between *S. mutans* and fissure decay was found, lesions could develop in the apparent absence of significant numbers of this species, while this species could persist in relatively high numbers for long periods without caries developing.

Table 2.8 The percentage viable count of *S. mutans* from a 'white spot' lesion and from adjacent sound enamel on the same tooth

Subject	Mean percentage viable count of S. mutans		Ratio S. mutans 'white spot'/ S. mutans sound enamel
	'White spot' lesion	Sound enamel	
1	1.30	0.03	43.3
2	0.01	0.002	5.0
3	0.06	0.002	30.0
4	0.06	0.02	3.0
5	0.8	0.01	80.0
6	63.2	0.5	126.4
7	1.4	0.2	7.0
8	0.2	0.07	0.3

Note: The viable counts are the mean value of several sites in the 'white spot' lesion and an equal number of sites on neighbouring sound enamel. Eight subjects were studied

The results of longitudinal surveys of approximal surfaces have proved equivocal. This may be due to difficulties of repeated, accurate sampling of the same site, problems of diagnosing the early lesion by radiographs, or it may mean that the aetiology of the initiation of approximal caries is less clear-cut than that of fissures. It should be remembered that fissures have a higher 'natural' concentration of *S. mutans* and are more streptococcal-dominated than approximal surfaces. No clear relationship between the presence of *S. mutans*, or any other organism, and caries initiation at approximal sites was found in a major study of English school-children. Indeed, it appeared that the isolation frequency and mean percentage viable count of *S. mutans* rose after, rather than before, the first radiographic diagnosis of a carious lesion. Frequently where this increase occurred, these lesions continued to progress through the enamel; increases in the number of lactobacilli at these sites were also common. This finding was in agreement with a study of Dutch army recruits in which the prevalence of *S. mutans* also correlated strongly with the clinical *progression* of a lesion. Caries progression occurred at 14 out of 55 sites; *S. mutans* was in excess of 5% of the total cultivable flora at 71% of these surfaces, while this species could not be detected on 51% of the tooth surfaces without caries progression. However, it is noteworthy that in both of these longitudinal studies of approximal caries, a small number of surfaces developed caries in the absence of detectable *S. mutans*, while *S. mutans* persisted in high numbers at sites that remained caries-free during the study.

Table 2.9 Percentage viable count and isolation frequency of bacteria recovered from progressive and non-progressive incipient carious lesions, and from sound, approximal enamel surfaces

Bacterium	Progressive lesion (n = 14)		Non-progressive lesion (n = 18)		Sound enamel (n = 32)	
	Percentage viable count*	Isolation frequency*	Percentage viable count	Isolation frequency	Percentage viable count	Isolation frequency
S. mutans	9.7	100	3.3	75	6.6	75
'S. mitior'	3.9	50	5.4	100	3.6	67
S. sanguis	6.1	100	8.5	87	6.4	100
S. salivarius	5.7	100	6.3	100	8.5	100
A. viscosus	28.9	100	32.8	100	32.3	100
A. naeslundii	0.3	50	4.5	50	2.3	80
A. odontolyticus	0.8	50	0	0	0	0
Lactobacillus spp.	0.7	75	0	0	0	0
V. alkalescens	10.6	100	8.9	100	9.4	100

*32 lesions from 22 children (aged 4–9 years) were diagnosed as incipient; 14 of the lesions progressed to a point requiring restoration; between 3 and 8 samples were taken from each site – the counts and isolation frequencies represent median values

One theory that emerged from these studies was that the flora associated with caries progression might differ from that associated with initiation. This theory has recently been tested in a study of incipient approximal lesions in Canada. Radiographically diagnosed lesions and control, sound surfaces were sampled microbiologically at regular intervals for 12 months. The flora associated with lesions that progressed to the point of requiring restoration were compared with that of non-progressive lesions and of control surfaces which, where possible, were the contralateral site in the same child (Table 2.9). Statistically positive correlations with progression were found with *S.*

mutans, Lactobacillus spp., *A. odontolyticus* and *V. alkalescens*, while '*S. mitior*', *A. naeslundii* and *A. viscosus* had negative associations. It was particularly striking that *A. odontolyticus* and *Lactobacillus* spp. were only found at sites where lesion progression occurred. These findings suggest that microbiology could prove a valuable adjunct to clinical diagnosis, particularly as radiographs were relatively insensitive in this respect – restoration of 'white spots' need only be contemplated when either or both of these bacteria are detected.

There have been some recent studies of nursing caries and of root surface caries. The upper anterior teeth of children with nursing caries were found to be heavily colonized by *S. mutans* and lactobacilli (particularly *L. fermentum* and *L. plantarum*) compared to control sites in the same mouth; *V. alkalescens* was also present in large numbers at diseased sites and it was considered that the presence of these bacteria might reflect environments with high concentrations of lactic acid. Early cross-sectional studies of root surface caries found high numbers (around 40% of the total cultivable flora) of *A. viscosus* in the plaque overlying lesions. In a recent longitudinal study the compositions of the flora from diseased sites were not statistically different from control sites and, in all sites, the flora was highly variable with time. Interestingly, *A. naeslundii* was isolated far less frequently than *A. viscosus* and was more associated with root surface health than disease. Also, the isolation of *S. mutans* and lactobacilli together from a site was a strong indicator of root surfaces at risk of decay, even though both bacteria were usually only minor components of the plaque flora.

In conclusion, bacterial species such as *S. mutans* and lactobacilli are more commonly associated with caries than with sound enamel. However, this association is not unique and, in a small number of cases, caries can occur in the absence of *S. mutans*, while *S. mutans* can sometimes persist in relatively high numbers without any apparent demineralization. This is not, perhaps, surprising when one considers the properties of bacteria that are associated with cariogenicity (Table 2.10). Many of these attributes are not unique to *S. mutans* or lactobacilli, with perhaps the exception of their acid tolerance. Although many bacteria may be able to lower the pH to below the 'critical pH' for enamel demineralization, the host may be able to cope and maintain the integrity of enamel through remineralization. However, if the diet changes and the frequency of sugar consumption is increased, then the pH in plaque will be lowered more often and aciduric (acid-tolerating) bacteria will be at a competitive advantage and thrive at the expense of other organisms. This shift in the composition of the flora could tip the balance in favour of demineralization. Just such a trend has been observed during *in vitro* studies of mixed cultures grown for several weeks in a chemostat. When the pH was lowered from 7.0 to 4.1 the proportions of *S. mutans, L. casei* and *V. alkalescens* rose; the glycolytic activity and the concentration of lactic acid produced by the community increased; while amino acid metabolism (and base production) was suppressed. Bacterial interactions can also modulate the cariogenicity of an organism. It has been demonstrated in gnotobiotic rats that *Veillonella* can form a food chain with streptococci by utilizing their lactic acid, converting it to the weaker acids acetic and propionic, and thereby reducing the number of carious lesions per animal. Also, other bacteria, particularly some of the Gram-negative anaerobes found in approximal plaque, can catabolize amino acids, urea and peptides and in doing so generate ammonia and other basic compounds. The importance of these reactions in plaque ecology should not be overlooked. It has been argued by some that caries results not so much from an over-production of acid but more from a deficiency of base production by plaque bacteria. Thus caries development will depend on the outcome of the interaction of diet, the plaque microbial community and host. It is not surprising, therefore, that direct correlations between single bacterial species and caries initiation are not always found.

Table 2.10 Properties of cariogenic bacteria

Property	Comment
Extracellular polysaccharide production from sucrose	Insoluble polymers are involved in plaque formation and may limit diffusion of acidic fermentation products
Intracellular polysaccharide production	Enables bacteria to make acid in the absence of exogenous carbohydrates
Rapid sugar transport	Sugar phosphotransferase uptake systems enable bacteria to scavenge for low concentrations of carbohydrates; under such conditions sugar transport and subsequent glycolysis is rapid
Acid production	The rate and type of acid formed are markedly influenced by environmental conditions
Acid tolerance	Although many plaque bacteria can produce a low environmental pH, few organisms are able to metabolize and grow under such conditions

PERIODONTAL DISEASES

The microbiology of periodontal diseases has undergone a reformation in recent years as a result of improvements in (a) sampling techniques, and (b) the taxonomy and identification of the isolates. Several distinct periodontal diseases are now recognized, and as more sophisticated and biochemical approaches are adopted in clinical diagnosis then groups of patients with more specific forms of disease will emerge. Evidence that bacteria are involved in periodontal diseases has come from gnotobiotic animal studies. Germ-free animals rarely suffer from periodontal disease although, on occasions, impacted food in the gingival crevice can give rise to an inflammatory response. However, when certain bacteria, particularly those isolated from human periodontal pockets, are used to infect these animals then inflammation is much more common and severe. These bacteria are predominantly Gram-negative (*Campylobacter, Actinobacillus, Eikenella,*

Bacteroides, Selenomonas, Capnocytophaga, Fusobacterium) although some streptococci and actinomyces can also be pathogenic in these animal models. Furthermore, when antibiotics active against these bacteria are administered to the infected animal, progression of the disease is arrested. In man, the evidence has come mainly from cross-sectional epidemiological studies (longitudinal surveys are not usually possible because of the chronic nature of the disease and the difficulties in predicting sites likely to become infected) and from the results of plaque-control studies. The bacteriology of the major types of periodontal disease will be described in the following sections; for simplicity it will be possible to describe only the principal organisms that have been implicated.

Gingivitis

Chronic marginal gingivitis is a non-specific inflammatory response to dental plaque involving the gingival margins. Many regard gingivitis as resulting from a non-specific proliferation of the normal gingival crevice flora due to poor oral hygiene. Certainly the total plaque mass increases, and this is associated with a marked increase in the numbers of facultatively anaerobic Gram-negative rods (these are mainly *Haemophilus parainfluenzae* and were not detected in one study of the healthy crevice, Table 2.7) and obligately anaerobic Gram-negative rods (including *Fusobacterium* spp. and asaccharolytic *Bacteroides* spp.); *Actinomyces* spp. also increase in proportions in gingivitis. However, results from one longitudinal study suggested that a more specific relationship might exist between certain bacteria (*A. viscosus* and black-pigmented *Bacteroides*) and cases of gingivitis that are associated with bleeding. In another longitudinal study of experimental gingivitis in four adult volunteers, in which the most comprehensive bacteriological analysis of plaque to date has been performed, 166 distinct bacterial groups (taxa) were detected. Of these, 73 taxa showed a positive correlation to gingivitis, 29 were negatively correlated while the remainder either showed no correlation or were regarded as being present as a result of gingivitis. The flora from different individuals was extremely variable, although certain trends did emerge. The flora became more diverse with time as gingivitis developed and progressed, and the most likely aetiological agents were *A. naeslundii, A. odontolyticus, F. nucleatum*, an unknown lactobacillus species, *Streptococcus anginosus* (similar to *S. milleri*), *V. alkalescens* and a non-typable *Treponema* sp. It is again interesting to note that the numbers and types of bacteria present appear to change with disease progression. The effect of bleeding on the composition of the flora is of great interest as the black-pigmented *Bacteroides* spp. require haemin for growth, and this can be obtained from the enzymic hydrolysis of blood proteins. The plaque micro-organisms do not invade the gingival tissues. Inflammation is induced by bacterial cell surface components and diffusible metabolic products. The nature of these toxic components will be discussed in a later section. There is also an exaggerated form of gingivitis that is associated with pregnancy, puberty, menstruation, stress, and the use of oral contraceptives. The factors responsible for gingivitis in pregnancy have been studied in detail. The composition of the sub-gingival flora fluctuates during pregnancy, and during the second trimester the proportions of *B. intermedius* increase significantly. Steroid hormones can be detected in crevicular fluid and, following laboratory studies, the rise in numbers of *B. intermedius* was attributed to the preferential ability of this species to metabolize progesterone and oestradiol; both hormones were able to replace the growth requirement for vitamin K by this species.

Chronic periodontitis

Chronic periodontitis is an inflammatory disease of the supporting tissues of the teeth. It can be distinguished from gingivitis in that not only are the gingivae involved but also the alveolar bone and the periodontal fibres. The nature of the stimuli that lead to chronic periodontitis is at present unknown but a subtle interaction between the bacteria, their products and the host defences is involved. Gingivitis is probably a precursor of chronic periodontitis but not all sites with gingivitis progress to more severe forms of periodontal disease. Bacteria believed to be implicated in periodontitis are located at the base of the pocket and, as discussed earlier, one of the major problems is to sample this area without recovering bacteria from other parts of the pocket. A number of studies have compared the flora of the healthy gingival crevice with diseased sites in the same mouth. Two general approaches have been adopted. The first attempts to analyse the whole of the pocket flora; the problems associated with identifying some of the bacteria together with the labour-intensive nature of plaque processing (Figure 2.1) means that only a small number of patients can be studied. Frequently, wide variations in the composition of the flora are found between different individuals with apparently the same clinical condition. The second approach, which is also the more common, screens plaque for the presence of only a few key bacteria, although this means that a larger number of samples and patients can be examined.

There is general agreement from studies using both approaches that the pocket flora is complex and is composed mainly of obligately anaerobic Gram-negative rod-shaped and filamentous bacteria, many of which are asaccharolytic (i.e. cannot make acid from sugars) and proteolytic, using amino acids and peptides as carbon and energy sources. However, the problems associated with this type of research, and which were alluded to above, have meant that there are confusing and contradictory reports in the literature concerning the actual micro-organisms present, and many clinically similar pockets have markedly dissimilar floras. For example, in a study of 'early periodontitis', peptostreptococci predominated in one pocket while black-pigmented *Bacteroides* spp. and *A. israelii* were recovered in large numbers from another. Dark-field microscopy has shown that many of the bacteria in plaque from patients with periodontitis are motile, and that spirochaetes can be present in large numbers. Indeed, for a long time it was believed that the numbers of these bacteria correlated with the severity of the disease process, but this association is now less clear. Improvements in sample collection and processing have resulted in the culturing and identification of some of these motile organisms, and species such as *Wolinella recta* and *Selenomonas sputigena* have been found more commonly and in higher numbers at diseased sites. Other studies have found a wide range of *Fusobacterium* spp., e.g. *F. nucleatum*, and *Bacteroides*, including pigmented and non-pigmented species. Cluster analysis of the complex microbiological data from pockets has shown that different *groupings* of a limited number of bacteria may be associated with particular stages or forms of periodontal disease. In some instances distinct groups of micro-organisms could produce a similar pathological response. Examples of these groupings include *B. intermedius*, *E. corrodens*, *F. nucleatum*, 'fusiform'-*Bacteroides* and *Actinomyces* spp. from 'minimally inflamed' periodontitis, while *F. nucleatum*, *B. gingivalis*, *W. recta*, 'fusiform'-*Bacteroides* and *Peptostreptococcus* sp. were found in different proportions in more severe cases of periodontitis (Table 2.11).

Table 2.11 Clusters of bacteria that were associated with periodontitis in man

Bacterium	*Percentage viable count (median value)*				
Cluster	*1**	*2*	*3*	*4*	*5*
A. actinomycetemcomitans	0	0	0	0	0
Actinomyces sp.	2	0	0	0	0
B. intermedius	12	0	0	0	0
B. gingivalis	0	3	0	39	21
'Fusiform' *Bacteroides*	3	1	7	4	15
E. corrodens	6	0	0	0	0
F. nucleatum	8	31	23	3	16
Peptostreptococcus sp.	0	7	0	1	0
W. recta	0	0	12	3	4

*Cluster 1 = "minimally inflamed" periodontitis;
clusters 2–5 = more advanced forms of periodontitis

The complexity and variability of the pocket flora can be further gauged from a recent comprehensive study of plaque from 38 sites in 22 subjects diagnosed as having 'moderate periodontitis"; 171 different bacterial taxa were recognized, of which only 22 bacteria and 5 types of treponeme were considered to be possible causative agents. Among the bacteria implicated in disease were *F. nucleatum*, *Peptostreptococcus* spp., six species of *Eubacterium*, *W. recta*, *Lactobacillus* spp., *Actinomyces* spp., *B. gingivalis*, *B. intermedius*, *Selenomonas sputigena* and *Staphylococcus epidermidis*, although many were present in very low proportions.

After considering the results of the studies outlined above, the following points can be made:

1.   Chronic periodontitis results from the activity of mixed cultures (consortia) of predominantly obligately anaerobic Gram-negative bacteria.

2.   The compositions of these consortia vary with the depth of the pocket and with the severity of the disease. However, until the criteria are standardized for the nomenclature of the different forms of periodontitis (i.e. 'early', 'moderate', 'advanced') it will be difficult to compare and interpret the results from different studies. Also it is now realized that destructive periodontal disease does not occur at a slow, continuous rate but progresses in bursts by recurrent acute episodes. Until methods are available to confirm whether a pocket is in an 'active' or 'inactive' phase it will again be difficult to make accurate assessments of the role of specific bacteria in disease.

3.   The composition of the flora varies markedly between studies. This might be due to differences in: (a) the plaque sampling or processing techniques, or in the levels of detection of key organisms due to the methods adopted; (b) the precise form of chronic periodontitis under investigation.
      The flora also varies widely within a study. This might be due to (a) lack of precision in diagnosing disease, (b) lack of precision in sampling individual pockets, (c) pockets being sampled during both active and inactive phases.

4.   Alternatively, different combinations of bacteria might give rise to similar pathological states, although it should be remembered that in cross-sectional studies it is difficult to distinguish between those bacteria that are responsible for disease and those which proliferate as a result of it. The concept of microbial specificity in terms of the aetiology of periodontitis need not be discounted; it should be redefined to include the role of *consortia* of bacteria in disease.

Juvenile periodontitis (periodontosis)

This is a rare condition that usually affects adolescents; it can have both a localized (restricted to the first permanent molars and the incisor teeth) or a generalized pattern of destruction. In contrast to chronic periodontitis, the plaque associated with localized juvenile periodontitis is sparse, containing few bacteria (approximately 10^6 colony-forming units per pocket) which are restricted to only a limited number of species. These bacteria are usually saccharolytic Gram-negative rods; in many early studies the predominant bacteria were not obligate anaerobes although they did require CO_2 for growth. The organisms found most consistently were *Capnocytophaga* spp. and *A. actinomycetemcomitans*. Both bacteria can produce a range of enzymes capable of destroying periodontal tissues but the most noticeable feature is the production of a powerful leukotoxin by *A.*

41

actinomycetemcomitans, enabling it to avoid one of the most important host defence systems in the periodontal pocket. These patients are also believed to have an impaired immune defence system. Mycoplasmas have been seen in immunocytological studies of patients with localized juvenile periodontitis, and they were also implicated, together with spirochaetes and a number of bacteria, in a recent bacteriological study. The role of *Capnocytophaga* spp. in juvenile periodontitis is now being questioned; several studies have found these bacteria in higher numbers in the flora of the healthy gingiva.

In one study of severe generalized periodontitis in 21 young adults, two unclassified *Treponema* species were closely associated with disease as were a number of bacteria including *F. nucleatum*, seven species of *Eubacterium*, lactobacilli, *Peptostreptococcus* sp., *B. intermedius* and *Selenomonas* spp. The precise role of these bacteria in disease has yet to be determined.

Acute ulcerative gingivitis

This disease is characterized by the formation of grey pseudomembranes on the gingivae which can easily slough off revealing an area of bleeding underneath. When smears are examined microscopically, spirochaetes can be seen as can Gram-negative filamentous bacteria. These bacteria were believed to be fusobacteria but a recent study of 22 ulcerative sites in eight patients has shown that these bacteria may also be *B. intermedius; Selenomonas* spp. and *A. odontolyticus* may also be involved in disease.

Only in the later stages of periodontitis, or in the more aggressive diseases such as juvenile periodontitis and acute ulcerative gingivitis, are bacteria found invading the tissues. These bacteria have been detected using scanning and transmission electron microscopy of sections of tissue and, on occasions, immunocytological techniques have been used to identify the invading organisms. In localized juvenile periodontitis, spirochaetes, mycoplasmas, *A. actinomycetemcomitans* and *Capnocytophaga sputigena* have been found in the periodontium, while a range of morphological types of Gram-positive and Gram-negative bacteria have been recognized in tissues in patients with advanced periodontitis.

VIRULENCE FACTORS IN PERIODONTAL DISEASES

Except in severe forms of periodontal disease, bacteria do not invade host tissues. Tissue damage is therefore mainly a result of enzymes and cytotoxins produced by plaque bacteria, and a damaging host inflammatory response to bacterial antigens and products. It should be remembered that although phagocytic cells play an important protective role in the defence of the pocket, the release of lysosomal enzymes will inevitably lead to the damage of epithelial cells. Virulence factors of periodontal pathogens are therefore related to:

1.   enzymes and cytotoxins causing direct damage to host cells,

2.   bacterial products that enable them to evade or modulate the host defences, and

3.   bacterial components that cause indirect damage to host cells by activating or enhancing an inflammatory response (Table 2.12).

Table 2.12 Bacterial virulence factors implicated in periodontal disease

1. *Substances causing inflammation*	
Polypeptides	Polysaccharides
Lipopolysaccharides	
2. *Substances causing tissue damage*	
Trypsin-like enzyme	Phospholipase A
Collagenase	Acid and alkaline phosphatases
Hyaluronidase	Butyric and propionic acids
Chondroitin sulphatase	Indole
Lipoteichoic acid	Ammonia
Lipopolysaccharide	Volatile sulphur compounds
Capsule-induced bone resorption	
3. *Substances modulating the host defences*	
Capsules	Proteases degrading:
Leukotoxin	Complement (C_3)
Polymorph-inactivating factors	Iron-binding proteins
Immunoglobulin-specific proteases	Proteinase inhibitors

Black-pigmented *Bacteroides* spp., *Capnocytophaga* spp. and *A. actinomycetemcomitans* can produce a number of enzymes that can destroy the integrity of the periodontal tissues; these include collagenase, hyaluronidase, and chondroitin sulphatase. Some bacteria also produce acid and alkaline phosphatases, which may be involved in alveolar bone breakdown, while phospholipase-A may produce prostaglandin precursors and so initiate prostaglandin-mediated bone resorption. These proteolytic enzymes, by reducing tissue integrity, facilitate the diffusion of cytotoxic substances such as indole, ammonia, butyric and propionic acids. Volatile sulphur compounds can also increase the permeability of the oral mucosa and inhibit protein synthesis. *Bacteroides gingivalis* has been shown to be more proteolytic than other species, and its potential virulence can be gauged from laboratory studies where it is the only species that, when injected in pure culture into mice, produces acute, rapidly spreading infections whereas other black-pigmented *Bacteroides* spp. produce only small, localized abscesses at the sites of inoculation.

Neutrophils, in association with specific antibodies against plaque bacteria, play a major protective role in the pocket. Therefore bacterial factors that interfere with these processes, or which enable organisms to evade the host defences, must make a significant contribution to the pathogenicity of these bacteria. Pathogenic black-pigmented *Bacteroides* spp. reduce the chemotaxis of polymorphs by (a) producing capsular material which can mask the chemotactic lipopolysaccharides (endotoxin) in their outer membranes, or (b) synthesizing as yet uncharacterized products which are themselves non-chemotactic but which compete for and block chemotactic receptors on polymorphs. *Capnocytophaga* spp. also elicit products that impair polymorph function, but by mechanisms distinct from those described above. Bacterial capsules have other properties too; in *B. gingivalis* the presence of a capsule correlates with a resistance to phagocytosis while capsular material derived from *A. actinomycetemcomitans* is a potent stimulator of bone resorption *in vitro*, being active at concentrations 1000-fold lower than purified lipopolysaccharides from the same organism. Antibodies against pocket bacteria might also protect the host by inhibiting the attachment of cells to host tissues, by exerting bactericidal or opsonizing effects, or by neutralizing toxins or enzymes. However, most black-pigmented *Bacteroides* and *Capnocytophaga* spp. produce IgA1, IgA2 and IgG proteases which will interfere with the protective actions of antibodies *in vivo*. Virulent strains of *A. actinomycetemcomitans* produce a powerful leukotoxin which primarily affects polymorphs, and to a lesser extent monocytes. It was found that 55% of isolates from localized juvenile periodontitis patients produced a leukotoxin compared with only 16% of strains from healthy sites. Also, serum anti-leukotoxin antibodies were detected in 94% of patients with disease but in only 19% of control subjects.

Other factors that can contribute to the severity of disease include a range of surface antigens that can produce an inflammatory response. These include lipoteichoic acid, polysaccharides and lipopolysaccharides (endotoxin). Lipopolysaccharides (LPS) from pocket bacteria can vary greatly in chemical composition and biological activity, although most will cause bone resorption in laboratory tests. The importance of lipopolysaccharides in disease is not clear since, in some pathogens, molecules that are more biologically active may actually mask LPS. Recently it has been shown that *B. gingivalis* has proteolytic enzymes that can inactivate proteinase inhibitors and pro-enzymes present in human plasma that enable the host to initiate and regulate the inflammatory response. It is not known yet whether other pocket bacteria have similar properties.

Another feature of the pathogenicity of black-pigmented *Bacteroides* spp. relates to their ability to degrade iron-binding proteins found in serum and hence crevicular fluid. These bacteria require haemin for growth; *B. gingivalis* is the most efficient species in the laboratory at degrading haeme-containing plasma proteins such as haptoglobin, haemopexin, transferrin, lactoferrin and albumin. The virulence of *B. gingivalis* in mice has been shown to be related to the availability of haemin in the original growth medium of the cells.

In summary, many bacteria implicated in the aetiology of periodontal diseases produce a wide range of factors that directly or indirectly damage host tissues and enable the organisms to modulate the host defences. Probably, no single species produces all of these factors at optimum concentrations. This may be one of the reasons, therefore, why consortia of bacteria are associated with most forms of periodontal disease (e.g. see Table 2.11). It may be that the combined actions of several bacteria are necessary to overcome the host defences, enabling other bacteria to multiply and produce toxins and enzymes which destroy gingival tissues resulting in the products of an even wider range of bacteria gaining access to underlying tissues. This is known as pathogenic synergism, and has been recognized in a number of other infections of man and animals.

FUTURE ROLE OF MICROBIOLOGY IN DIAGNOSIS OF PLAQUE-MEDIATED DISEASES

The key to the effective management of infectious diseases, including those mediated by dental plaque, is early diagnosis and appropriate therapeutic intervention. The preceding sections have shown that the plaque microflora associated with caries and periodontal diseases is complex, and often consortia of bacteria are implicated. The composition of these consortia can vary markedly between individuals and with the severity and type of disease. In periodontal disease, many of the key bacteria are slow-growing or are difficult to cultivate and identify. Is it possible, therefore, to use any of the above microbiological information in the clinic:

1.   to identify susceptible sites or patients,

2.   as a diagnostic aid to assess the success or failure of therapy, particularly in periodontal disease?

In Sweden, the levels of *S. mutans* and/or lactobacilli in the saliva of schoolchildren are monitored regularly. High carriage rates of either organism are considered to indicate a high caries risk for the individual. Preventive measures applied to these children can reduce selectively the numbers of *S. mutans* leading to a subsequent reduction in caries incidence. These preventive measures include professional tooth cleaning and oral hygiene instruction, dietary counselling, and the application of antimicrobial substances such as fluoride and/or chlorhexidine. This type of programme has also been applied to mothers with young babies. When salivary counts of *S. mutans* were reduced in heavily infected mothers, there was a significant reduction in the incidence of its transmission from mother to baby, resulting in a delay in both the acquisition of this species and the time of the appearance of the first carious lesion.

It has already been shown that it may be possible to predict the progression of incipient lesions merely on the basis of the presence of lactobacilli or *A. odontolyticus* at a site (Table 2.9). A similar approach has been made to assess treatment efficacy in periodontal disease. In a pioneer study the presence of *B. gingivalis*, *B. intermedius*, spirochaetes and motile rods in sub-gingival plaque samples was related to post-treatment periodontal disease activity in 20 adults with moderate-to-severe periodontitis. To simplify the techniques involved, plaque was obtained using paper points and was dispersed using vortex mixing; *B. gingivalis* and *B. intermedius* were identified by indirect immunofluorescence, while the spirochaetes and motile rods were detected by phase contrast microscopy. It was found that the presence of *B. gingivalis* and spirochaetes at sites correlated strongly with continued loss of periodontal attachment; no associations were found with motile rods or *B. intermedius*. However, these bacteria were not detected at several active lesions and so treatment decisions based solely on the absence of these organisms could result in the omission of necessary therapy. It was concluded, though, that treatment should be continued as long as *B. gingivalis* and spirochaetes are detectable in samples of sub-gingival plaque.

These studies suggest that, in the future, it may be possible to use the presence of selected key bacteria in plaque as diagnostic predictors of sites at risk of further disease activity. However, before such a possibility becomes reality, it will be necessary to refine clinical diagnostic methods and to determine the role of a wider range of plaque bacteria in disease.

FURTHER READING

Bowden, G. H. W., Ellwood, D. C. and Hamilton, I. R. (1979). Microbial ecology of the oral cavity. In Alexander, M. (ed.) *Advances in Microbial Ecology*. Vol. 3, pp.135–217. (New York: Plenum Press)

Boyar, R. M. and Bowden, G. H. W. (1985). The microflora associated with the progression of incipient carious lesions in teeth of children living in a water-fluoridated area. *Caries Res.*, **19**, 298–306

Loesche, W. J., Syed, S. A., Laughon, B. E. and Stoll, J. (1982). The bacteriology of acute necrotizing ulcerative gingivitis. *J. Periodontol.*, **53**, 223–30

Marsh, P. D. and Keevil, C. W. (1986). The metabolism of oral bacteria in health and disease. In Hill, M. J. (ed.) *Microbial Metabolism in the Digestive Tract*. pp.155–81. (Boca Raton: CRC Press)

Moore, W. E. C., Holdeman, L. V., Smibert, R. M., Good, I. J., Burmeister, J. A., Palcanis, K. G. and Ranney, R. R. (1982). Bacteriology of experimental gingivitis in young adult humans. *Infect Immun.*, **38**, 651–67

Moore, W. E. C., Holdeman, L. V., Cato, E. P., Smibert, R. M., Burmeister, J. A. and Ranney, R. R. (1983). Bacteriology of moderate (chronic) periodontitis in mature adult humans. *Infect. Immun.*, **42**, 510–15

Silverstone, L. M., Johnson, N. W., Hardie, J. M. and Williams, R. A. D. (1981). *Dental Caries. Aetiology, Pathology and Prevention*. (London: MacMillan)

Slots, J. and Genco, R. J. (1984). Black-pigmented *Bacteroides* species, *Capnocytophaga* species, and *Actinobacillus actinomycetemcomitans* in human periodontal disease: virulence factors in colonization, survival and tissue destruction. *J. Dent. Res.*, **63**, 412–21

Slots, J., Emrich, L. J., Genco, R. J. and Rosling, B. G. (1985). Relationship between some subgingival bacteria and the periodontal pocket depth and gain or loss of periodontal attachment after treatment of adult periodontitis. *J. Clin. Periodontol.*, **12**, 540–52

3
Dental Caries in Humans and Animal Models

S. J. CHALLACOMBE

Introduction

Dental caries is one of the most prevalant diseases of man. In spite of recent reductions in the rate of decay in Western societies, the prevalence of caries in developed countries remains at greater than 95% of the population. Caries is still increasing in the developing countries. Thus for practical purposes it can be considered as ubiquitous in developed countries. The cost of treatment of dental disease is probably the most expensive of bacterial infections and it also results in considerable loss of time and productivity.

Dental caries may be defined as the localized destruction of tooth tissue by bacterial action. Dissolution of the hydroxyapatite crystals seems to precede the loss of organic components of both enamel and dentine, and this demineralization is thought to be caused by acids resulting from the bacterial fermentation of dietary carbohydrates. It is important to note that not all surfaces of tooth are equally afflicted, and that areas which are protected from cleansing, such as the fissures and areas between the teeth, are much more susceptible to decay.

The concept of immunity to caries depends on the demonstration that caries is a bacterial infection. Although vaccination against dental caries was attempted in the 1930s, the real impetus for development of vaccination against caries came with the demonstration, using germ-free animals, that caries could not occur in the absence of bacteria, and that specific bacteria were needed. No amount of refined carbohydrate would produce caries in the absence of bacteria. These early experiments established caries as an infective disease, and are discussed in further detail below.

With regard to host defences, the tooth sits in a unique position between the secretory immune system and the systemic immune system (see Chapter 1). The majority of the tooth surface would seem to be accessible to saliva, though the most caries-susceptible sites around the gingival margin and between the teeth (approximally) are bathed in crevicular fluid which is

47

derived from serum (Figure 3.1). Thus either serum or salivary antibodies could play a role in protection against caries, and both these mechanisms have been examined for natural immunity in man, and for the protective effects in vaccination experiments in animal models. It is possible that, to achieve 100% protection by immunological methods, effective induction of antibodies in both serum and salivary systems would be necessary.

This chapter examines the microbiological basis of caries in man and in animals, on which immunity is based. The evidence for any natural immunity in man, and the possible role of serum or salivary antibodies, is examined, as well as models of immunization against caries in animals.

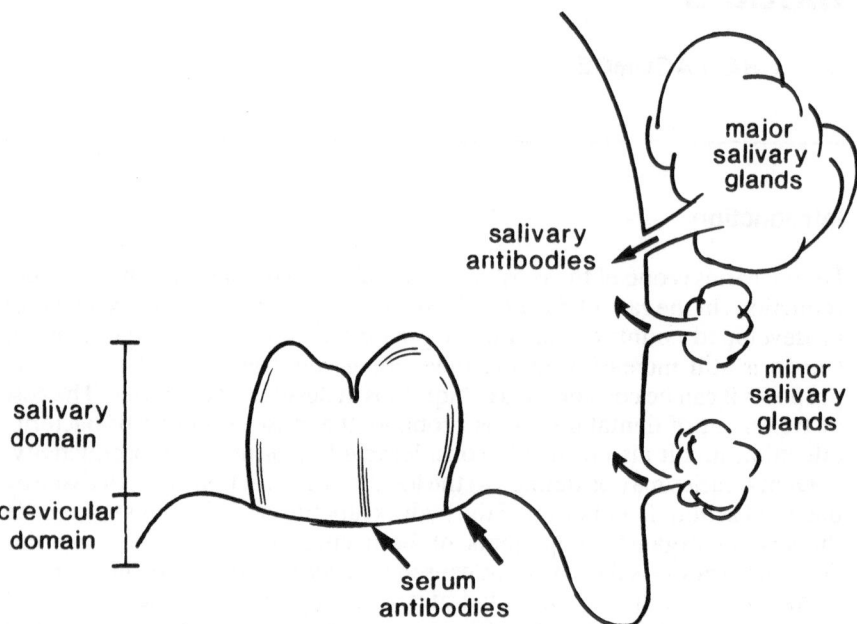

Figure 3.1 Relationship of secretory and systemic immune systems to the tooth surface. The crevicular domain is the area of the tooth exposed predominantly to serum antibodies via the gingival crevice, and the salivary domain the area exposed predominantly to salivary antibodies

The concept of dental caries as an infective disease

The concept of vaccination against caries depends on the disease being shown to be a specific bacterial infection rather than a non-specific infection. This evidence can be derived like any other infectious disease by applying Koch's postulates (Table 3.1) which essentially examine the association of bacteria with caries in man and extends this to examining the cariogenic potential of specific bacteria in animal models. Thus for an organism to be realistically considered to be cariogenic, it must both be associated with caries in man and be able to produce caries in animal models.

Table 3.1   Koch's postulates

1. The micro-organism must be present in every case of the disease
2. The micro-organism must be isolated from the diseased host and grown in pure culture
3. The specific disease must be reproduced when a pure culture of the organism is inoculated into a healthy susceptible host
4. The micro-organism must be recovered from the experimentally infected host
5. Under normal circumstances the micro-organism induces a rise in specific antibodies

Note: The fifth postulate has been added some time after Koch, but is used in diagnosis of disease

ESTABLISHMENT OF DENTAL CARIES AS AN INFECTIVE DISEASE

Association of bacteria with caries in humans

Identification of bacteria involved in the pathogenesis of dental caries has proved difficult because of the complex flora of the oral cavity. Earlier this century, lactobacilli and streptococci were identified as two of the organisms associated with dental decay, and a streptococcus was isolated which appeared rod-like in an acid environment and was called *Streptococcus mutans*. However, firm evidence that bacteria caused caries came only in the 1950s and 1960s following the germ-free experiments, and the definitive association of *S. mutans* and dental caries occurred even later.

The germ-free and gnotobiotic model enabled individual organisms to be tested for their ability to produce caries, but the model has the disadvantage that some pure cultures only cause caries in the absence of competition from the rest of the oral flora and thus may not reflect its cariogenic potential in the mouth of humans.

Transmissibility of caries in animals

In the 1960s, a number of closely related strains of streptococci were isolated from carious lesions in hamsters. These were able to produce typical lesions when inoculated in the mouth of caries-free animals. This clearly demonstrated that caries could be transmitted. The infectious nature of the disease was also demonstrated, since when animals with caries lesions were caged with hamsters that were caries-free and thought to be resistant, these latter animals also developed caries. However, strains of bacteria shown to cause caries in one animal species are not always able to induce caries in other species.

Transmissibility of caries in humans

It has not been possible ethically to determine whether caries can be transmitted in humans, but there is strong circumstantial evidence to suggest that this is the case, based on studies with transmissibility of strains of *S*.

49

mutans. An interesting series of experiments by Rogers (1977), who studied the biotypes of *S. mutans* in families, showed that the biotype of children closely matched that of the maternal strains, suggesting that these organisms had been derived from the mother. Since *S. mutans* is not found in edentulous children and babies, but is present after teeth erupt, then this organism must be derived from carriers. The evidence of Rogers suggests that the mother is the most likely source.

Association of specific bacteria with caries: microbiological evidence

The specific bacteria which have been associated with caries in man are outlined in Table 3.2 and given in detail in Chapter 2. It should be noted that the term 'dental caries' encompasses different types of caries lesions – notably those on smooth surfaces, those in pits and fissures and those on root surfaces. The aetiologies of these different types of caries may all be different, since the conditions pertaining in fissures and on smooth surfaces are clearly different, and root surface caries is decay of cementum and then dentine rather than enamel. In addition, rampant caries, which is the production of many new carious lesions over a short period of time, differs clinically from the more common slower type of caries and may possibly be more non-specific in aetiology.

Table 3.2 Micro-organisms associated with dental caries in humans

Species	Type of caries
S. mutans	Smooth surface, fissure, rampant root
L. casei	Smooth surface, fissure, rampant
L. acidophilus	Fissure
A. viscosus	Root surface
A. naeslundii	Root surface

The main genera which have been associated with dental caries in man are the lactobacilli, streptococci and actinomyces. Representative strains of each of these species have been shown to cause caries in animal models. There are problems in interpretation of most microbiological studies since these are cross-sectional, and do not distinguish between flora which has arisen as a result of a lesion, and flora which has caused the lesion. In addition the bulk of plaque may be irrelevant to the caries process and may obfuscate real differences in cariogenic flora of the tooth surface. Nevertheless, these studies have provided valuable data with regard to differences between carious lesions and sound surfaces.

Lactobacilli

Although many species of lactobacilli are found in plaque (see Chapter 2), *L. acidophilus* and *L. casei* are two strains which have shown to be cariogenic in animal models. It has been found that the numbers of lactobacilli in saliva or on the tooth surface broadly correlate with caries activity, but not always in individual subjects. Some authors have found that the numbers of lactobacilli in the mouth increase prior to clinically detectable carious lesions, though the majority view is that the number increases in plaque subsequent to the initiation of caries. The number of lactobacilli in saliva seem to be influenced by the quantity of dietary carbohydrate ingested.

The collective data indicate that lactobacilli are not of major importance in the initiation of human carious lesions. Their presence within the lesion and their recognized acidogenic properties, along with the ability to cause caries in animal models (see below), suggest that they may be important secondary invaders which contribute to the progression of tooth decay and may be important contributors to the overall acid production in rampant caries. With regard to the species a number of authors have found that *L. casei* rather than *L. acidophilus* is associated with caries both in children and adults.

Actinomyces

Actinomyces appear to be the predominant species in plaque from sound enamel surfaces, from carious lesions and from plaque samples from tooth surfaces. Strains of both *A. viscosus* and *A. naeslundii* can cause root surface caries in animals, and it is possible that actinomyces may contribute to root surface caries in man (see below) and also in rampant caries, though it does not seem to be a major contributor to smooth-surface caries.

Streptococci

Strains of *S. mutans, S. sanguis, S. faecalis* and *S. salivarius* can cause caries in animals. It is highly unlikely that *S. faecalis* or *S. salivarius* play a role in the aetiology of caries in man, since neither of these species are found in any appreciable numbers in plaque and no numerical association with caries has been found.

S. sanguis is cariogenic in some animal models (see below) and is universally present in plaque. However, the prevalence of *S. sanguis* in plaque is not greater in subjects with carious lesions, nor over carious lesions in comparison in smooth surfaces. An inverse relationship has been found between the number of *S. sanguis* and the presence of carious lesions both in human and animal experiments. At the present time there is little evidence to suggest that *S. sanguis* is a major contributor to caries in man, though involvement in rampant caries, and perhaps also in caries of pits and fissures, is possible.

Streptococcus mutans – There appears to be substantial evidence in favour of a pathogenic role of *S. mutans* in caries in man. This organism can produce copious amounts of extracellular polysaccharide from sucrose, much of which is insoluble in water. It is also very acidogenic and can cause caries in all animal models so far, including studies in rats, hamsters, monkeys and gerbils.

Many investigators around the world have attempted to relate the number of *S. mutans* in plaque with the presence of carious lesions. There has been an impressive degree of concordance in the results with a consistent finding that the number of *S. mutans* in plaque over carious lesions is greatly increased in comparison with that over sound surfaces, and in addition that *S. mutans* is more commonly isolated from those subjects with carious lesions. In our own studies (Figure 3.2) we have compared the numbers of *S. mutans* in plaque in three groups of subjects: those with low caries experiences, those with high past caries experience but no lesions, and those who have one or more carious lesions.

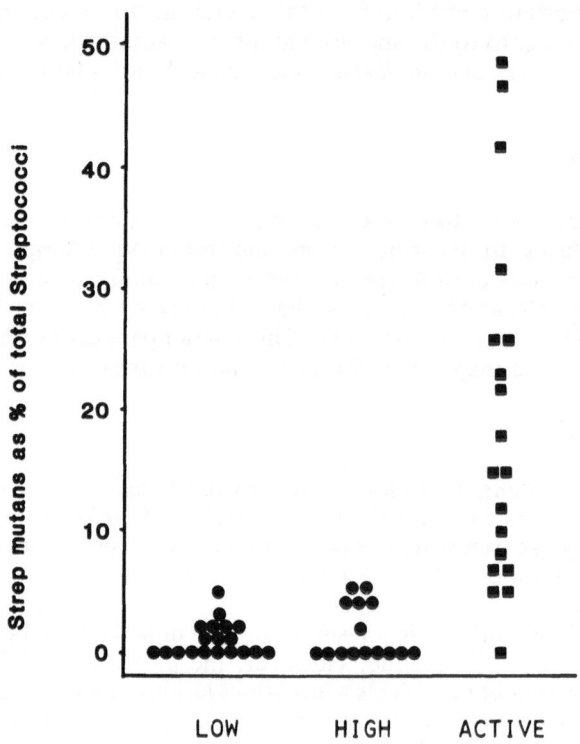

Figure 3.2   Numbers of *Streptococcus mutans* in plaque from three groups of subjects. Low = low MF (no carious lesions), high = high MF (no carious lesions), active = carious lesions and high DMF

In the absence of detectable caries, the numbers of *S. mutans* in plaque were very low, but in those with carious lesions the numbers were substantially raised in nearly all subjects. In addition, there is no correlation between the numbers of caries-inducing streptococci and past caries experience. Such cross-sectional studies do not provide proof that *S. mutans* causes the caries, since the numbers may increase once a carious lesion has been initiated. The strong association of *S. mutans* and caries is, however, confirmed by longitudinal surveys which have shown a strong relationship between the numbers of *S. mutans* and the initiation of caries.

However, an important point from microbiological studies in man is that although there is a very strong association between *S. mutans* and caries, some lesions can develop in the absence of *S. mutans*, particularly in fissures. In addition there are occasions on which there are large numbers of *S. mutans* present in plaque which do not necessarily lead to the initiation of caries.

Root surface caries

The strong association between *S. mutans* is with smooth surfaces, and microbiological studies have not shown a convincing relationship with regard to root surface caries. Indeed early cross-sectional studies suggested that increased numbers of *A. viscosus* were found with root surface lesions, but since this organism already contributed some 30% of the plaque flora on sound root surface, the increase to 40% or so is not convincing. More recent studies have not been able to confirm this association, and suggest that the isolation of *S. mutans* and lactobacilli together was a strong indicator of root surfaces and risk of decay. Interestingly, numbers of *Veillonella* are raised in root surface caries, and this may reflect the lactic acid environment (see Chapter 2).

Antigens of S. mutans

To date eight different serotypes of *S. mutans* have been recognized (a–h) on the basis of cell wall carbohydrate antigens. Recent studies suggest that serotypes c, e and f, where the cell wall serotype-specific carbohydrate is a polymer of glucose and rhamnose, should alone be designated as *S. mutans* (see Chapter 2). Serotype c is the most prevalent in human dental plaque taken on a worldwide basis. In addition to the serotype carbohydrate, the cell walls of *S. mutans* contain lipoteichoic acid and protein interspersed throughout the peptidoglycan layer of the cell wall, and which also present at the cell surface (Figure 3.3).

The *S. mutans* cell surface possesses a coat of filamentous structures commonly termed fimbriae, mainly composed of protein. Several cell surface proteins have recently been characterized and designated I/II and III. Antigen I/II is a protein antigen with two antigenic determinants. It has a molecular weight of 185 000, and has been used in several immunization experiments (see below). Glucosyltransferase enzymes are present in the cell wall, which also contains dextran binding proteins. Both these groups of proteins seem to be important in adherence of *S. mutans* to hard surfaces, and adherence and aggregation is enhanced in the presence of sucrose and dextrans. All the major components of *S. mutans* cell walls could be of potential importance in caries immunity.

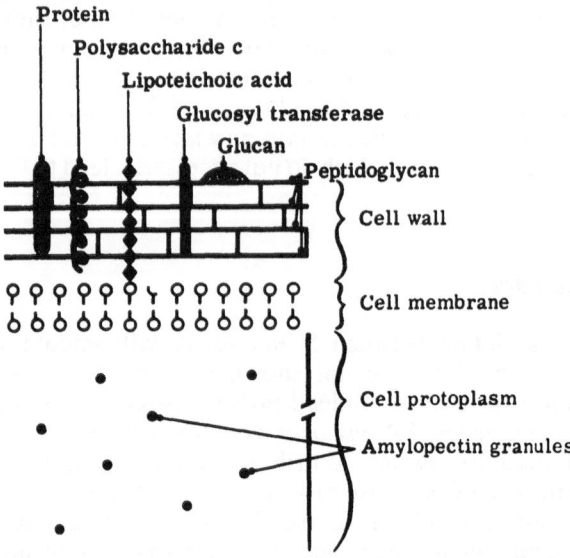

Figure 3.3 Diagrammatic representation of cell wall antigens of *S. mutans* (with permission from Lehner, 1982)

Immunological evidence for association of specific bacteria with caries

There have been few studies assaying antibodies to a range of oral bacteria and relating these to caries experience. In one study antibodies against a wide range of bacteria (Table 3.3) were assayed, and relationships with caries were only found with antibodies reactive with *S. mutans*. This clearly suggests some specificity for *S. mutans* with the process of dental caries.

Table 3.3 Immunological association of oral bacteria with caries in humans

Strain	? rise in antibodies in disease
S. mutans	Yes
S. sanguis	No
S. salivarius	No
S. mitior	No
L. casei	No
L. acidophilus	No
A. viscosus	No

CARIOGENIC POTENTIAL OF SPECIFIC BACTERIA IN ANIMAL MODELS

It cannot be assumed that, because an organism causes caries in an animal model, this has any relevance to decay in humans. Nevertheless, the demonstration that an organism is capable of producing caries is important if taken in association with data from man.

There have been three separate approaches to the study of cariogenic potential of bacteria in animal models. The most productive has been the gnotobiotic systems using rats and hamsters and, more recently, mice. The gnotobiotic model has the disadvantage that some pure culture may only cause caries in the absence of competition from the rest of the oral flora, and this may not reflect its cariogenic potential in the mouth of man.

Two methods have been developed which overcome this problem. Strains of bacteria can be made resistant to an antibiotic and superimposed on the normal flora of conventional animals with the organisms being isolated on media containing antibiotic, or animals may be exposed to antibiotic in their drinking water to suppress the normal flora and then infected with a strain which has been made resistant to the antibiotic.

Summary of cariogenic activity

A summary of cariogenic activity of different species of bacteria in a variety of animal experiments is given in Table 3.4. This table has been constructed to emphasize the different types of caries, and indicates the differing caries potentials of various strains of bacteria examined. Thus lactobacilli in general have been found capable of causing pit and fissure caries, and *Actinomyces viscosus* capable of causing root surface caries. By far the most cariogenic organism in a number of different animal models is *S. mutans*, which has been shown to be capable of producing smooth surface caries, pit and fissure caries, and root surface caries.

Table 3.4 Summary of cariogenic activity of different species of bacteria in animal experiments

	Type of caries			Animals
	Smooth surface	Pit and fissure	Root surface	
S. mutans	+++	+++	++	Rat, hamster, mouse, monkey, gerbil
S. sanguis	+	++		Rat
S. salivarius		+		Hamster
S. faecalis		+		Rat
L. casei		+		Rat
L. acidophilus		+		Rat
A. viscosus	±		++	Hamster, rat
A. naeslundii			+	Hamster

However, as emphasized above, to fulfil Koch's postulates, data from animal experiments should be taken in conjunction with microbiological studies in man. Thus *S. salivarius* and *S. faecalis*, though capable of causing caries in animals, are unlikely to be major contributors to caries in man, whereas *S. mutans* is found in carious lesions in man, can cause carious lesions in animals, and can be reisolated from those lesions.

IMMUNITY TO CARIES IN HUMANS

Non-specific immunity

Defence mechanisms in the mouth can be either non-specific or specific (see Chapter 1). The non-specific defence mechanisms include the mucosal barrier and saliva in terms of its lubricating and buffering capacities and the constituents of saliva such as lactoferrin, lactoperoxidase and lysozyme. The general properties of these proteins have been discussed in Chapter 1. A number of workers have tried to detect differences in the salivary components between subjects with high and low caries experience. However, a consistent and meaningful pattern has not been detected, though the recent observation that secretory IgA antibodies may act synergistically with lysozyme and lactoferrin has led to renewed interest in the possibility that combinations of these may still be important in immunity to caries in humans.

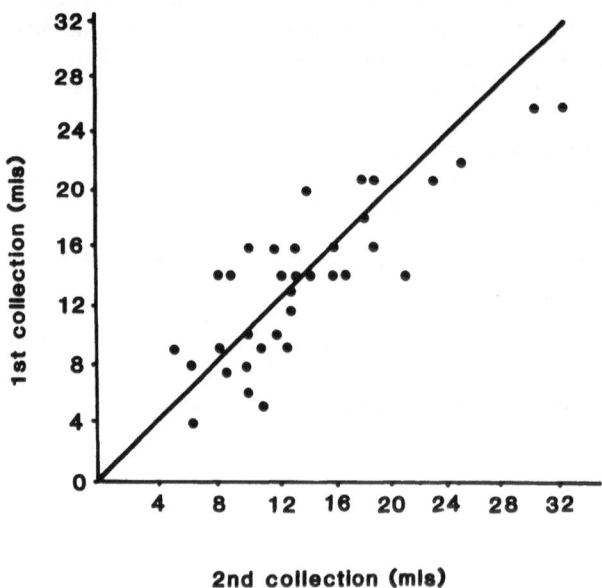

Figure 3.4 Relationship between the volume of parotid saliva collected on two separate occasions, 6 months apart. Saliva was collected under standard conditions of partial stimulation

Total immunoglobulin levels have also been examined with regard to caries, and can be regarded as non-specific. No consistent pattern has emerged with regard to the concentration of salivary IgA. A number of studies have claimed raised IgA concentrations in subjects of low caries experience, but many studies have not been able to detect differences and two studies have found higher IgA levels in subjects with increased caries experience.

Many of these studies have not taken the secretion rate of saliva into account. This is important, since in healthy subjects the secretion rates may vary 8-fold. However the secretion rate of an individual may be quite consistent. In one study, as seen in Figure 3.4, there was a good correlation between the volume of saliva obtained on one occasion under standardized conditions compared with that taken 6 months later under the same conditions of partial stimulation with 2% citric acid.

The IgA secretion rate (micrograms of IgA per gland) in subjects of high caries experience seems to be significantly lower than that of subjects with low caries experience. However, it is likely that specific antibodies are much more important than total IgA.

Specific immunity

Principles and objectives of investigations

In general, immunological investigations of bacterial diseases in man have two main objectives: (a) to determine if there is a specific association of any particular organism with the disease, and (b) to determine whether there is any evidence of natural immunity and if so, whether this is humoral or cellular, secretory or systemic, or related to specific isotype, etc. Comparisons have usually been made between populations identified as being resistant to a particular disease with populations being identified as susceptible to the same disease.

Table 3.5 Principles of immunological investigations in caries epidemiology

Question	Group	Bacteria
Is there natural immunity?	Compare caries-resistant with caries-susceptible	Those bacteria associated from microbiological studies
Is there an immune response to caries?	Compare subjects with lesions with matched group without lesions	Bacteria and antigens thought to be associated with the caries process

It is recognized in most infective diseases that actual infection leads to a stimulation of the immune system with an increase in specific antibodies or cell-mediated immunity. In fact, this is a useful test in the diagnosis of many infective diseases. If this important principle is applied to dental caries, this means that in order to detect any role of immunity in protection against caries, then comparison must be made between subjects of low caries experience and those who are identified as being caries-susceptible (by high DMF) but with no carious lesions. This comparison should, as with other infectious diseases, allow the question of any role of immunity in resistance to be determined (Table 3.5).

The second question of identifying specific organisms can be determined by comparing a group of subjects who have lesions with subjects of similar caries experience but without lesions. A rise in specific antibodies against a particular organism will provide evidence that this organism might be involved in the caries process.

These principles have been derived from studies of other infectious diseases but there may be some difficulty in the application to dental caries since the time of onset of decay is often not known. There are also difficulties in controlling for other known associated factors such as diet, fluoride intake, etc. Nevertheless, studies using these principles have provided useful information. In contrast, comparisons between subjects of low DMF and those with rampant caries are generally not helpful. Unfortunately, this is an approach which has been used by several investigators on the basis that subjects with rampant caries indicate a susceptible group, but the possibility that the infecting organism may induce an antibody response has been overlooked.

Types of immunity

As discussed in Chapter 1, it is clear that the secretory (mucosal) immune system can be stimulated quite independently from the systemic immune system. The induction of antibodies in saliva may be achieved by either local or central stimulation (Table 3.6). For local production, antibodies may be applied topically or injected around the salivary glands. For central immunization, antigen is delivered to the gut and stimulates the release of antibody precursor cells from the Peyers patches. These cells migrate not only to salivary glands, but to all secretory tissues where they secrete dimeric IgA. This attaches to secretory component receptor on the epithelial cells (Figure 3.5), becomes intracellular, and is then secreted into the salivary ducts.

Table 3.6 Method of induction of salivary antibodies

Local
   Topical application of antigen
   Instillation of antigen into salivary ducts
   Injection of antigen in salivary gland vicinity

Central (by gut-associated lymphoid tissue)
   Ingestion of antigen in diet
   Intragastric or intraduodenal immunization

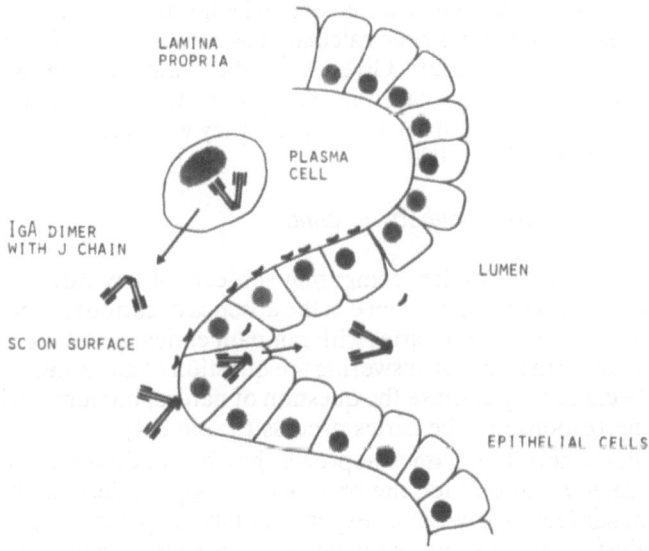

Figure 3.5 Secretion and transport of dimeric IgA to salivary glands. Plasma cells in the lamina propria secrete dimeric IgA. This binds to SC acting as receptors on the surface of epithelial cells. The SIgA is internalized, transported across the cell and secreted into the ducts. The precursor of the plasma cell may have originated in the gut-associated lymphoid tissue

It should be noted that for the most effective salivary antibody responses, two signals may be required: a primary signal resulting in the localization of antigen-sensitive cells in the mucosa and a secondary signal from the local application of antigen.

Systemic serum antibodies in crevicular fluid

The tooth sits in a fluid collar of crevicular fluid (Figure 3.1). Antibodies in crevicular fluid are largely derived from serum, though there is on average a local contribution, particularly of IgG, up to about 20% of the total antibody content. This may be considerably greater in individual sites. Passage of IgG, IgA and IgM from serum to crevicular fluid can be shown by injecting radiolabelled immunoglobulins intravenously. Such experiments in primates have indicated that the passage of IgG and IgA is maximal ½–1 hour after injection, whereas IgM is maximal at approximately 2 hours after intravenous injection. The differences are probably related to the molecular size. Interestingly, the migration of radiolabelled polymorphonuclear leukocytes (PMN) is very rapid indeed, and these can be found in crevicular fluid some 10 minutes after injection intravenously.

Effective protection against caries may require the combination of specific and non-specific factors (see below). The immunoglobulin concentration in crevicular fluid seems to be between one-half and three-quarters that of serum. The flow rate of crevicular fluid into the oral cavity is difficult to estimate but has been calculated as between 1 and 2 ml per day or 0.3 µl per tooth per hour. Given that the total volume of saliva is approximately 750 ml per day, this would indicate that serum antibodies could play a role in the oral cavity at large if they were effective at a dilution between 1 : 500 and 1 : 1000.

Relationship of serum antibody to caries

There have been few studies comparing subjects of low caries experience with those of high caries experience in the absence of carious lesions. Several studies have compared low caries with rampant caries, and these studies are of dubious value in terms of answering the question of any natural immunity in caries because they confuse the question of natural immunity with that of an immune response to the caries process (Table 3.4).

In studies where the former approach has been adopted, and subjects carefully selected to exclude the presence of incipient lesions, it has been found that subjects of low caries experience have high serum IgG antibody titres against *S. mutans* and the mean levels are significantly greater than those in subjects of high caries experience (Figure 3.6). Serum IgG antibodies showed the greatest differences, though serum IgM and IgA antibodies were also highest in subjects of low caries experience. The finding of raised IgG antibodies to whole cells of *S. mutans* in the subjects of low caries experience has been confirmed using a variety of different immunological tests including haemagglutination, complement fixation, enzyme-linked immunosorbent assay (ELISA) and radioassay. This relationship seems to be specific to *S. mutans* and has not been found with strains of *S. sanguis, S. salivarius, L. casei, L. acidophilus*, or *Actinomyces viscosus* (Table 3.3). A similar finding of raised antibody levels in subjects with low caries experience has recently been reported with regard to the surface protein antigen I/II. This protein has been used in immunization experiments in animals, and inhibition studies indicate that this is a major antigenic component of the *S. mutans* cell wall.

Recent studies which have examined IgG subclasses indicate that this raised response in subjects of low caries experience is due to IgG1 and IgG2 antibodies directed against *S. mutans* and predominantly IgG1 antibodies directed against streptococcal antigen I/II. These studies would be consistent with the interpretation that serum IgG antibody contributes to the protection against caries in these subjects.

Effect of dentinal carious lesions on serum antibody

A comparison of subjects of high caries experience with and without dentinal lesions indicates a raised antibody titre in subjects with carious lesions (Figure 3.6). This raised antibody titre seems to be specific to *S. mutans*, and this implicates *S. mutans* in the pathogenesis of this disease.

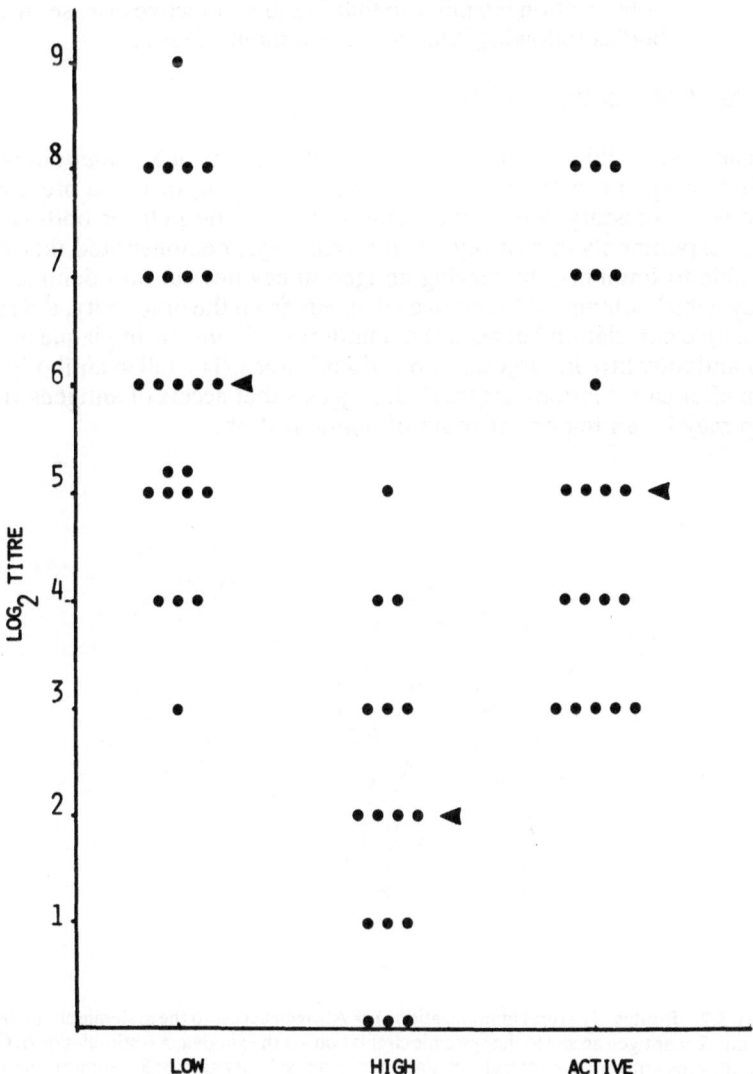

Figure 3.6 Serum IgG antibodies to *S. mutans* in relationship to the caries experience. Low = low MF group, high = high MF group, active = high DMF group with one or more carious lesions. Serum IgM antibodies followed a similar though less significant pattern. The relationship was not found with various other oral bacteria examined, including *S. sanguis*

This raised antibody titre has been reported with serum IgG and IgM, though not with serum IgA antibody.

Raised serum antibody titres in subjects with carious lesions (Figure 3.6) is consistent with the view that infection with *S. mutans* and the development of carious lesions is associated with a rise in specific antibodies to *S. mutans*.

This type of observation is similar to that found in infective diseases where a rise in antibodies following infection is commonly found.

Route of natural immunization

It is not clear if this response is to increased numbers of *S. mutans* in plaque with consequent immunization through the gingiva, or if the presence of lesions is necessary with immunization through the pulp or both (Figure 3.7). Experiments in monkeys, many years ago, demonstrated that it was possible to immunize by placing antigen in cavities cut into dentine. One study, which attempted to remove all plaque from the oral cavity, did report a positive correlation between the numbers of *S. mutans* in plaque and the IgG antibody titre in subjects with carious lesions. The fall in antibody titre, seen after caries lesions are treated, suggests that access of antigens via the pulp may be an important route of immunization.

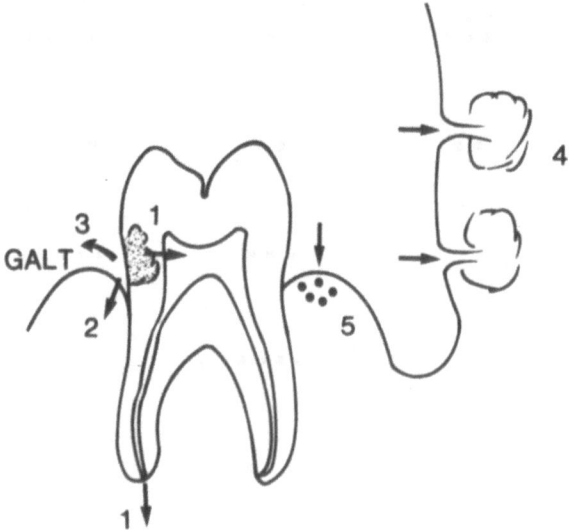

Figure 3.7 Routes of natural immunization. 1 = Antigen access to the systemic circulation via the pulp; 2 = antigen access to the systemic circulation via the gingiva; 3 = stimulation of GALT by swallowing antigen; 4 = topical stimulation of minor salivary glands; 5 = topical stimulation of local gingival lymphocytes

Conversely there is no doubt that antigens in plaque can induce systemic effects. In experiments where plaque was allowed to accumulate over a 4-week period in student volunteers, an increase in cell-mediated responses to *S. mutans* was found, which returned to baseline when oral hygiene was reinstituted.

Relationship of salivary antibodies to caries

Many studies have attempted to examine the relationship of salivary antibodies to dental caries on the same basis as studies of serum antibodies.

Unfortunately, salivary antibody levels appear to be more variable than serum antibodies, and the secretion rate of antibodies has been taken into account in few studies, even though the great variation in salivary secretion rates is well known. No consistent patterns have emerged and raised levels of salivary IgA antibodies to *S. mutans* have not been found in subjects of low carious experience. In fact it seems that the salivary IgA antibody levels may increase with the degree of caries experience, and may reflect the cumulative carious experience.

An inverse relationship between serum IgG and salivary IgA antibodies has been reported, and this raises interesting questions as to the relationship between the secretory and systemic immune systems (Figure 3.8). It should be noted that the presence of antibodies does not in itself indicate protection, since in certain circumstances antibodies may be in fact damaging.

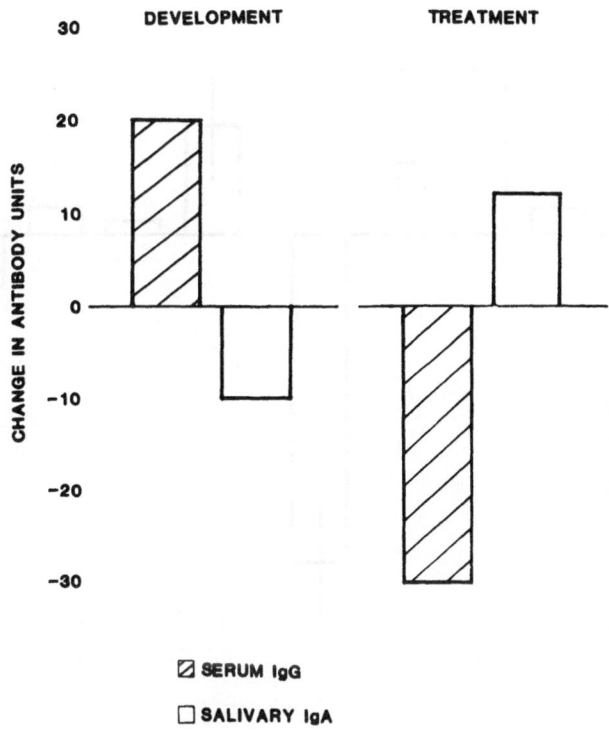

Figure 3.8 Change in serum and salivary antibodies to *S. mutans* following development or treatment of dental caries, showing inverse relationship between serum IgG and salivary IgA antibodies

Induction of salivary antibodies in humans

It has been shown that salivary IgA antibodies in man may be induced by ingestion of capsules filled with *S. mutans* organisms. No long-term studies have been performed to see the effect of such antibody in caries. At present it seems that longer-term immunization would be necessary, since the salivary antibody response is short-lived. Salivary antibodies may prove to be effective since a reduction in number of *S. mutans* has been reported in such immunized subjects.

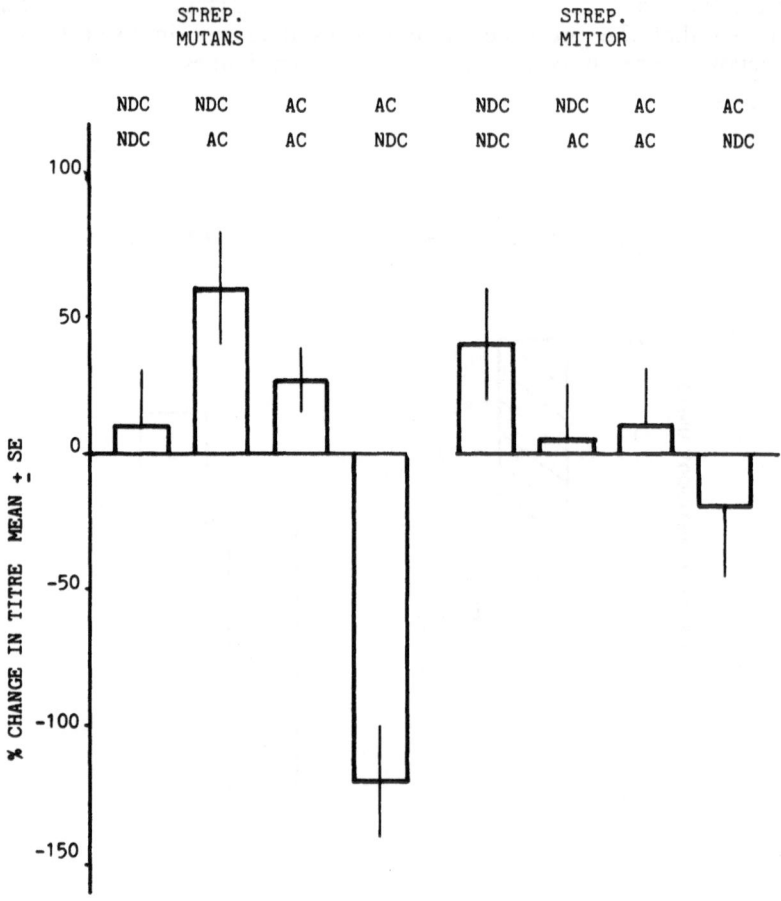

Figure 3.9 Sequential changes in serum IgG antibody titre against *S. mutans* in relation to treatment or development of dental caries. Development of caries was associated with a rise in the antibody titre to *S. mutans* and treatment with a fall. Antibodies to other oral bacteria did not show any relationship. NDC–NDC = No detectable caries on either visit; NDC–AC = patients with caries lesions on second visit; AC–AC = patients with caries lesions on both visits; AC–NDC = patients who have had their lesions treated

Sequential studies

The objective of sequential studies is to determine whether any change in caries status is accompanied by changes in antibody status in either serum or saliva. These studies are of necessity long-term, and to date only one such study has been reported. The results of this study are summarized in Figure 3.9, and indicate that the antibody levels against *S. mutans* in subjects whose caries status is stable, remained consistent over the period of examination, which was greater than 2 years. The development of carious lesions was accompanied by a rise in serum IgG and IgM antibody levels and, interestingly, treatment of carious lesions was accompanied by a fall in serum antibody levels, particularly of the IgG class, over the next year or so. Analysis of antibodies to a control organism – *S. mitior* – showed no such association.

With regard to salivary antibodies, no obvious relationship with caries emerged, but responses seemed to follow the opposite pattern to serum antibody.

Interpretation of immunological studies in humans

The results of sequential studies are consistent with the interpretation that immune responses to dental caries are similar to those in other infective disease. Development of caries is associated with a rise in serum antibodies, and treatment of caries is associated with a fall in caries. Subjects who do not develop caries have a stable antibody level, whether this is high or low.

Taking the cross-sectional and sequential studies together, one interpretation would be that on exposure to *S. mutans* antigens subjects develop an antibody response which is individually high or low. If high, this may contribute to protection against caries, but if low, the subjects are susceptible. In this group, if caries develops they are capable of mounting an immune response since high levels of antibodies are found in subjects with lesions. It appears, however, that these subjects may not be capable of maintaining a high response since treatment of caries is followed by a fall in the serum antibody titre. Thus the essential immunological defect may be an inability to maintain high antibody levels following antigenic challenge.

There is a paradox in that the highest levels of antibody are found in those with least caries experience, and presumably those with least exposure to the cariogenic organism *S. mutans*. This raises the question of whether the ability to mount a high serum antibody response to low amounts of antigenic challenge is genetically determined.

Genetic factors

An attempt has been made to examine the question of whether the ability to mount and maintain a high serum antibody response to *S. mutans* is genetically linked. Earlier investigations had shown that T lymphocytes from caries-free subjects had a greater potential for proliferation on stimulation with *S. mutans* antigen than caries-prone subjects. This was consistent with the findings with serum antibodies.

When such lymphocytes are cultured in the presence of antigen derived from *S. mutans*, factors are given off from the cells which can be assayed in a variety of *in vitro* systems. T helper factor is such a lymphokine, which can augment the immune responses of unrelated and unsensitized lymphocytes.

In one study of caries-prone and low caries subjects using streptococcal antigen I/II, it was found that specific helper factor was released optimally by a dosage of between 1 and 10 ng of SA I/II from lymphocytes from low caries subjects but that the optimal for caries-prone subjects was 1000 ng (see Figure 3.10). This indicated a marked difference in responses, and certainly supported the suggestion that caries-resistant and caries-prone

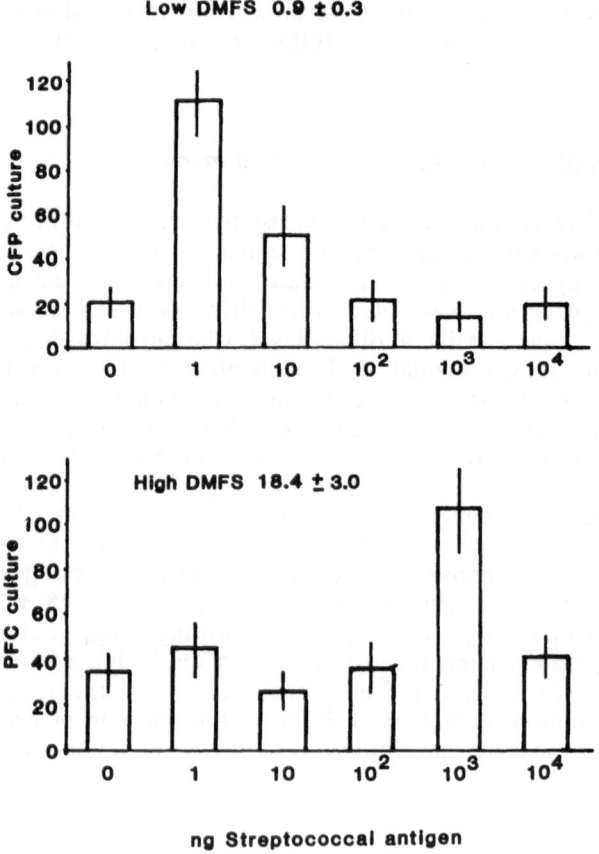

ng Streptococcal antigen

Figure 3.10 T helper function in subject of high and low caries experience. The subject's lymphocytes are incubated with streptococcal antigen and the production of T **helper** factors assayed separately using mouse cells. The optimal antigen concentration in subjects of low caries experience was considerably lower than in subjects of high caries experience

66

subjects differed in their ability to mount and maintain serum antibody responses to *S. mutans*. The response to antigenic stimulation using SA I/II was related to the histocompatibility antigens of the subjects, and in particular to the HLA-DR locus. The helper activity, which was optimal as a low dose, was found in HLA-DRW6-positive subjects, whereas subjects who showed an optimal response at the high antigen dose were found to be HLA-DRW6-negative.

These findings suggest that the ability to respond to very small amounts of streptococcal antigens may be the reason for the high antibody levels to *S. mutans* in low caries subjects. However, the immunoregulation of such responses is complex and this is an area requiring further study.

IMMUNIZATION AGAINST CARIES IN ANIMAL MODELS

Animal models

Rodents

There have been two main models used in studies of caries immunity in animals and these have been in rodents and in primates. Probably the most widely used model has been the gnotobiotic rat, in which the animals have been infected with *S. mutans*. Usually, in these studies, the animals are fed on a diet containing sucrose, immunized and then challenged with the same *S. mutans* from which the vaccine was derived. Any immunity to caries can be assessed by comparing the salivary or serum antibody responses and caries development in immunized animals with those of sham-immunized controls.

Germ-free rats offer probably the simplest model for caries immunity since non-infected animals remain caries-free but have the disadvantage that the cariogenic organisms are acting without a normal flora. Thus it can not be assumed that findings derived from this model will necessarily be applicable to the situation when *S. mutans* is imposed on a normal flora. The rodent model also has the disadvantage that the tooth structure and form is not analogous to that in man, and although there are great similarities between the immune systems, there are differences also. For example, the rat saliva contains approximately 50% IgG, whereas human saliva contains less than 1% IgG. The model has the advantage of being relatively cheap, and variables such as diet and flora can be easily controlled.

Primate model

In recent years much attention has focused on the primate model of caries immunity. Two main models have been used – rhesus monkeys and fascicularis monkeys. The primate model has several advantages over the rodent model (Table 3.7). In particular the teeth are very similar to humans;

the systemic and secretory immune systems are virtually identical to those of man, with known differences only in the half-lives of immunoglobulins; and when they consume a diet based on that in humans the number of *S. mutans* rises without the need to implant.

Table 3.7   Features of animal models of dental caries

	Primates	*Rodents*
Tooth form similar to humans	+	−
Systemic immune system analogous to humans	+	+
Secretory immune system analogous to humans	+	±
Oral flora analogous to humans	+	−
Increase in *S. mutans* without implantation	+	−
Ease of control of variables	±	+
Cheapness to maintain	−	+
Length of time per experiment (months)	12	2

It seems, therefore, that initiation and progression of caries in the monkey model is very analogous indeed to that in humans. Caries develops over a period of several months, which is thought to be similar to that in man. The disadvantages of the model are that it is extremely expensive to maintain, and that each experiment must, of necessity, last for many months. In most circumstances this has meant that the experimental groups of animals are smaller than would be ideal for most statistical analyses.

Passive immunization

Early attempts at passive immunization, when hamsters were treated with rabbit hyperimmune antisera against cariogenic streptococcus gave no protection. Passive immunization has not been generally accepted as a viable method of protection against caries, and very few animal experiments have been performed. Passive transfer of IgG antibodies to *S. mutans* has been shown in rhesus monkeys to give protection against dental caries (see below).

Very recently the use of monoclonal antibodies against streptococcal antigen has allowed this concept to be re-examined. It has been shown that the administration of monoclonal antibody directed against antigen I/II to the gingival area of rhesus monkeys results in a reduced number of *S. mutans* and a decreased incidence of caries. Since monoclonal antibodies can be produced in large amounts, this raises the possibility that administration of such specific antisera in a carrier such as toothpaste might be an effective way of immunization.

Active immunization

Experiments in rodents

The first convincing evidence that local injection of killed *S. mutans* into the salivary gland region of rats could induce a local antibody response was by Taubman and Smith in 1974. These workers showed a marked reduction in the level of dental caries in immunized animals, and also showed significant levels of serum and salivary antibodies to *S. mutans*. A number of studies since then have shown that injection of antigens derived from *S. mutans* suspended in complete Freund's adjuvant and injected around the salivary glands will indeed induce a salivary IgA response as well as serum, and can result in protection against caries. However, injection of antigens in adjuvant around salivary glands is not an ideal immunization regime for humans.

Oral immunization in rodents

The concept of a common mucosal immune system (see Chapter 1) has stimulated research into the possibility of central (GALT) immunization and its role in the induction of salivary antibodies. The selective induction of secretory IgA antibodies to *S. mutans* in saliva in the absence of serum antibodies is also attractive because the possibility of side-effects from serum antibodies is diminished.

Some 10 years ago, it was demonstrated that oral immunization led to IgA antibodies in saliva and also in colostrum and milk with no serum response. If these animals were challenged with *S. mutans* a reduced caries incidence was found in immunized animals. Further work has shown that the concentration of antigen is important, and that the secretory system may become hyporesponsive if the antigen concentration is too great, and non-responsive if the antigen concentration is too low. It should be noted that these studies not only provide evidence of the role of secretory IgA in caries immunity in the rodent model but also provide supportive evidence for the concept for a common mucosal immune system.

The hamster has been a useful model in caries immunity and studies have indicated that hamsters orally immunized with an impure glucosyl transferase (GTF) produced salivary anti-GTF antibodies and reduced carious lesions in comparison with controls. In contrast to the experiments reported with oral immunization in rats, immunization in hamsters seems to be accompanied by low titres of serum IgG and IgM antibodies.

It is clear that the nature of the antigen, particularly whether it is particulate or soluble, may influence both the observed IgA response and any serum immune response. As a general rule, administration of soluble proteins by the intragastric route can result in the induction of antibodies in secretions, but may give rise to.antibodies in serum also. Administration of

69

particulate antigens such as whole bacteria seem to be more effective in inducing antibodies in secretions, but less effective in inducing antibodies in serum by this route.

Summary of caries immunity studies in rodents

The results of caries immunization studies in rodents clearly suggest that the salivary IgA response can be effective in reducing caries in this model. There is no doubt salivary IgA responses can be induced by oral administration of particulate or soluble *S. mutans* antigens. It is assumed that the secretory IgA may protect either from inhibition of GTF activity or reaction with cell surface components, resulting in decreased adherence of bacteria.

Studies in other animal models suggest that the most effective secretory responses are induced by a two signal system – a primary signal resulting in the distribution of IgA-sensitive cells to mucosal tissues and a second signal derived from the presence of antigen in a mucosal region. With respect to caries, this would indicate that the presence of *S. mutans* on the tooth surface in sensitized animals would allow for further local recruitment and proliferation of IgA antibody-producing cells. The role of serum antibodies in protection against caries in rodents is less clear. Many of these successful immunization programmes have induced serum as well as salivary antibodies. Whereas salivary antibodies alone may result in caries protection, studies using serum antibodies alone have been equivocal. It remains possible that, even in the rodent model, serum antibodies could contribute to protection.

Immunization experiments in primates

The experimental model

Experimental caries experiments in the rodent model have been the basis for establishing that caries was an infective disease (see above). The first successful experimental caries model in monkeys was established by Bowen, who demonstrated in the mid-1960s that, if fascicularis monkeys were kept on a high sucrose diet, the bacterial flora was very similar to that found in man. In addition, he showed that rampant dental caries could be induced successfully and reproducibly in this model.

The rhesus monkey (*Macaca mulatta*) has also been established as a suitable model for immunological studies using a human-type diet.

Implantation of S. mutans – Early experiments attempted to implant *S. mutans* which had been made antibiotic-resistant onto the normal flora of the animals. It was soon realized in experiments with the rhesus monkey, and later with the fascicularis monkey, that implantation was not necessary.

70

Soon after the animals had been put on a high-sucrose diet, natural *S. mutans* began to increase in the plaque. The origins of this *S. mutans* are not entirely clear, since they could either be part of the normal flora which is usually undetectable but increases to detectable levels on a sucrose diet, or they could be derived from the handlers of the animals. The majority of the *S. mutans* strains have been serotype c, though some are of serotype e. In addition, a strain of *S. mutans* has been described which is of serotype h and appears to be restricted to monkeys.

Systemic immunization

Successful immunization against dental caries was first reported in the primate model by Bowen in 1969. In a preliminary communication on immunization of fascicularis monkeys he showed a reduction in caries in deciduous teeth in the three animals which had been immunized intravenously with whole live cells of a strain of *S. mutans*. High titres of agglutinating antibody were induced in the test group and in addition precipitating antibodies against glucosyltransferase (GTF) were found. The implication was that serum antibodies may have been responsible for this reduction in caries.

Lehner and his colleagues have described many experiments in the rhesus monkey model, and have demonstrated unequivocally that caries can be reduced by immunization (Table 3.8). In early experiments animals were immunized either subcutaneously or submucosally with whole cells of *S. mutans* in Freund's incomplete adjuvant (FIA). Antibodies were detected in both serum and saliva against whole cells or cell wall extracts of *S. mutans*. Significant reductions in the caries in deciduous teeth were seen following immunization by either route in the order of 75–80%.

Although salivary antibodies were detected, the reduction in caries correlated with serum antibodies to *S. mutans* antigens. Results also indicated that, for antibodies to be effective, they should be present before *S. mutans* has reached appreciable proportions in dental plaque. Further experiments extended these findings to permanent teeth where subcutaneous injections of whole cells of *S. mutans* in FIA elicited high titres of serum antibodies and protection against caries. These studies seem to confirm the suggestion that serum antibodies were responsible for protection. Such systemic immunization elicits not only serum antibodies but also a cell-mediated response. Skin hypersensitivity and increased lymphoproliferation against *S. mutans* can be detected after such systemic immunization. The immunoregulation of immune responses has been the subject of much further research and is discussed below.

Glucosyltransferase – The demonstration that *S. mutans* produced glucosyltransferase which, in turn, produced insoluble polysaccharide which was a mixture of alpha 1–3 and alpha 1–6 linkages, raised the questions (a)

Table 3.8 Immunization against dental caries in primates

Streptococcus mutans antigen	Route	Adjuvant	Caries reduction	S. mutans reduction	Antibodies in	
					Serum	Saliva
Whole cells	i.v., s.c.	FIA, Al (OH)$_3$	Yes	Yes/no*	Yes	No
	s.m.		Yes	Yes/no	Yes	Yes
	In diet	None	No	No	No	Yes
Cell walls	s.c.	FIA	Yes	No	Yes	No
GTF	s.c.	FIA, Al (OH)$_3$	No	No	Yes	No
Ag I/II	s.c.	FIA, Al (OH)$_3$	Yes	Yes/no	Yes	No
Ag I	s.c.	FIA, Al (OH)$_3$	Partial	No	Yes	No
Ag B	s.c.	FIA, Al (OH)$_3$	Partial	No	Yes	No
Ag A	s.c.	FIA, Al (OH)$_3$	Yes	No	Yes	No

Key: FIA = Freund's incomplete adjuvant; s.c. = subcutaneous; s.m. = submucosal; i.v. = intravenously; GTF = glucosyltransferase
*Reduction in *Streptococcus mutans* in some experiments

whether this enzyme was important to the cariogenic potential of the organism and (b) whether immunization against GTF might be effective. It seems that, in the rodent model, immunization with GTF may produce protection against caries, and it was shown that purified GTF injected in adjuvant around the salivary glands may induce effective protection. However, in the primate model immunization with GTF has been less effective, and this has been examined in both the fascicularis and rhesus monkey models (Table 3.8). Interestingly, immunization with *S. mutans* would result in serum antibodies against GTF, but whereas the IgG antibodies would inhibit the activity of GTF, IgM and IgA antibodies could have an enhancing effect on GTF. Thus a large IgM or IgA response would overcome any inhibitory effect of IgG, and could result in an increased incidence of caries following immunization rather than a decrease.

Passive transfer experiments

The experiments described above clearly indicated that serum antibodies were responsible for the protection against caries, and thus antibodies in serum must reach the tooth surface. Experiments using radiolabelled IgG, IgA and IgM showed that serum immunoglobulins can pass to the oral cavity of monkeys when injected intravenously.

Convincing evidence that serum antibodies could reach the oral cavity, and be effective, were provided by passive transfer experiments where serum and purified immunoglobulin preparations from animals immunized with *S. mutans* were injected intravenously into non-immunized animals. The short half-life of immunoglobulins, which in the case of IgG in the rhesus monkey is approximately 8 days, meant that serum or immuno-globulin had to be injected every 3 weeks or so over a period of up to a year. Animals given purified IgG containing antibody activity against *S. mutans* showed a reduction in caries. Animals injected with IgA or IgM containing antibodies to *S. mutans* did not show any significant reduction in comparison with controls given non-immune serum, but IgA and IgM have shorter half-lives than IgG and it is difficult to maintain high levels of serum antibodies by passive immunization.

These studies clearly indicate that serum IgG can pass to the oral cavity and protect unimmunized animals. Interestingly, transfer of whole immune serum did not result in protection, and it is possible that this was due to the inhibitory effect of IgA antibodies on the IgG activity. This observation raises the important point that effective immunization may depend on a high IgG to IgA ratio, since IgA antibodies have been found in a number of systems to inhibit the actions of IgG.

Oral immunization

The observation that serum antibodies can protect against dental caries does not obviate the possibility that salivary IgA antibodies could also be protective. Salivary antibody responses in rhesus monkeys immunized with *S. mutans* by a variety of routes, including the oral submucosal or subcutaneous routes, have been reported. Although salivary antibodies can be detected after any of these routes of immunization the most effective way seems to be by intragastric immunization. Thus intragastric immunization with capsules filled with *S. mutans* over 13 days led to a detectable haemagglutinating and agglutinating antibody response in saliva. A second series of immunizations over 11 days gave a similar type of response.

These findings were similar to those reported in man and raised the important question of the duration of secretory responses. In both instances the salivary antibody titre had fallen to baseline levels within a few weeks, and the duration of the response after the second series of immunizations was also only a few weeks. It should be noted that although intragastric immunization has been reported to induce salivary antibodies in a number of animal models and in man, two groups have reported failure to detect antibody responses in saliva after intragastric immunization in primates.

An alternative method of inducing salivary IgA antibodies by central (GALT) immunization is to apply the antigen in drinking water. This also results in a detectable salivary antibody response, but when the antigen is withdrawn from the diet the salivary antibody level returns to baseline values. Nevertheless, this method seemed more appropriate for longer-term immunization than did intragastric immunization with capsules. With respect to caries in rhesus monkeys, the daily addition of 10^{11} cells of *S. mutans* in drinking water for 18 weeks did not result in a reduction in caries (Table 3.7) and in addition no decrease in the colonization of *S. mutans* was detected.

Thus to date there is no convincing evidence in the primate model that oral immunization can lead to a reduction in caries, though this has not been excluded. It is possible that application of antigen in adjuvant intra-gastrically may provide a longer-lasting salivary antibody response which may allow the question of protective salivary IgA antibody to be addressed.

It does seem that salivary IgA antibodies in the primate may interfere with adherence of *S. mutans*. In a series of experiments in *Macaca fascicularis*, *S. mutans* was first injected in the vicinity of the parotid gland, and this injection was followed by intraductal instillation of antigen into the parotid duct. Although no salivary antibodies were detected after the injection around the salivary gland region, the subsequent intraductal immunization resulted in both salivary and serum immune responses. When animals were infected with *S. mutans* significantly lower numbers were noted in the immunized animals, and if this were true in the longer term, this might allow salivary IgA mediated protection from caries.

Protein antigens of *S. mutans*

Clearly purified antigens would be more acceptable as a human vaccine than whole bacterial cells. The observation that cell walls of *S. mutans* induced antibodies protective against caries, but that this protection was lost if the cell walls were treated with trypsin or pronase, suggested that the protective antigens were protein. Several protein antigens have subsequently been isolated from the cell walls of *S. mutans*. The characterization of protein antigens of *S. mutans* has been followed by analysis of purified proteins as protective antigens in caries immunization.

Three main protein antigens (I, II and III) have been identified in extracts of culture supernatants from *S. mutans*. Streptococcal antigen I/II has two antigenic determinants present in a single molecule with a molecular weight of 185 000, whereas antigen I has a molecular weight of 150 000 and antigen II is 48 000.

Recently it has been shown that subcutaneous injection of one or two doses of 1 mg of SA I/II in FIA or in aluminium hydroxide would elicit serum IgG, IgA and IgM antibodies and, in addition, skin delayed

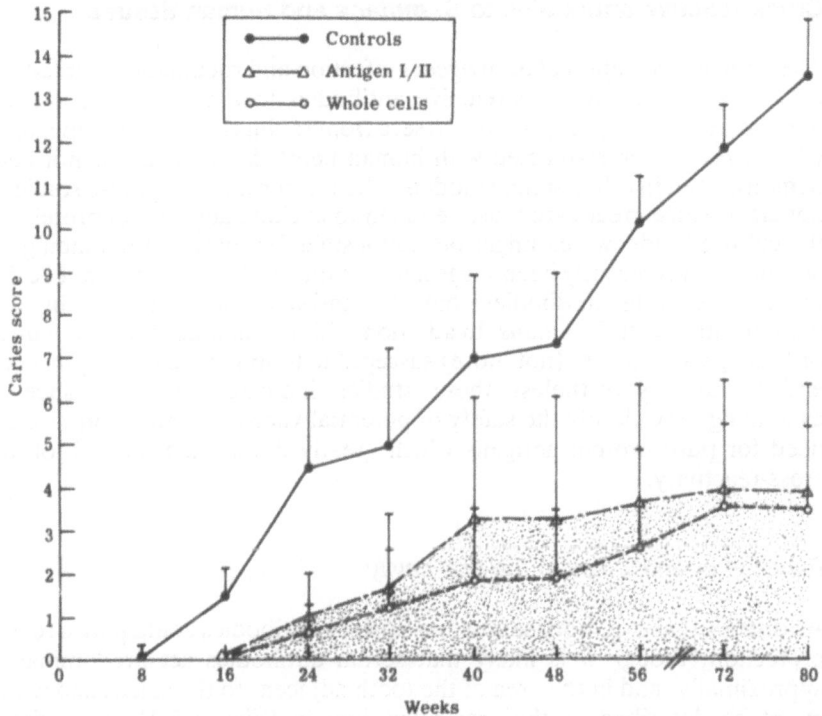

Figure 3.11 Immunization against dental caries in rhesus monkeys. Immunization was subcutaneously with whole cells of *S. mutans* or with purified protein antigen. A similar reduction in dental caries was found with both antigen preparations examined (from Lehner *et al.*, 1982, with permission)

hypersensitivity reactions to *S. mutans*. More importantly the reduction in caries seen in the animals immunized with antigen I/II was equivalent to the reduction seen in animals immunized with whole cells of *S. mutans* (Figure 3.11). This reduction in caries was accompanied by a reduction in numbers of *S. mutans* detected in immunized animals in comparison with controls.

Interpretation of immunization studies

It seems that purified antigens from *S. mutans* can induce protection against dental caries in the primate model. Effective immunization has been induced by one subcutaneous injection of antigen in aluminium hydroxide, which is an adjuvant acceptable and in common human use. Taking into account the similarities of the primate model to man (Table 3.7), these studies indicate that there is a real prospect for immunization in humans, although a comprehensive series of safety tests is necessary before immunization can be started in humans.

Cross-reactive antibodies to *S. mutans* and human tissues

The known association of *S. pyogenes* infection and rheumatic fever led to a close analysis of any cross-reactive antibodies to antigens of *S. mutans*. Some years ago it was reported that sera from rabbits immunized repeatedly with *S. mutans* cross-reacted with human heart tissue. This has not been demonstrated in other animal models. The interpretation of these studies is not clear, since great care must be taken to exclude any animal proteins in the culture fluids, which might be responsible for some of the binding. In addition, it has recently been suggested that the binding seen may not be due to cross-reacting antibodies but to anti-idiotypes induced by the immunization with *S. mutans*. In addition rabbits immunized with *S. mutans* or *S. sanguis* were less (not more) susceptible to induction of streptococcal endocarditis. Nevertheless these studies indicate the importance of examining very closely the safety of potential vaccines, and emphasize the need for pure protein antigens which greatly diminished the risk of any cross-reactivity.

Function of antibodies in the oral cavity

As discussed above, both serum and salivary antibodies could play a role in protection, though it is likely that serum antibodies act predominantly approximally, and in the area of the tooth adjacent to the sulcus and which might be described as the crevicular domain (Figure 3.1) and salivary antibodies which act predominantly on exposed surfaces of the tooth which might be described as the salivary domain (Figure 3.1).

There seems no doubt, from studies on immunization against dental caries in primates, that serum IgG antibodies can act on the tooth surface. It is known that there is rapid passage of serum antibodies to the oral cavity, and that such antibodies in the gingival fluid retain biological activity. In addition, it is estimated that between 1 and 2 ml of crevicular fluid come into the oral cavity per day. It is thus theoretically possible that serum antibodies could act through the oral cavity if they are shown to be effective in inhibition of bacterial functions at a dilution of between 1 : 500 and 1 : 1000.

MECHANISMS OF ACTION OF ANTIBODIES IN CARIES IMMUNITY

Some of the possible ways in which antibodies could act upon cariogenic bacteria are listed in Table 3.9. It should be noted that several different mechanisms could be operative simultaneously, or that some mechanisms are operative in one site, e.g. the fissure, whereas they are not important in another site, e.g. the smooth surface.

Many workers have examined the number of *S. mutans* in plaque in immunized compared with control animals. The results have been very variable, even from the same laboratories. Many studies have found a reduction in the numbers in immunized animals, including results from both the rat and the primate model. In other experiments reductions in numbers have not been found. There are technical difficulties in interpretation of such data since the bulk of plaque may be irrelevant in the caries process and only those organisms against the enamel surface itself might be important. Theoretically, it is not necessary for there to be a reduction in numbers of cariogenic bacteria for immunization to be effective. As outlined in Table 3.8, inhibition of various metabolic activities could result in the neutralization of cariogenic bacteria without there being reduction in numbers.

Table 3.9 Some possible mechanisms of action of antibodies in caries immunity

1. Inhibition of adherence	4. Complement-dependent lysis
2. Inhibition of enzyme activities	5. Agglutination
3. Opsonization	6. Interaction with non-specific mechanisms

Inhibition of adherence

It is generally accepted that adherence of an organism to the host is a prerequisite for infection. The elegant studies of Williams and Gibbons in 1972 demonstrated that purified parotid IgA could inhibit the adherence of *Streptococcus salivarius* to human buccal epithelial cells. Since then, several workers have shown that secretory IgA could inhibit the adherence of various other species of bacteria including *Escherichia coli, Vibrio cholera* and *Neisseria gonococcus*. Inhibition of the adherence of *S. mutans* by salivary IgA has been shown in monkeys and in rats. Serum antibodies, particularly of the IgG class, have also been shown to be effective in the inhibition of adherence. There are three main possible mechanisms thought to be responsible for the inhibition of adherence:

1. reducing the hydrophobicity of bacteria by binding with surface antigens including lipoteichoic acid and thus reducing the negative charge;

2. direct interference with glucosyl transferase (GTF) activity preventing the formation of adhesive extracellulose polysaccharides; and

3. blocking cell surface antigens which act as receptor sites for cell-bound GTF.

These latter surface protein binding sites (adhesins) of *S. mutans* seem to mediate the sucrose-independent binding of these organisms to salivary pellicle which coats the tooth. Antibodies against the cell surface protein antigens of *S. mutans* I, I/II and III will bind to hydroxyapatite and have been shown to inhibit the subsequent adherence of the organism. Treatment of *S. mutans* cells with anti-I/II antibody will reduce glucan-dependent cell to surface adherence and also cell to cell adherence. The mechanism may be by steric hindrance rather than by direct blocking of adhesin sites. It is unlikely that this is the sole mechanism in protection against caries, since anti-GTF antibody almost completely abolishes glucan-dependent adherence of *S. mutans* cells to hard surfaces, but the same antigen has been unable to protect monkeys against caries in immunization experiments (Table 3.8) though it has been successful in rodent experiments. This raises the possibility that glucan-dependent adherence may not have a major role in caries.

Inhibition of enzyme activity

One of the best-studied mechanisms of action of salivary IgA is the inhibition of GTF activity. It should be noted, however, that under certain circumstances enhancement of enzyme activity can also occur, and this raises the interesting possibility that in some conditions the induction of antibodies may be harmful rather than helpful. Indeed experiments discussed above have indicated that immunization with GTF occasionally results in an increase in caries in animals, and that serum IgA antibodies may enhance GTF activity.

Elegant experiments over a number of years using radiolabelled sucrose have demonstrated that serum IgG antibodies may inhibit this enzyme activity. Inhibition of GTF leading to a lack of production of insoluble extracellular polysaccharide was a most attractive hypothesis for the action of antibody in caries immunity. Certainly immunization of rats or hamsters with purified GTF is effective in reducing caries, and this indicates that inhibition of GTF activity may be effective in this model. In these experiments reduction in colonization of *S. mutans* has been shown, and the

78

antibodies induced in serum are active in inhibition of GTF activity. The failure to achieve successful immunization with GTF in the primate model may indicate that any inhibitory effect of IgG is neutralized by an enhancing effect of other serum or salivary antibodies.

GTF is not the only enzyme which might be inhibitable. Various authors have examined the possibility that antibodies may result in a reduction in acid production of *S. mutans*, but this has not been established. Nevertheless, inhibition of various metabolic activities of the *S. mutans* organisms by antibodies remains an attractive possibility.

Opsonization

As discussed above, IgG is the major immunoglobulin in blood and gingival crevice, and there is no doubt that serum IgG can be effective on the tooth surface, as demonstrated in successful passive immunization studies in monkeys. Crevicular fluid also contains a high concentration of polymorphonuclear leukocytes (PMN), and over 65% of these crevicular PMNs are functionally competent. However, since most of the PMNs in saliva are non-functional in terms of their ability to phagocytose and kill *S. mutans* it seems likely that effective opsonization is limited to the gingival crevice.

Opsonization enhancing phagocytosis by PMNs and macrophages may be a powerful way in which antibody combats micro-organisms either directly or in combination with complement activation. The binding of specific IgG and IgM antibody in the crevice, as elsewhere in the systemic system, will activate the classical pathway of the complement activation, resulting in chemotactic C3a and C5a fragments, which may have the effect of attracting more polymorphs and monocytes to the site, and amplify the effectiveness of the antibody–PMN interactions.

Gingival crevice PMN are effective in phagocytosing *S. mutans*, and crevicular fluid antibodies are effective as opsonins. Indeed crevicular fluid is able to support an impressive increase in phagocytosis compared with saline, and the active factors seem to be both complement- and antibody-dependent. It should be noted that the release from PMN of lysosomal enzymes extracellularly could be an effective way of damaging bacteria, as has been shown for some periodontopathic bacteria, which then have an effect extracellularly.

Complement-dependent lysis

All the components of complement are present in crevicular fluid, and complement-dependent lysis has been shown to be effective against Gram-negative bacteria and viruses. It is less likely that activation of the complement pathway is directly involved in defence against Gram-positive bacteria such as *S. mutans*. However, the abundance of PMN in the crevice, which are maintained by the chemotactic properties of C3a and C5a, makes it likely that complement activation plays a role in opsonization and killing. It remains possible, however, that a combination of the attack sequence of complement (C6–C9) may act in synergistic fashion with other antibacterial factors in the gingival crevice area to induce lysis.

Agglutination

Theoretically, agglutination of bacteria by salivary IgA, or indeed serum IgG, could either enhance or inhibit bacterial plaque accumulation. Enhancement could occur when agglutinins are already attached to the tooth surface or to other bacteria, and thus the attachment of bacteria would be facilitated (coadhesion). Inhibition could occur when the agglutinins are free in saliva and when aggregates of bacteria are formed which lead to enhanced removal of these bacteria from the oral cavity and inhibition of attachment. These processes could occur equally well with specific agglutinins such as IgA or non-specific agglutinins, including mucins and glycoprotein.

Experimentally there is much evidence to support the view that salivary IgA could, depending on the conditions, enhance or decrease bacterial colonization, particularly with regard to *S. sanguis* or *S. mutans*. It has been found that some 80% of samples of whole saliva will agglutinate *S. sanguis*. Removal of IgA leads to a decrease in agglutination and decrease in adherence by hydroxyapatite. Interestingly, if the hydroxyapatite were coated with salivary IgA, then an increase in adherence was found.

There appear to be both specific and non-specific agglutinins present in whole saliva, and up to three different agglutinin systems in saliva have been reported, two of which were not immunoglobulin. It is difficult to see a role for serum IgG in agglutination, and it is more likely that if agglutination is effective at all then salivary IgA is the mechanism.

Interaction of salivary IgA with non-specific mechanism

Saliva contains mucin, lactoferrin, lysozyme and lactoperoxidase, all of which may interact with salivary IgA.

Salivary IgA and mucin – Secretory IgA will bind to mucins through cysteine residues. Salivary IgA can be found in complexes of very high molecular weight, which have agglutinin activity and presumably reflect IgA–mucin complexes in the oral cavity. Elsewhere in the secretory system release of mucins by antibody–antigen complexes has been shown, and it remains possible that a similar mechanism could be operative in the oral cavity and lead to enhanced mucus release and mucin–IgA interactions.

Salivary IgA and lactoferrin – Lactoferrin is an iron binding protein which has bacteriostatic activity and this can be enhanced, or under some circumstances reduced, by secretory IgA antibodies. There is preliminary evidence *in vivo* to suggest that salivary IgA antibodies and lactoferrin may be effective in reducing bacterial activity, and this is an area which merits much more research.

Salivary IgA and lysozyme – Some years ago it was shown that purified secretory IgA from colostrum could lyse *E. coli* in the presence of complement and lysozyme, whereas neither component on its own was effective. This has been confirmed in more recent studies, and these observations suggest that similar mechanisms might be operative in the oral cavity. The concentrations of complement in whole saliva would seem too small for this to be a major defence mechanism except if inflammation is present. It has also been shown that salivary mucins can inhibit lysozyme activity, and thus the effectiveness of lysozyme as an antibacterial mechanism in the oral cavity would be dependent on a number of interactions.

Salivary IgA and lactoperoxidase – A recent study has reported that salivary IgA can enhance the anti-microbial effect of lactoperoxidase. The IgA may give bacterial specificity to an effective non-specific mechanism. Interestingly, either IgA1 or IgA2 was effective, but serum IgG or serum IgM had no effect. This suggests a specific relationship between IgA and lactoperoxidase, which may be of great importance at mucosal surfaces.

Growth and survival

It is difficult to investigate the effect of antibodies upon growth and survival of oral bacteria *in vitro* in any way which might be relevant to conditions prevailing *in vivo*. More work is needed in this area to see whether antibody will inflict subtle changes in metabolism which make the organism less able, for instance, to survive low pH conditions, or whether acid production is inhibited whilst numbers remain the same. It should also be noted that certain strains of bacteria, including *S. sanguis*, can secrete a protease capable of cleaving secretory IgA, and it is possible that inhibition of this enzyme or similar enzymes may be important in the effectiveness of antibodies at the tooth surface.

CONCLUSIONS

Dental caries has been established as an infective and transmissible disease. There is a strong association between the numbers of *S. mutans* in plaque and dental caries in humans, though some caries may occur in the absence of *S. mutans*. *S. mutans* has been linked immunologically with dental caries. Root surface caries, fissure caries and rampant caries may differ microbiologically from smooth surface caries. *S. mutans* is very cariogenic in animal models, but *L. casei, S. sanguis* and *A. viscosus* can also cause different types of caries in animal models.

In humans, low caries prevalence is associated with high serum IgG antibodies to *S. mutans* and to the protein antigen I/II, but not to other oral bacteria. Salivary IgA antibodies do not appear to be raised in subjects of low caries experience. The presence of caries lesions is associated with increased antibodies to *S. mutans* and the development of caries with a rise in specific antibodies. There appear to be genetic differences, linked to the HLA-DR, in the ability to respond to streptococcal antigen. Subjects of low caries experience appear able to respond to very low amounts of antigen.

Caries in animal models can be inhibited by immunization against *S. mutans*. In the rodent model the induction of salivary antibodies can lead to protection against caries, whereas in the primate model the induction of serum IgG antibodies is protective. Protection can also be demonstrated by the passive transfer of IgG antibodies, showing that serum antibodies must be able to act at the tooth surface. Protein antigens have been isolated from *S. mutans*, and streptococcal antigen I/II is as effective as whole cells in inhibiting caries. Local immunization with this antigen in the gingiva may also be effective, and local passive immunization with monoclonal antibodies to SA I/II can also protect against caries.

FURTHER READING

Bowen, W. H. (1969). A vaccine against dental caries. *Br. Dent. J.*, **126**, 159–60

Bowen, W. H., Cohen, B., Cole, M. and Colman, G. (1975). Immunisation against dental caries. *Br. Dent. J.*, **139**, 45–58

Challacombe, S. J. (1980). Serum and salivary antibodies to *Streptococcus mutans* in relation to the development and treatment of human dental caries. *Arch. Oral Biol.*, **25**, 495–502

Challacombe, S. J., Bergmeier, L. A. and Rees, A. S. (1984). Natural antibodies in man to a protein antigen from the bacterium *Streptococcus mutans* related to dental caries experience. *Arch. Oral Biol.*, **29**, 179–84

Huis in't Veld, J. H., van Palenstein Helderman, W. H. and Backer Dirks, O. (1979). *Streptococcus mutans* and dental caries in humans: a bacteriological and immunological study. Antonie van Leeuwenhoek. *J. Microbiol. Serol.*, **45**, 25–35

Lehner, T. (1982). Regulation of immune responses to streptococcal protein antigens in dental caries. *Immunology Today,*, **3**, 73–7

Lehner, T., Challacombe, S. J., Wilton, J. M. A. and Caldwell, J. (1976a). Cellular and humoral immune responses in vaccination against dental caries in monkeys. *Nature*, **264**, 69

Lehner, T., Russell, M. W., Caldwell, J. and Smith, R. (1982). Immunisation with purified protein antigens from *Streptococcus mutans* against dental caries in rhesus monkeys. *Infect. Immun.*, **34**, 407–15

Lehner, T., Russell, M. W., Challacombe, S. J. *et al.* (1978). Passive immunisation with serum and immunoglobulin against dental caries in rhesus monkeys. *Lancet*, **1**, 693–5

McGhee, J. R. and Michalek, S. M. (1981). Immunobiology of dental caries: microbial aspects and local immunity. *Ann. Rev. Microbiol.*, **35**, 595–638

Rogers, A. H. (1977). Evidence for the transmissibility of human dental caries. *Aus. Dent. J.*, **22**, 53–6

Russell, M. W. and Lehner, T. (1978). Characterisation of antigens extracted from cells and culture fluid of *Streptococcus mutans* serotype c. *Arch. Oral Biol.*, **23**, 7–15

Russell, R. R. B. and Colman, G. (1981). Immunisation of monkeys (*Macaca fascicularis*) with purified *Streptococcus mutans* glucosyl-transferase. *Arch. Oral Biol.*, **26**, 23–8

Smith, D.J., Taubman, M.A. and Ebersole, J.L. (1979). Effect of oral administration of glucosyltransferase antigens on experimental dental caries. *Infect. Immun.*, **26**, 82–9

4
Periodontal Diseases

L. IVANYI and H. N. NEWMAN

CHRONIC PERIODONTITIS

General considerations

Diseases of the periodontium are among the most frequently occurring human afflictions. Based on the age of onset, distribution of lesions and rate of progression, most patients can be classified as having mild or severe periodontitis. In juveniles the distribution of the disease may be either localized or generalized and may progress rapidly or slowly in either case. Clearly the generalized rapidly progressive is the most severe form. The forms of juvenile periodontitis are described later in this chapter.

Amongst young adults it is possible to recognize both mild and severe forms of the disease, the former usually characterized by slowly progressing horizontal bone loss and the latter by rapidly progressing vertical bone loss which is invariably generalized but often irregular. In middle-aged and older individuals the same forms of mild and severe periodontitis can be recognized, the mild disease being more common.

There have been advances in the knowledge of the microflora associated with chronic periodontitis and some of the specific bacterial species which can destroy periodontal tissues have been identified. As a result of the application of improved methods for isolation and classification of oral micro-organisms, certain groups of bacteria have been associated with various forms of the disease. These include *Bacteroides intermedius, Eikenella corrodens, Fusobacterium nucleatum* and *Actinomyces* species in mild periodontitis, while *F. nucleatum, B. gingivalis, Wolinella recta* and *Peptostreptococcus* species are among those associated with the severe form of the disease (see Chapter 2).

Bacterial plaque is firmly established as the major aetiological factor in the initiation and development of the early stage of periodontitis, chronic gingivitis. Epidemiological data suggest that untreated gingivitis generally progresses to periodontitis. However, this assumption remains unproven and it appears that in many cases a progression may not occur. In general, gingivitis is common in the primary and permanent dentition in children and adults. Although loss of attachment is rarely found in children, the prevalence of periodontal pockets and alveolar bone loss is increased in teenagers. Since periodontal destruction progresses with increasing age after the age of 20, chronic periodontitis is considered a major cause of tooth loss in adults. Despite a variety of experimental approaches using populations with divergent cultural and socioeconomic backgrounds, the results of cross-sectional epidemiological surveys have shown remarkably consistent positive correlations between periodontitis and both age and the presence of microbial plaque; differences in disease prevalence are related to levels of oral cleanliness, utilization of dental services and educational status.

The pattern of periodontal destruction may reflect episodic bursts of activity over short periods of time at individual sites. These bursts appear to occur randomly throughout the mouth. Some sites demonstrate a brief active destructive burst before going into a period of remission, whilst other sites remain free of disease throughout the individual's life. The sites which demonstrate destructive activity may show no further activity or could be subject to one or more bursts of activity at later time periods.

Chronic periodontitis involving long-term interaction between host and bacteria is characterized by a spectral pattern possibly attributable to temporal development in clinical manifestations and immunological parameters. For more than a decade periodontal research has focused on the nature of the interaction between bacterial substances and various host defence mechanisms in order to understand the basis of the soft tissue destruction and alveolar bone resorption that are characteristic of periodontitis. Considerable attention has been given to the immunological mechanisms which may play a part in these diseases. With the exception of acute necrotizing ulcerative gingivitis and some cases of juvenile and severe progressive periodontitis, bacteria do not normally invade the gingival connective tissue. However, bacterial antigens activate the immune responses of the host, resulting in various manifestations. The immunologically competent cells, such as lymphocytes and plasma cells, predominate in affected gingival tissues. Immunoglobulins with antibody specificity for oral bacterial antigens are present in human sera, in gingival crevicular fluid and in gingival tissues. Peripheral blood lymphocytes and gingival lymphocytes are sensitized to oral bacterial antigens as detected by *in vitro* tests. Hence the concept of hypersensitivity to oral micro-organisms as a major factor in the pathogenesis of chronic periodontitis has gained wide support. Both antibody-mediated and cellular hypersensitivity may contribute to the inflammatory reactions in periodontal lesions. On the other hand, evidence is accumulating that the immunological reactions towards bacteria and their products primarily represent a manifestation of the host defence to infection. These immune responses can be affected by bacterial immunomodulatory substances resulting in a spectrum of both 'T' cell and antibody-mediated reactions.

Immunopathology

Plaque accumulation experiments have been used extensively to elucidate the pathogenesis of chronic inflammatory periodontal disease both in humans and animals. These studies showed that chronic periodontitis develops in four stages. The initial lesion is an acute inflammatory response occurring within 1–4 days following plaque accumulation. During this stage the gingival vessels become engorged and dilated, and large numbers of neutrophils migrate into the junctional epithelium and into the gingival crevice. The early lesion, which occurs within 4–7 days, is characterized by the formation of a soft tissue infiltrate containing small and medium-sized lymphocytes and macrophages. The established lesion, consisting of predominantly plasma cells, develops within 2–3 weeks. This lesion may remain stable or convert to an aggressive state with the destruction of alveolar bone. The aggressive phase, termed the advanced lesion, is characterized by the presence of large numbers of infiltrating plasma cells and lymphocytes. Subsequently it has been shown that gingivitis is a lymphocyte-dominated lesion, while periodontitis is a plasma cell-dominated lesion.

Based on immunohistochemical investigations of experimental gingivitis and chronic gingivitis in children and adolescents, there is general agreement that T lymphocytes predominate in the inflamed soft tissues with a smaller number of B lymphocytes and macrophages. In chronic periodontitis the nature of the infiltrate varies widely. Some authors observed predominantly plasma cells, others found that the number of lymphocytes was equivalent or even exceeded that of plasma cells. Studies of Ig isotypes associated with these plasma cells and lymphocytes revealed the presence of variable proportions of IgA, IgG as well as IgM-producing cells. Macrophages and certain lymphocytes have cytophilic antibodies attached via the Fc receptor which could mimic antibody-producing cells. Thus, monospecific $F(ab')_2$ reagents specific for each immunoglobulin class were used to prevent non-specific binding of antibody via the Fc receptor. The results showed that the largest proportion of the cells in tissue sections was positive for IgG with smaller proportions positive for IgA and IgM. These findings are in agreement with *in vitro* studies which have shown that the predominant immunoglobulin produced by gingival lymphocytes is IgG. Around 20% of immunoglobulin present in the gingival tissue reacts with oral microbial antigens but immune complexes were not detected. The proportion of T cells in the infiltrate in progressive periodontitis is a matter of controversy. Initial studies showed a prevalence of B cells with only a small number of T cells being present. More recently, studies with monoclonal antibodies demonstrated that T lymphocytes accounted for 30% of the infiltrating cells. Of the remaining cells, 50% were identified as B cells and 13% as macrophages. T lymphocytes and macrophages were found to be localized in the connective tissue subjacent to the pocket epithelium, in an area which is most intensely exposed to bacterial antigens.

A number of workers examined suspensions of cells extracted from diseased periodontal tissues. Using formation of spontaneous sheep red blood rosettes (E rosettes) or monoclonal antibodies as markers for T cells and surface membrane immunoglobulin for B cells, 50–70% T cells and 30% B cells were identified. Using monoclonal antibodies against T lymphocyte subsets, aberrations in the T cell subset distribution were observed. Several authors reported decreased T4/T8 lymphocyte ratios (T4 = helper/inducer and T8 = suppressor/cytotoxic subsets) in young adults and middle-aged patients with severe periodontitis.

Current evidence indicates that periodontitis is not a simple B cell lesion as initially claimed. Instead, the infiltrated region contains numerous sets of infiltrating cells organized in an unusual way, with a region rich in T lymphocytes and macrophages immediately subjacent to the pocket epithelium and a region in the central lamina propria, located further away from the bacterial agents, which is rich in B cells and plasma cells and poor in T lymphocytes.

Neutrophil functions

Neutrophils are, most likely, defensive cells providing continuous protection for the periodontal tissues. These inflammatory cells migrate into the junctional epithelium and gingival crevice in response to local chemotactic substances elaborated by plaque bacteria. The majority of crevicular neutrophils from healthy sites are viable and capable of phagocytosis. Ultrastructural studies have shown that neutrophils come into direct contact with dental plaque in the sulcus and actively phagocytose plaque micro-organisms. The protective effects of neutrophils include phagocytosis and killing of bacteria as well as inactivation of potentially destructive bacterial products. Opsonizing antibody and complement play a role in the interaction of neutrophils with certain micro-organisms. The protective function of these cells is also demonstrated by the fact that patients with neutrophil disorders often present unusually rapid severe periodontitis (see Chapter 9). However, neutrophils may also participate in the local tissue destruction as they contain lysosomal enzymes and potentially toxic oxygen radicals which are capable of degrading tissue components. Localized tissue damage by antigen–antibody complexes also depends on the presence of neutrophils (see Chapter 12).

Recently it has been reported that gingival crevice neutrophils recovered from lesions of severe periodontitis have reduced phagocytic capacity when compared to cells recovered from lesions of mild periodontitis. Furthermore, the viability of neutrophils has a tendency to decrease in deep pockets when compared to control sites. Several oral pathogens have been shown to have the potential to cause neutrophil dysfunction or even destruction. In summary, the reduced defensive function of neutrophils results in rapidly progressive periodontal tissue destruction.

Macrophage mediators

Macrophages are engaged in phagocytosis, antigen presentation to T lymphocytes and in immunoregulatory functions in both humoral and cellular immunity. Cytokines derived from macrophages play an important role in initiation and regulation of immune responsiveness. Some of these inducer functions may be mediated by interleukin-1 (IL-1), whilst the suppressor activities may be mediated by prostaglandin E_2 (PGE_2). Distinctive functions may be ascribed to various macrophage subpopulations; there is some evidence that IL-1 and PGE_2 are produced by separate macrophage subsets. The secretion of IL-1 can be induced by a variety of stimuli, such as activated T cells, lymphokinin (colony-stimulating factor), immune complexes, C5a complement component, lipo-polysaccharide (LPS) and cell wall components from Gram-positive bacteria. However, one has to bear in mind that several other cell types after stimulation can also produce IL-1. The release of IL-1 from keratinocytes *in vitro* is spontaneous with no apparent requirement for other stimuli, although LPS increases its production and is also a stimulant of IL-1 production by B lymphocytes.

IL-1 appears to be responsible for many effects such as stimulation of T helper and B lymphocyte responses, fibroblast proliferation, interferon production and collagen type IV production by epidermal cells. The finding of enhanced osteoblast proliferation, alkaline phosphatase production and bone resorption by osteoclasts suggests that IL-1 may be a regulatory factor in bone remodelling. Gingival fluid from subjects with clinically healthy gingiva was shown to contain IL-1, but the IL-1 levels were found to be greater in gingival fluid from inflamed gingiva. IL-1 might be produced by macrophages, or gingival epithelial cells, or both. Within the gingival environment IL-1 enhances the production of other lymphokines including interleukin-2 by T lymphocytes or natural killer cells, and enhances the activity of B cells, thus promoting both cellular and humoral immunity.

Certain products of Gram-negative bacteria, such as lipids or lipopolysaccharides, stimulate a subpopulation of macrophages to secrete prostaglandins (PGs) of the E series. PGs are also produced by other cells and tissues, such as gingiva. The most obvious role of PGs is in inflammation. PGE_1 and PGE_2 cause local vasodilation, increased vascular permeability, potentiation of the action of histamine and bradykinin and accumulation of oedema fluid. PGE_2 has also been shown to stimulate bone resorption and to inhibit bone collagen synthesis. Another important role of PGs lies in immunosuppression. PGE_1 and PGE_2 inhibit mitogen- and antigen-induced lymphocyte stimulation, depress macrophage inhibitory factor activity and direct cytolysis by activated lymphocytes and antibody formation. In contrast, PGE_2 may stimulate some functions of macrophages, such as collagenase production and Fc-mediated phagocytosis. Moreover, PGE_2 may reduce chronic inflammation by inhibiting the production of oxygen radicals. PG-mediated suppression of mitogen/antigen-induced lymphocyte proliferation may operate through activation of T suppressor cells, which possess PG receptors, or by interference with IL-2 production and action, but the relationship between PGE_2 and IL-1 functions is not yet fully understood.

Prostaglandins have been detected in gingival fluid from patients with chronic gingivitis. Furthermore, an immunohistochemical study demonstrated a number of macrophages containing PGE_2 in gingival sections from patients with severe periodontitis. Thus PGE_2 produced at a local site may contribute to the suppression of both T and B cell-mediated functions in severe periodontitis.

It has been demonstrated that patients taking anti-inflammatory drugs which inhibit PG synthesis (such as indomethacin) had less gingival inflammation, reduced depth of periodontal pockets, loss of attachment and less bone loss compared with a control group of subjects. Indomethacin also diminished alveolar bone destruction in a canine model of rapidly progressing periodontitis.

T lymphocyte responses

T (thymus-derived) lymphocytes are engaged in cell-mediated immunity. When sensitized lymphocytes interact with an antigen they proliferate and secrete a variety of lymphokines, such as IL-2, γ-interferon, skin-reactive factor, chemotactic factor, migration inhibition factor and cytotoxic factor. However, some lymphokines have tissue-damaging potentials; for example, osteoclast activating factor (bone resorbing factor). Distinctive functions may be ascribed to helper/inducer ($T4^+$) and to suppressor/cytotoxic ($T8^+$) subsets. $T4^+$ lymphocytes are engaged in proliferation and lymphokines secretion, whilst $T8^+$ lymphocytes mediate cytotoxicity and immuno-regulation of cellular and humoral immunity. $T4^+$ lymphocytes help B cells to make antibodies to the majority of antigens (T cell-dependent antigens) although some antigens (T cell-independent) may stimulate B cells directly to secrete antibodies. IgG responses are generally more T cell-dependent than IgM production. B cells can also be activated polyclonally by stimuli such as lipopolysaccharide, teichoic acid, dextran, levan and peptidoglycan. Activated B cells are capable of secreting osteolytic mediators as well as other potentially destructive lymphokines. *In vitro* T cell reactions to oral micro-organisms used as lymphocyte stimulants have been used to investigate the immune status of individuals with chronic periodontitis. The 'lymphocyte transformation' test, which measures the blastogenic (proliferative) response of peripheral blood lymphocytes to sensitizing antigens, has been used most frequently. Although a direct correlation between the magnitude of the response to putative periodontal Gram-negative pathogens and severity of the periodontal disease has been reported, this relationship has not been confirmed in other investigations. Other studies demonstrated that lymphocytes from patients with chronic gingivitis and mild periodontitis responded to bacterial antigenic extracts, while the majority of patients with severe periodontitis failed to demonstrate lymphocyte stimulation. Although essentially all studies have shown responsiveness in patients with gingivitis and mild periodontitis, conflicting results have been reported in the periodontally healthy groups.

Selection of healthy subjects who received stringent tooth cleaning and dental hygiene instruction to assure minimal plaque accumulation may possibly explain the unresponsiveness reported in some studies. Hence the 'super-healthy' controls may not be representative of normal periodontally healthy subjects. Their gingival tissue may contain an inflammatory cellular infiltrate upon histological examination, suggesting antigen penetration and systemic sensitization. Furthermore, differences in lymphocyte culture conditions may also account for the discrepancies between the various studies.

The finding of low *in vitro* lymphocyte proliferative responses to periodontopathic bacteria in patients with severe periodontitis is of particular interest. Depletion of cell cultures of T suppressor cells enhanced lymphocyte responses in these patients. It has also been shown that after periodontal therapy lymphocytes from the same subjects responded significantly to bacterial antigens. Moreover, the spontaneously occurring blastogenic activity and the incidence of Ia^+ T cells in unstimulated cultures were both lower in patients with severe periodontitis than in controls. The results suggest an abnormal T cell regulation in these patients. It may be argued that findings in the 'blood are not necessarily representative of immune reactions within the gingival environment. However, investigations of T lymphocyte subsets in periodontal tissues showed decreased T4/T8 lymphocyte ratios in patients with severe periodontitis. Furthermore, the lack of response to oral bacterial antigens was observed in cultures of mononuclear cells extracted from periodontal tissues of patients with severe periodontitis. All these results suggest increased functional activity of T suppressor cells in inflamed periodontal tissues. The mechanisms which lead to enhanced activity of T suppressors are complex and not fully understood. However, high antigen concentration, antigen–antibody complexes and prostaglandins may play a role. The suppressed host defence mechanism may contribute to the progression of the disease to its severe form. However, patients with immunodeficiences and patients on immuno-suppressive drugs do not suffer from, nor are they more susceptible to, severe periodontitis.

Although immunosuppressive agents prevent the immune system from rejecting a grafted kidney, other aspects of the host defence mechanisms are probably preserved to adequately control infection. Indeed, these patients have a normal level of T cells in their blood and unimpaired responses to mitogens and antigens from dental plaque.

Experiments on thymectomized hamsters and congenitally athymic rats have both demonstrated increased alveolar bone loss. Cyclophosphamide suppression of lymphocyte functions produces severe bone loss in ligature-induced periodontitis in rats. Finally, in rats monoinfected with an oral Gram-negative bacterium (*Eikenella corrodens*) the increase in severity of bone loss corresponded to a marked decrease in cell-mediated immune responses to this antigen. Taken together, these results indicate a protective role of T cell-mediated immunity in periodontitis.

B lymphocyte responses

B lymphocytes (bone marrow derived) are engaged in antibody formation. After interaction with the antigen, B cells differentiate into blast cells and plasma cells, secreting large amounts of antibodies.

The potential of antibodies to inhibit the adhesion of bacteria to mucosal surfaces is well established. Antibodies to *Actinomyces viscosus* will inhibit its coaggregation with *Streptococcus sanguis*; such bacterial interactions may be of importance in the colonization of the subgingival area by periodontopathic organisms. Antibodies of the IgA and IgG classes (local and serum derived) can limit the entry through epithelial surfaces and spread of bacterial antigens. In the periodontal area this function is maintained by antibodies present both in the gingival crevice fluid and in the gingival tissues. IgA particularly is conducive to health in this respect because of its inability to initiate complement reactions and to cause a release of lytic enzymes from inflammatory cells. It has also been shown that the salivary immune response can be protective in experimental periodontal disease in rats after local immunization with *Streptococcus mutans, Actinomyces naeslundii* or *A. viscosus*. Bone loss was reduced in animals that demonstrated high salivary antibody responses, while bone loss was increased in animals demonstrating a weak salivary response. In another experiment, immunization of dogs with dental plaque which was followed by increased serum antibodies to plaque, antigens reduced the lesions of gingival connective tissue caused by plaque accumulation. The reduced connective tissue lesions were attributable to the formation of immune complexes which inhibited antigen penetration through the junctional epithelium. These results appear to be at variance with experiments in which the application of ovalbumin to the gingival sulcus of squirrel monkeys immunized to this protein promoted the development of gingival lesions. This damage, however, could be initiated only when the junctional epithelium was mechanically disrupted, thereby giving the antigen access to the connective tissue. However, other workers failed to extract immune complexes from tissues taken from either humans or dogs with chronic periodontitis. These studies indicate that immune complexes may not contribute significantly to periodontal pathology.

It would appear that an intact junctional epithelium provides an effective barrier to antigen penetration. Such an hypothesis is further supported by the findings of other investigators who applied the tracer protein, horseradish peroxidase, to the gingiva of rabbits immunized to this antigen. In non-immunized control animals peroxidase rapidly penetrated the junctional epithelium and entered the connective tissue, but in immunized rabbits only very small amounts of the antigen penetrated the epithelium. It was suggested that the antiperoxidase antibodies present in the intercellular spaces of the epithelium reacted with the penetrating antigen, to form antigen–antibody complexes which activated complement. It was argued that the release of chemotactic factors was responsible for the epithelial infiltrate of neutrophils which engulfed the complexes, allowing only small amounts of peroxidase to reach the connective tissue. Thus, a less pronounced inflammatory reaction was found in the gingival connective tissue of immunized than that of the non-immunized experimental animals. Furthermore, suppression of B cell functions by cyclophosphamide produces severe bone loss in ligature-induced periodontitis in rats. All these results indicate that humoral immunity to plaque antigens represents a defence mechanism within the junctional epithelium and the underlying connective tissue.

The level and distribution of crevicular fluid antibody was studied in patients with chronic periodontitis. Elevated antibody levels were demonstrated in approximately 9% of periodontal test sites. The elevated responses were shown to be limited to particular bacterial specificity at any one site, particularly to *A. actinomycetemcomitans*, *B. gingivalis* and *B. intermedius*, rather than to clinical categorization. Those sites yielding elevated antibody levels exhibited no obvious differences in clinical parameters of probeable depth or attachment level as compared with sites in which antibody levels were similar to serum levels. Thus, elevated antibody levels in crevicular fluid may relate to change in disease activity that is not detectable by normal clinical criteria. Other studies demonstrated suppressed local antibody synthesis to *B. gingivalis* in patients with severe periodontitis. It is possible that *B. gingivalis* colonizing the subgingival area can induce degradation of immunoglobulins by powerful proteases.

The presence of antibodies to periodontopathic organisms in the sera of periodontal patients has been well documented. Elevated levels of serum IgG antibodies to anaerobic oral bacteria were observed in patients with mild periodontitis. Antibody titres to *Veillonella*, *Fusobacterium* and *Eikenella* significantly increased in serum after successful therapy, and a relationship between the high antibody titres'to *Actinobacillus* and reduced disease activity has been reported recently. Sera from patients with mild periodontitis frequently contain elevated levels of antibodies to putative periodontal pathogens not found in their pocket floras. These observations are suggestive of sequential infection and of induction of protective immunity against reinfection by the same organism. In accord, patients with high serum antibody titres have a simple bacterial flora compared to those with low serum antibody titres. All these results are consistent with the hypothesis that the antibodies have a protective effect.

In severe periodontitis of young and adult patients the serological findings are variable. Some authors reported increased IgG antibody titres to putative periodontal pathogens, others reported an absence of elevated antibody titres, or even decreased antibody titres when compared with normal subjects. Evidence is accumulating that these patients have indeed low serum IgG antibody levels to *Bacteroides intermedius*, *B. ochraceus*, *Fusobacterium nucleatum*, periodontitis-associated treponemas, *Veillonella parvula*, *Actinobacillus actinomycetemcomitans* and *Bacteroides gingivalis*. However, others reported increased serum antibody titres to *B. gingivalis* in about 50% of patients with severe periodontitis and their decrease after periodontal therapy. In all these studies whole bacterial cells or crude extracts were used as the antigenic stimulants. Such preparations include a variety of antigens, some of which may be associated with protective functions, while others merely reflect infection with the micro-organisms. One study examined antibody levels to lipopolysaccharide extracted from *B. gingivalis* and found an inverse relationship between pocket depth and the level of IgG antibody in patients with severe periodontitis. Overall, these results agree with a protective effect of humoral immunity in periodontitis.

Protective and pathogenic interactions

Periodontal disease involving long-term interaction between host and bacteria is characterized by a spectral pattern possibly attributable to temporal development in clinical manifestations and immunological parameters. In the mild form of the disease peripheral blood and gingival lymphocytes extracted from periodontal tissues respond by *in vitro* cell-mediated immunity to oral bacterial antigens. The interpretation of these findings could be as follows.

Sensitization with oral bacterial antigens results in systemic immunity. T lymphocytes become sensitized in the lymph nodes and probably also in the spleen, which is followed by their recirculation, as detected by their presence in peripheral blood. The finding of sensitized T cells within the gingival tissues indicates that they return to the site of antigenic challenge where they carry out functional activities which localize the bacterial antigens and facilitate their phagocytosis by macrophages.

Serum-derived and locally secreted antibodies have the potential to inhibit initial adhesion and bacterial interactions which may be of importance in the colonization of the subgingival area by periodontopathic organisms. They also restrict the penetration of antigens into the gingiva by the formation of immune complexes. Other activities of antibodies include opsonizing, neutralizing and/or killing the bacteria. Thus the 'relative' integrity of periodontal tissues is maintained by the interplay of cell- and antibody-mediated immunity to oral bacteria and their products.

Dysfunction of immune responses of various degrees of specificity frequently occurs in severe periodontitis. It is plausible that suppressed host defences, particularly those induced by oral pathogens themselves, may contribute to the disease process. Immunosuppressive factors of bacterial origin could lead to colonization by the initiating organism or by other opportunistic organisms and to subsequent bacterial invasion of gingival connective tissue. Several micro-organisms have been shown to suppress cellular and humoral immune responses. These include *Veillonella parvula, Actinobacillus actinomycetemcomitans*, oral treponemas, *Capnocytophaga ochracea* and *Fusobacterium nucleatum*. Previous studies proposed the role of *V. parvula* and *A. actinomycetemcomitans*-induced suppressor T cells in the mechanism of T cell anergy. Apart from activation of suppressor T cells, some bacteria mediate their suppressive effects by other mechanisms including suppressor macrophages (*C. ochracea*, oral treponemas) and by altering T helper cell activity (*F. nucleatum*). Suppressor T cells may also be responsible for low antibody levels in patients with severe periodontitis.

As a result of defective cellular and humoral immunity bacteria and their toxic products may gain entrance into the periodontal tissues. The presence of bacteria in gingival connective tissue from patients with severe periodontitis has been reported by several authors. Of particular importance are *Bacteroides* species which have the potential to degrade antibodies in the area, thereby facilitating the spread of toxic products of bacterial origin. The virulence factors of periodontal pathogens and their mode of action are described in Chapter 2. As the critical aspect of inflammatory periodontal disease is a loss of alveolar bone, the bone-resorbing capacity of bacterial products deserves particular attention. Amongst these, surface capsules, slimes and lipopolysaccharides possess significant bone-resorbing potentials. Although lipopolysaccharides (LPS) from periodontopathic bacteria vary in chemical composition and biological activities, most of them have been shown to cause bone resorption *in vitro*. LPS and other bacterial products can also bring about bone resorption indirectly by activating lymphocytes and macrophages to secrete mediators of bone resorption, such as osteoclast-activating or bone-resorbing factor, interleukin-1 and prostaglandins. Bone-resorbing activity has been found in 50% of culture supernatants of lymphocytes isolated from chronically inflamed periodontal tissues, but the levels were not related to the severity of periodontal disease.

JUVENILE PERIODONTITIS

General considerations

Juvenile periodontitis is a disorder of the supporting apparatus of the teeth which occurs in adolescents. It can be distinguished from adult periodontitis not only by its early onset, but also by the poor relationship between the amount of plaque on one hand and the degree of tissue destruction on the other. Initially, the disease appears to be confined to the periodontium around the first molars and incisors (localized juvenile periodontitis) with characteristic vertical or irregular bone loss. The localized lesions of juvenile periodontitis may progress rapidly and may also spread to other parts of the dentition causing generalized alveolar bone destruction (generalized juvenile periodontitis). A few case reports have provided evidence for such progression, whilst other investigators reported that 39% of patients with juvenile periodontitis aged between 21 and 30 years still had only molar/incisor involvement. There is increasing evidence for the hereditary nature of juvenile periodontitis. X-linked inheritance has been suggested but both sexes are affected. Therefore an autosomal recessive model of inheritance seems more likely. Studies on the association of the disease with HLA have so far produced equivocal results.

The importance of *Actinobacillus actinomycetemcomitans* in the aetiology of localized juvenile periodontitis (LJP) is based on the following findings. There is an increased prevalence of oral *A. actinomycetemcomitans* in LJP patients as compared to control subjects. In LJP patients this organism is found in large numbers in periodontal pockets, but is either not present or is found only in small numbers in healthy sites. There is an indication that *A. actinomycetemcomitans* may enter the gingiva adjacent to periodontal pockets, where it may produce potent toxic factors. There is a good correlation between elimination of *A. actinomycetemcomitans* from subgingival plaque and successful treatment of this disease.

Immunological findings

Patients with juvenile, in contrast to adult, periodontitis, frequently show depressed neutrophil chemotaxis and phagocytosis. In most of these patients monocyte chemotaxis appears normal, although occasionally depressed monocyte as well as neutrophil chemotaxis was observed. Some LJP patients have serum factors which may inhibit neutrophil chemotaxis. *A. actinomycetemcomitans* also produces a polymorphonuclear leukocyte chemotaxis-inhibiting agent. Furthermore, several strains of *A. actinomycetemcomitans* produce a leukotoxin which is capable of lysing human neutrophils. These factors may function in the periodontal pocket to exacerbate the systemic neutrophil chemotaxis defect seen in many patients with LJP. However, sera from LJP patients contain antibodies which neutralize the leukotoxin. Furthermore, both leukotoxin-producing and non-producing strains were isolated from these patients. The observation that non-leukotoxic strains could be recovered at one point in time as sole *A. actinomycetemcomitans* organisms from LJP lesions suggests that leukotoxin is neither unique nor necessary for the development of LJP. Alternatively, the infecting *A. actinomycetemcomitans* strain may have converted from a leukotoxin-producing to a non-leukotoxin-producing strain. Results from several laboratories demonstrate a strong relationship between serum IgG antibody titres to both leukotoxic and non-leukotoxic strains of *A. actinomycetemcomitans* and LJP. Elevated serum IgM and IgA responses and salivary IgA antibodies to this organism were also observed in the LJP patients. However, *Bacteroides gingivalis* is rarely found in these patients and the antibody titres to this organism are low. Conceivably, the antibodies to *A. actinomycetemcomitans* develop after the disease is initiated and some destruction has occurred, but then exert a protective effect against further spread and destruction, leading to a 'burn-out' state of the disease. Antibodies to *A. actinomycetemcomitans* are also found in gingival fluid at levels comparable to those found in serum. In patients demonstrating ongoing loss of probing attachment, antibody levels in gingival fluid to *A. actinomycetemcomitans* may exceed those present in the serum during the period of no bone loss. In one interesting experiment a periodontal probe was inserted into deep periodontal pockets containing large numbers of *A. actinomycetemcomitans* and then placed into a healthy gingival sulcus in the same LJP patient. The results showed that the organisms did not colonize the healthy sites and were eliminated within 3 weeks. It appears most likely that the antibodies (opsonizing and/or preventing attachment) or activated macrophages eliminated the organisms from the recipient site. Taken together, antibodies specific for *A. actinomycetemcomitans* probably act protectively against periodontal destruction in LJP.

In contrast with LJP, patients with generalized juvenile periodontitis (GJP) show high serum IgG antibody titres to *B. gingivalis*. These antibodies have been shown to merely reflect infection with the micro-organism without a protective function. Hence, spreading of the disease to teeth other than the incisors and molars could be due to colonization with *B. gingivalis* succeeding the initial *A. actinomycetemcomitans* infection. Indeed, *B. gingivalis* has been shown to be more proteolytic than other species and its virulence was demonstrated by an acute, rapidly spreading infection and bone resorption after being injected into mice. However, even in GJP the extent of bone resorption was found to be dependent on the presence of precipitating antibody to *A. actinomycetemcomitans*. Within the disease group there were significantly fewer involved teeth in subjects with precipitating antibody (antibody positive) than amongst those in whose sera precipitins were not seen (antibody negative).

In conclusion, high antibody levels specific for *A. actinomycetemcomitans* may have a protective effect against further periodontal destruction. Monitoring of these antibody levels may prove to be a useful test in the prediction of the arrest or further progression of the disease in patients with juvenile periodontitis.

NECROTIZING ULCERATIVE GINGIVITIS (NUG)

This condition generally presents as an acute gingivitis of rapid onset, characterized by discrete ulceration and destruction of affected papillae, painful residual gingivae and a characteristic halitosis. The lesions may spread extensively orally and facially in malnourished patients to produce 'cancrum oris'. If untreated, a chronic form of the disease may supervene, which is thought to predispose to further acute episodes.

The clinical features are characteristic but are usually substantiated by smears of the lesions which by phase-contrast or dark-ground microscopy reveal large numbers of fusiform rods and spirochaetes.

For many years this condition has been considered as an infection produced by oral bacteria, principally spirochaetes and fusiform rods. *Bacteroides* and, to a lesser extent, protozoa were also implicated. Current evidence indicates that an immune defect produces the rapid gingival tissue breakdown that allows these commensal oral organisms to grow in excessive numbers. Early work suggested that lowered tissue resistance was a factor. Severe colds and stress were cited as examples. More recently, both humoral and cellular factors have been implicated. Salivary IgM appears not to be affected but decreases have been demonstrated in salivary IgG, IgA and SIgA, which to some indicate a hypogammaglobulinaemia as an aetiologic factor. Within 1–4 days of clinical onset, others have noted increases in serum IgM and decreases or increases in serum IgG which may reflect the presence of many plasma cells in tissues previously affected by chronic gingivitis. Higher IgG and IgM titres to intermediate-size spirochaetes have been noted. Complement levels appear to be normal. Spirochaete endotoxin activity has been proposed as a mechanism to explain the increase in serum IgM. Stress may also be relevant in this context, as excessive hydrocortisone activity may inhibit antibody production by directing amino acids from protein production to carbohydrate metabolism.

The polymorphonuclear leukocytes in the NUG lesion tend to concentrate in large numbers between epithelium and bacteria, which is similar to the less marked PMN accumulation in the same location in chronic gingival and periodontal inflammation. It has been suggested that the typical surface ulceration of the lesion is due to the release of hydrolytic enzymes from the large numbers of accumulated PMN. The presence of an intact basal layer in the affected epithelium suggests, however, that tissue destruction originates within the epithelium and not in the subjacent connective tissue. It may be observed that extensive gingival ulcers resembling those of NUG can occur in chronic neutropenia, infectious mononucleosis and leukaemia, and there has been a suggestion of PMN dysfunction in NUG in terms of both chemotaxis and phagocytosis.

No patterns of transformation of lymphocytes different from those of chronic gingivitis occur in NUG, although there has been a suggestion of the NUG lesion being attributable to a local Schwartzman reaction to Gram-negative species, particularly fusiforms.

PERIAPICAL PERIODONTITIS

Acute periapical periodontitis is manifested by exquisite pain by light contact with the affected tooth. The periodontal space is widened and the tooth hypermobile. Chronic periapical periodontitis presents usually without symptoms, but the affected tooth is non-vital and there may be a (minimal) area of periapical rarefaction evident radiographically.

Inflammatory changes ranging from acute to chronic characterize the periapical periodontitis lesion. Plasma cells are common with immuno-globulins being produced in the order IgG>IgA>IgE>IgM. Many PMN, lymphocytes and mast cells are also present. It has been found that capillary endothelial pericytes of the lesion show increased lysosomal activity and may form foreign body giant cells. Mast cells in the affected tissues may contribute to connective tissue breakdown. No evidence has been found to implicate immune complex formation in periapical periodontitis. Acute periapical lesions contain a dense polymorphonuclear infiltrate with a few lymphocytes and plasma cells.

DRUG-INDUCED GINGIVAL HYPERPLASIA

Drug-induced gingival hyperplasia generally presents with marked tissue enlargement due basically to fibrous hypertrophy, with varying levels of inflammation which may produce changes from increased redness and oedema to gross granulomatous change.

Oral contraceptives

Perhaps the commonest drug-induced gingival enlargement is that attributable to oral contraceptives, although the increase in tissue volume is almost entirely due to inflammation. Progesterone, progestin and oestrogen have each been shown to be capable of increasing the adhesion of granulocytes and platelets to small vessels resulting in microthrombus formation. Mast cell disruption has been observed, as have vascular proliferation and increased permeability and gingival exudate formation, probably due more to oestrogen than to progesterone. The features described appear to be most evident during the initial 6 months of taking the contraceptive, although some have noted more inflammation in those taking the pill for more than 5 years compared with those taking it for a lesser period. The mechanism of increased inflammation has not been established, but it is possible that the effects of progesterone are due to its effect of increasing prostaglandin synthesis.

Anticonvulsants

The use of several anticonvulsant drugs is associated with marked fibrous gingival enlargement. The principal drug implicated is phenytoin, although primidone and phenobarbitone have been found to produce very similar effects. So does the anti-angina drug nifedipine, a calcium channel blocker, which is thought to have similar effects at the cellular level despite differences in target tissue, which in its case is cardiac and smooth muscle. The affected tissue is hypertrophic rather than hyperplastic, the enlargement being due to increased amounts of both collagen and ground substance. This may reflect a decreased rate of breakdown of extracellular material within fibroblasts. Depression of cellular and humoral immune responses has been described including IgA reduction, although epilepsy itself may predispose to IgA deficiency, which would then be evident if and when phenytoin or other anticonvulsants were taken. There have been contradictory reports concerning similar changes with phenytoin in serum IgG and IgM levels, some showing increased, some decreased, and some unchanged, serum levels. Comparison of gingival levels of immunoglobulin revealed higher IgG in phenytoin hyperplastic tissue but not in tissue affected by idiopathic gingival hyperplasia. IgM also appears to be more abundant in the phenytoin-affected tissue. The higher IgG level in the latter has been attributed to the greater level of associated inflammation. There is a report of increased lysozyme, lactoperoxidase and lactoferrin in unstimulated whole saliva of affected patients.

Non-steroidal anti-inflammatory drugs

Diminished periodontal inflammation has been observed in patients receiving immunosuppressive drugs. Steroids do not appear to have a predictable periodontal effect, although a suppressive effect has been attributed to inhibition of prostaglandin synthesis. Indomethacin and flurbiprofen are non-steroidal anti-inflammatory drugs which can delay the onset and reduce the level of inflammatory reaction and bone resorption, again due probably to their effects on prostaglandin synthesis, blocking lymphocyte activation.

Cyclosporin

The immunosuppressive drug cyclosporin, now used so widely in patients who have received organ transplants, is associated with a generalized gingival enlargement with both fibrous and oedematous components similar to, or even indistinguishable from, that induced by phenytoin. The inflammatory infiltrate in the affected gingiva contains mainly plasma cells, although some tissue areas are relatively non-inflamed. Cyclosporin appears to affect T-cells, mainly T-helper and to a lesser extent T-suppressor. In patients with uncontrolled gingival hyperplasia and poor plaque control, bone and then tooth loss may occur.

FURTHER READING

Davies, R. M., Smith, R. G. and Porter, S. R. (1985). Destructive forms of periodontal disease in adolescents and young adults. *Br. Dent. J.*, **158**, 429–36

Genco, R. J. and Slots, J. (1984). Host responses in periodontal diseases. *J. Dent. Res.*, **63**, 441–51

Ivanyi, L. (1980). Stimulation of gingival and blood lymphocytes by antigens from oral bacteria. In Lehner, T. and Cimasoni, G. (eds) *Borderland between Caries and Periodontal Disease.* pp. 125–34. (London: Academic Press)

Lehner, T. (1982). Cellular immunity in periodontal disease: an overview. In Genco, R. J. and Mergenhagen, S. E. (eds) *Host–Parasite Interactions in Periodontal Diseases.* pp. 202–16. (Washington, DC: American Society for Microbiology)

Loe, H., Anerud, A., Boysen, H. and Smith, M. (1978). The natural history of periodontal disease in man. The rate of destruction before 40 years of age. *J. Periodontol.*, **12**, 607–19

Newman, H. N. (1982). Infection and the periodontal ligament. In Berkovitz, B. K. B., Moxham, B. J. and Newman, H. N. (eds) *The Periodontal Ligament in Health and Disease.* pp. 335–57. (Oxford: Pergamon)

Page, R. C. and Schroeder, H. E. (1982). *Periodontitis in Man and Other Animals: a Comparative Review.* (Basle: Karger)

Socransky, S. S., Haffajee, A. D., Goodson, J. M. and Lindhe, J. (1984). New concepts of destructive periodontal disease. *J. Clin. Periodontol.*, **11**, 21–32

Wilton, J. M. A. and Lehner, T. (1980). Immunological and microbial aspects of periodontal disease. In Thompson, R. A. (ed.) *Recent Advances in Clinical Immunology.* pp. 145–81. (Edinburgh: Churchill-Livingstone)

Zambon, J. J. (1985). *Actinobacillus actinomycetemcomitans* in human periodontal disease. *J. Clin. Periodontol.*, **12**, 1–20

5
Infectious Diseases with Oral Manifestations

D. M. WALKER

HERPES SIMPLEX

General considerations

Herpes simplex hominis Type 1 (less frequently Type 2) is the commonest viral infection of the oral cavity. Herpes zoster not infrequently affects the face or mouth. Other vesicular eruptions such as hand, foot and mouth disease and herpangina, due to the Coxsackie A group of viruses, occur as occasional epidemics among children of nursery-school age.

Viral replication

Herpes simplex is a DNA virus. The double-stranded DNA encloses a protein core. The virus has an outer shell of geometrically arranged subunits or capsomers making up a capsid in the shape of an icosahedron. This is in turn surrounded by a bilayered membrane. Viral DNA replication takes place within the nucleus of the host cell and as the virus particles burst out of the nucleus they acquire an outer envelope derived from the nuclear membrane by budding (Figure 5.1). During infection the herpes virus adsorbs, possibly by specific binding sites, to the surface of the oral epithelial cell which it penetrates, shedding its envelope. The DNA genome of the uncoated virus first transcribes messenger RNA which is translated in the host cell ribosomes to form viral proteins. Certain early genes code for proteins which shut down normal synthesis of the host cell's DNA and protein. Other early gene products include enzymes concerned in herpes virus replication. The late proteins to be translated are of structural type necessary for the complete viral particle (virion).

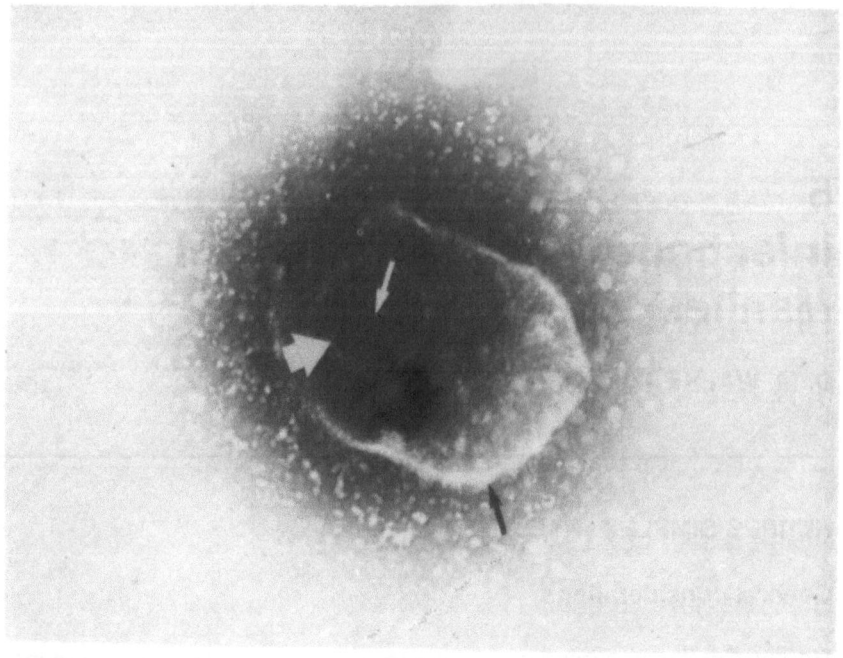

Figure 5.1 Transmission electron micrograph of the herpes simplex-type 1 virus with a DNA core (narrow white arrow), protein capsid (broad white arrow) and cell envelope (black arrow) (× 80 000)

Immunological aspects of pathogenesis

Antigens in herpes infection

During infection, herpes virus antigens appear in the nucleus, cytoplasm and cell membrane of the infected cells. Intriguingly there is also virus-determined expression of new host antigens on the cell surface.

Antibody formation

Seven to 10 days after the primary infection there is a diagnostic rise in the titre of complement-fixing and neutralizing serum antibody to herpes simplex which is initially of IgM class and then superseded by a sustained rise in IgG antibody. Secretory IgA (SIgA) antibody appears in saliva.

Protective effect of antibody

IgG antibody helps to eliminate the virus by its opsonizing action, promoting phagocytosis of the antibody-coated virus by polymorphs and macrophages via their membrane Fc–IgG receptors (Figure 5.2). The virus may strike back. For example, virus-determined Fc receptors developing on the surface of cells infected by herpes simplex and the varicella zoster virus can bind IgG non-specifically and interfere with the recognition of adjacent viral antigens (Figure 5.3). Fc receptors for IgG recently discovered on the surface of the herpes virus itself could similarly hamper the action of neutralizing antibody. Virus-coded C3 receptors appearing on herpes-infected cells could deplete the local supply of complement. Virus antigen appearing on infected cells could likewise mop up the available antibody.

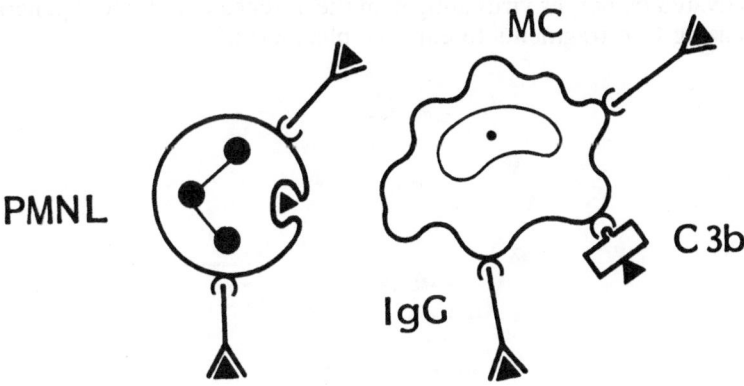

Figure 5.2 Phagocytosis of virus by polymorphs (PMNL) and macrophages (MC) via their Fc-IgG and C3b receptors

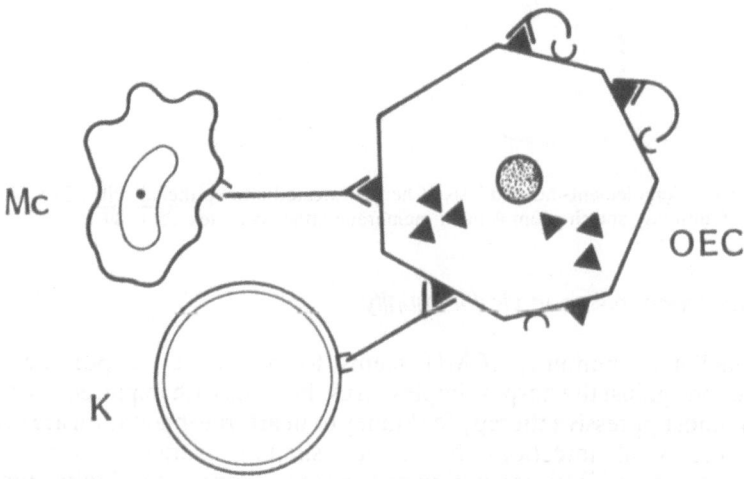

Figure 5.3 Effect of antibody on virus-infected cells. Virus determined Fc receptors (⋎) for IgG appearing on the surface of infected epithelial cells (OEC) may block binding to adjacent viral antigens (▲) by opsonizing antibody promoting killing of viral-infected cells by macrophages (MC) or K cells (K)

Secretory IgA antibody in saliva may prevent infection by blocking viral binding sites on host cells. SIgA clumping of virus effectively reduces the number of infective units.

Complement

The major antiviral effect of complement occurs in combination with IgG antibodies, causing lysis of herpes-infected cells which release the virus which is subsequently inactivated (Figure 5.4). The alternative pathway can be activated by herpes virus antigen in the absence of antibody, generating opsonizing C3b fragments to enhance phagocytosis.

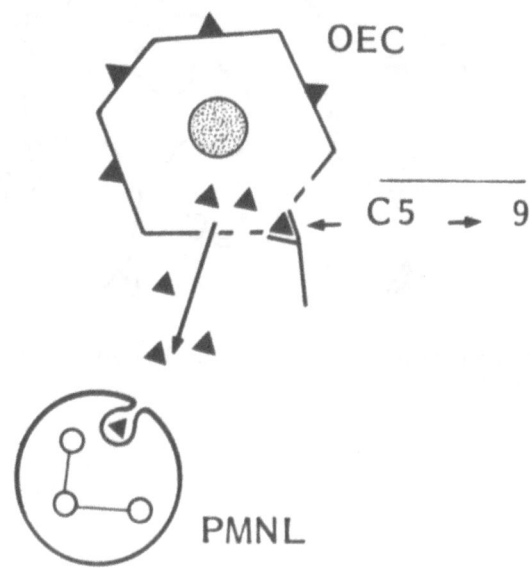

Figure 5.4 Complement-induced lysis of herpes-infected oral epithelial cells (OEC) by the action of antibody and the complement membrane attack complex C5b6789

Cellular mechanisms in viral immunity

Cell-mediated immunity (CMI) seems to be of key importance for protection against the herpes simplex virus. Patients with impaired CMI due to immunosuppressive therapy for kidney or heart transplantation are prone to severe viral infections by herpes simplex, varicella zoster and cytomegalovirus. Patients prescribed cytotoxic drugs for leukaemia or lymphoma are similarly at risk. Mice undergoing neonatal thymectomy which impairs T cell immunity have a reduced resistance to herpes infection. Cytotoxic T lymphocytes, natural killer cells and macrophages are all involved in this cellular protection. Cytotoxic T lymphocytes lyse virally infected cells, releasing the virus into the extracellular environment for disposal by antibody, complement and phagocytes (Figure 5.5). T cells recognize the virus-coded antigens expressed on the cell surface. In addition the cytotoxic T lymphocytes and the infected target cells need to have in common the same major histocompatibility complex (MHC) Class 1 antigen. Presumably, therefore, the T cell has either two receptors for the HSV and MHC antigens respectively, or a single combined receptor. Cytotoxic T cells with restriction for MHC – Class 2 antigens have been discovered but their clinical significance is as yet undetermined. Herpes simplex viruses can replicate within T lymphocytes, which may make the latter functionally defective.

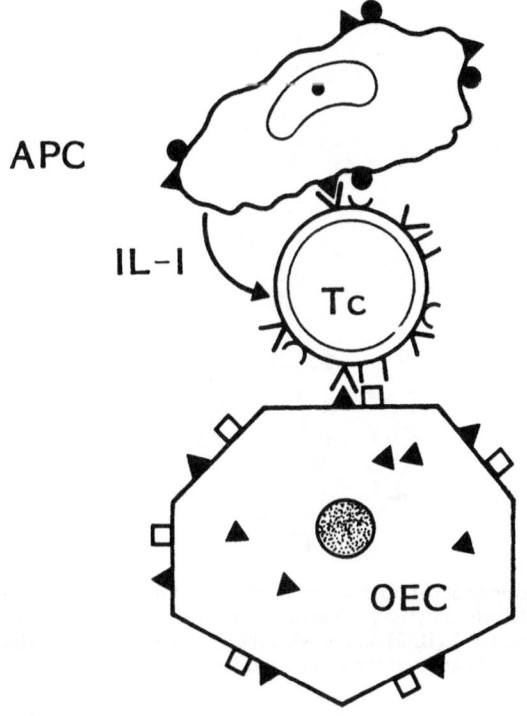

Figure 5.5 MHC-restricted killing of virus-infected oral epithelial cells (OEC) by cytotoxic T cells (Tc). The viral antigen (▲) is presented on the surface of the antigen-presenting cell (APC), e.g. a Langerhans cell. This activates the T cell, with the help of interleukin-1 (IL-1). The cytotoxic T cell must also have the same MHC-1 (□) and MHC-2 (●) determinants as the target cell and antigen-presenting cell respectively

Natural killer (NK) cells show spontaneous cytotoxicity towards virus-infected cells. Their importance in natural immunity to viral infections stems from the fact that their killing activity is not MHC-restricted and is efficient in unimmunized subjects. Their activity can be boosted by interferon

(IFN-1) produced by infected cells (Figure 5.6). IFN-1 induces the expression of interleukin-2 receptors on inactive precursor NK cells. An IL-2 signal from helper T cells induces NK cell proliferation, generating cytolytic NK cells. Interferons, a group of glycoproteins produced in infected host cells, also have the effect of making adjacent cells more resistant to viral replication by inhibiting viral DNA and protein synthesis, limiting the spread of infection. Interestingly, NK cells are also capable of making interferon, which may make them resistant to infection by the invading virus. Macrophages can produce prostaglandin (PGE_2) which tends to damp down NK cell activity.

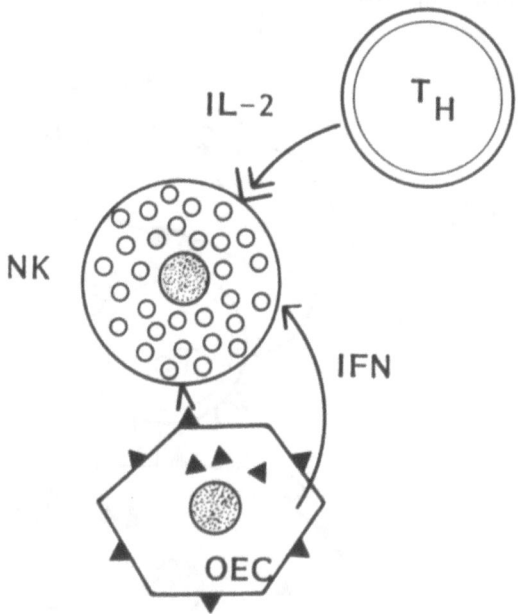

Figure 5.6 Cytotoxicity of natural killer cells (NK) for oral epithelial cells (OEC) infected by the herpes virus. Interferon (IFN) released by the infected cells induces the expression of receptors for interleukin-2 (IL-2) on the NK cells. IL-2 released from helper T lymphocytes (T_H) then causes proliferation of these activated NK cells

Macrophages can digest virions intracellularly and also selectively destroy virus-infected cells, particularly when antibody is present. *In vitro*, macrophages can prevent cell-to-cell spread of the herpes simplex virus without destroying the cells. Interleukin-1 is a soluble product (monokine) of macrophages which initiates and amplifies all T cell-dependent immune responses. The secretion of another useful monokine, interferon, has already been mentioned. Macrophages, the Langerhans cells in the oral mucosa and dendritic cells in the regional lymph nodes, are concerned in antigen presentation to T helper cells and B cells, an MHC-Class 2 restricted function. Antibody-dependent cellular cytotoxicity mediated by K cells may also occur (Figure 5.7).

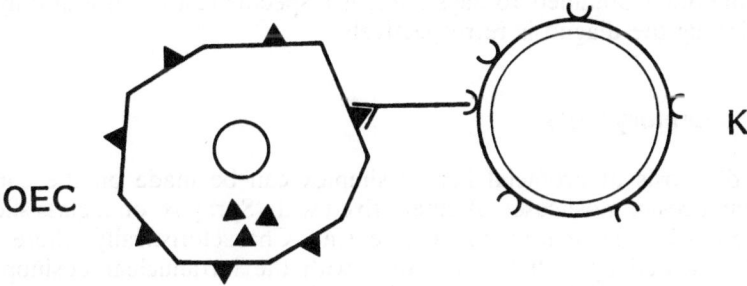

Figure 5.7 Antibody-dependent cell-mediated cytotoxicity by killer (K) cells. The K cells bind to the infected target oral epithelial cells (OEC) by an Fc receptor for the antiviral IgG antibody

Systemic manifestations

These are rare. A herpes meningoencephalitis may complicate a primary infection or possibly originate from the dormant virus in the trigeminal ganglion. Eczema herpeticum is a severe, sometimes fatal, generalized skin eruption in children with chronic eczema. In visceral herpes simplex, which is often fatal, newborn infants contract the virus from the genital tract of their mothers. Necrotizing lesions are found in the liver, spleen, kidneys, adrenal glands and brain.

Oral manifestations

The primary oral herpes simplex infection usually affects young children although it may be delayed until adult life, as a vesicular eruption of the oral mucosa, with swelling of the gingivae and enlargement of the submandibular lymph nodes. In about half the population the virus is not subsequently completely eradicated but persists in a latent state in the trigeminal ganglion. Despite its apparent dormancy, the herpes simplex virus may be constantly reactivated, travelling down the peripheral branches of the trigeminal nerve to the skin and oral mucosa where the organisms are promptly killed by the immune system.

It is proposed that recurrent herpes labialis ('cold sores') results when the local host defences are temporarily deficient. For example, the recrudescence of herpes simplex lesions is associated with reduced MIF production by T lymphocytes. A fall in NK-like activity occurs before each attack, later to rebound to above normal levels.

Immunological diagnosis

A rise in the serum-neutralizing, or complement-fixing, antibody as demonstrated in paired serum samples, one taken at the onset of symptoms and the other obtained 10 days later, is a specific test but useful only for confirming the diagnosis retrospectively.

Key laboratory tests

The diagnosis of orofacial herpes simplex can be made on the clinical appearances in most cases. A smear fixed with 'Sprayfix' on a glass slide is stained with haematoxylin and eosin. Characteristically there are multinucleated epithelial cells, some with the intranuclear eosinophilic inclusion bodies of Cowdry Type A. Similar appearances occur in herpes zoster and in chickenpox. Tissue culture of swabs from the lesions conveyed in viral transport medium detects the virus rather more sensitively but this test takes 48 hours. The addition of serum-containing antibody to HSV-1 inhibits the cytopathogenic effect of the virus, giving the test its specificity. Transmission electron microscopy of unfixed samples of vesicle fluid (transported between two glass slides) takes only a few hours but this facility is only available in specialized centres.

Vaccination against herpes simplex

The association between carcinoma of the uterine cervix and chronic cervicitis with HSV-Type 2 has prompted the preparation of a vaccine using formaldehyde-treated viral glycoprotein combined with an adjuvant. Similar work is in progress to develop a vaccine against HSV-1 which might protect children against encephalitis, or immunocompromised individuals against severe recurrent infection.

HERPES ZOSTER

The DNA varicella zoster virus (VZV) causes the generalized vesicular skin rash chickenpox, usually in childhood. The VZV virus subsequently persists in a latent state in the dorsal root ganglia. Although almost all adults harbour the virus, it only becomes reactivated to cause shingles in a small proportion of subjects, usually in middle age or later. An acquired immunodeficiency may be responsible, as shingles is relatively common in immunocompromised individuals, for example patients with Hodgkin's disease or other lymphomas. One or more branches of the trigeminal nerve may be affected, involving the corresponding dermatome, and its intra-oral mucosal counterpart. The usually unilateral segmental distribution of the grouped skin vesicles or oral erosions and the severe pain usually make the clinical diagnosis straightforward. If there is any doubt, the confirmatory laboratory tests are essentially similar to those described for herpes simplex.

CANDIDOSIS

General considerations

Candida albicans is the most important species of this genus of unicellular fungi or yeasts. It can be isolated in small numbers from the healthy mouth, particularly from the tongue, in almost 50% of the normal dentate population. Approximately 55% of denture-wearers harbour the yeast, particularly if the prostheses are worn continuously day and night. The blastospore form of the dimorphic fungus predominates in the healthy carrier state, whereas hyphae and blastospores are usually found in smears of the lesions in infections (candidosis).

Immunological aspects of oral candidosis

In healthy immunocompetent dentate adults the local defensive mechanisms are sufficient to prevent infection by the feebly pathogenic *Candida albicans*. This protection takes a number of forms:

Non-specific immunity

Candida species cannot usually be isolated from healthy skin but can be cultured from the skin of patients with various dermatoses. The normal oral mucosa presents a similar barrier to infection and when the mouths of healthy volunteers are inoculated with *C. albicans* the organisms are speedily eliminated. The continuous shedding of surface epithelial cells helps to limit the surface flora.

Salivary flow

By its flushing effect, salivary flow dislodges bacteria and yeasts from the surfaces of teeth and the oral mucosa, and thus limits oral microbial populations. Patients with a frank xerostomia, such as in Sjögren's syndrome, are susceptible to dental caries and candidal infections. Saliva contains specific candidal antibodies of predominantly secretory immunoglobulin A class (SIgA) and other inhibitory factors such as lactoferrin, a chelating agent which competes with oral micro-organisms for the free iron essential for their multiplication. Salivary lysozyme and lactoperoxidase also have useful antimicrobial actions.

Competition from oral commensal bacteria

The normal resident bacterial flora of the oral cavity checks the proliferation of *Candida albicans* by competition for essential nutrients or by lowering pH due to acids produced by lactobacilli or streptococci. Alternatively, bacteria may block receptor sites for candidal colonization on the surface of oral epithelial cells. Suppression of oral bacteria by broad-spectrum antibiotics disturbs the balance of this ecosystem in favour of candidal proliferation, resulting in 'antibiotic sore mouth' (acute atrophic candidosis).

Phagocytosis

Polymorphonuclear leukocytes (PMNL) and monocytes (MC) can phagocytose and kill fungi such as *Candida* even in the absence of the specific opsonizing antibodies available in blood and saliva (see below). Candidal hyphae may be more difficult to ingest than spores. In secondary immunodeficiency states, for example the agranulocytosis due to cytotoxic drugs used in the treatment of malignancy, the small number of circulating PMNL renders patients liable to thrush involving the mouth, pharynx and oesophagus. These patients with advanced malignancy, including leukaemia, are also at risk from disseminated candidosis.

In some primary immunodeficiencies (see Chapter 11) qualitative rather than quantitative defects in polymorphs or macrophages predispose to candidosis of skin or mucous membrane. Defective PMNL phagocytosis partly explains the susceptibility of diabetics to thrush. Impaired PMNL and monocyte migration is a factor in chronic mucocutaneous candidosis. Alternatively, the leukocytes may phagocytose *Candida* quite normally but intracellular killing is faulty due to NADPH oxidase deficiency or myeloperoxidase deficiency. A shortage of either enzyme results in defective generation of free oxygen metabolites necessary for killing within the cell's lysosomes. Intractable candidosis in the mouth can be the result.

Virulence factors

Can any strain of *C. albicans* infect the mouth given a susceptible host, or are the chances of infection determined by variations in the virulence of the yeast? *C. albicans* mutants which are unable to produce extracellular proteinase which seems to be important for tissue invasion show reduced virulence of mice when injected intravenously. There is also some relationship between the ability of *C. albicans* and other *Candida* species to adhere to the mucosal epithelial cells and their pathogenicity. Conditions favouring germ tube formation promote adherence to buccal cells. Mannose-containing binding sites on the surface of the organisms and receptor sites on the epithelial cells are involved in this attachment. Blocking of these sites by lectins might prevent oral colonization and infection.

Specific immunity

Serum antibody – Although specific antibodies to *C. albicans* of all the major isotypes are present in serum, most antibody is of IgG class. These antibodies have been detected by a variety of techniques such as agglutination, precipitation, complement fixation, indirect immuno-fluorescence and, latterly, enzyme-linked immunoassay. The antibodies are predominantly directed against mannan carbohydrate antigens in the yeast cell wall. Acting alone, antibody and complement cannot kill *Candida*. They act by speeding up phagocytosis by PMNL and macrophages, which are attracted by the chemotactic C3a and C5a generated by complement activation by IgG antibody. PMNL and MCs are equipped with membrane receptors for the Fc end of IgG and complement C3b serving to attach the bacteria to the cell surface (immune adherence) (Figure 5.8).

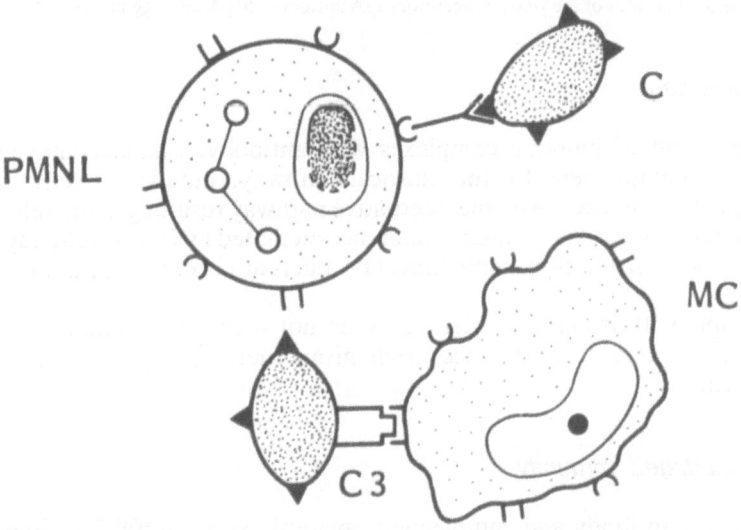

Figure 5.8 Opsonization of *Candida* (C) by IgG antibody and complement for phagocytosis by polymorphs (PMNL) and macrophages (MC) via their Fc-IgG and C3b receptors

Non-immunological factors have been found in normal serum capable of killing (candidacidal factor) or clumping *Candida*. Iron deficiency induces a cell-mediated immune defect to *Candida*. Endocrine disorders, such as diabetes mellitus, hypoadrenocorticism, hypoparathyroidism or hypo-thyroidism, have also been associated with chronic candidal infection.

Salivary antibodies – Salivary antibody is of predominantly secretory IgA class. By agglutinating the organisms, and by blocking their receptor sites for oral epithelium, secretory IgA plays a part in restricting candidal adherence and colonization of the mouth (Figure 5.9). IgA can also opsonize the yeast for phagocytosis. IgA deficiency has been observed in patients with chronic mucocutaneous candidosis. Some subjects with an isolated IgA deficiency enjoy good health, however, and they may be protected by a compensatory production of secretory IgM.

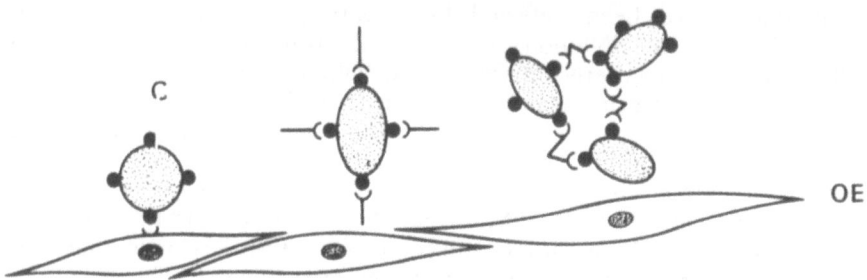

Figure 5.9 Inhibition of adherence of *Candida* (C) for oral epithelium (OE) by blocking of surface binding sites of the yeast by secretory IgA antibody. SIgA also agglutinates the *Candida*

Complement

In the form of immune complexes with antibody, *Candida* antigen can activate complement by the classical pathway, but whole cells trigger complement activation by the alternative pathway resulting in the release of chemotactic C3a. The immune adherence mediated by C3b has already been mentioned. In addition, some fungal products are chemotactic in their own right.

People with isolated C3 deficiency do not seem to be unduly prone to candidosis, and other defence mechanisms therefore appear to be more important.

Cell-mediated immunity

Although antibody and complement obviously serve useful functions, the normal or elevated levels of serum and salivary antibody in some patients with intractable infections suggests that humoral immunity is insufficient on its own. An impaired T cell-mediated delayed hypersensitivity response to *Candida* seems to be the basic defect in many patients with chronic mucocutaneous candidosis. The skin delayed hypersensitivity response to intradermal infection of *Candida* antigens may be negative (cutaneous anergy). The *in vitro* lymphocyte transformation test in response to *Candida* antigen, or other antigens or mitogens, may be subnormal due to a serum inhibitory factor, possibly a mannan cell constituent of the yeast cell wall. There may be reduced production of lymphokines, such as leukocyte or macrophage migration inhibitory factor (LMIF or MMIF) when the patient's lymphocytes are stimulated.

Faced with an unexplained or atypical form of chronic oral candidosis, the dental surgeon should remember that occasionally this is an oral manifestation of the acquired immunodeficiency syndrome (AIDS) (see Chapter 11). Cell-mediated immunity is deficient in AIDS due to a selective reuction in the number of T helper cells which are specifically infected and eradicated by the HTLV-3 virus.

Systemic manifestation

Most forms of candidosis are superficial infections of the mucous membranes or the skin. In immunocompromised patients, such as those with advanced malignancy, particularly when receiving cytotoxic or immunosuppressive therapy, a disseminated, sometimes fatal, form of candidosis can occur in which the fungus is carried in the blood stream to sites such as the heart valves, lungs, kidney or brain. An indwelling venous catheter is often the portal of entry for this deep-seated infection (see Immunological diagnosis).

Oral manifestations

Candidal infections of the mouth may be classified as follows (see also Tables 5.1–5.3):

Acute pseudomembranous candidosis (thrush)

This is a common infection in babies or elderly or debilitated people. The white plaques resembling milk curds contain candidal hyphae and spores, epithelial cells and polymorphs, and are easily detached from the oral mucosa.

Acute atrophic candidosis

This is also known as 'antibiotic sore mouth' because it frequently complicates antibiotic therapy. There is a stomatitis with a widespread generalized depapillation of the tongue (see the section on Oral candidosis).

Chronic atrophic candidosis ('denture sore mouth')

This asymptomatic confluent inflammation of the entire denture-bearing mucosa of the palate results from candidal colonization of the fitting surface of the maxillary denture, usually in patients wearing their prosthesis continuously day and night. Only these local factors are usually involved.

Chronic hyperplastic candidosis (candidal leukoplakia)

This speckled or nodular leukoplakia found in middle-aged or elderly patients carries a significant risk of malignant transformation. Tobacco smoking and continuous denture wearing are important local factors promoting this type of candidosis, although one report found limited immune defects in this group of patients.

113

Table 5.1 Oral candidosis

	Type of candidosis	Synonym	Age of onset	Associated factors
(i)	Acute pseudomembranous candidosis	Thrush	Any age	Non-specific or specific (immune)
(ii)	Acute atrophic candidosis ('antibiotic mouth')	Antibiotic sore mouth	Any age	Broad-spectrum antibiotic therapy
(iii)	Chronic atrophic candidosis	Denture stomatitis	Adults	Dentures worn continuously
(iv)	Chronic hyperplastic candidosis	Candidal leukoplakia	Usually middle-aged or elderly	Tobacco smoking Denture wearing
(v)	Median rhomboid glossitis		Third or later decades	Tobacco smoking Denture wearing

The infection is confined to the mouth. There are usually obvious local and/or systemic predisposing factors. Genetic factors are not involved.

Table 5.2 Classification of candidoses of skin and mucous membranes
Group 1: Oral candidosis as part of a mucocutaneous candidosis in patients with a general profound immunodeficiency

Syndrome	Inheritance	Distribution	Onset	Prognosis
Di George syndrome Hereditary thymic aplasia (Nezelof) Swiss type agammaglobulinaemia Chronic granulomatous disease of childhood	Congenital or genetically determined	Skin, mouth, nails	Early childhood	Usually die young of associated disease

Table 5.3 Classification of candidoses of skin and mucous membranes
Group 2: Chronic mucocutaneous candidosis is the major presenting complaint. All patients have chronic hyperplastic oral candidosis

	Type	Inheritance	Distribution	Associated features	Onset
(i)	Familial chronic mucocutaneous candidosis	Autosomal recessive	Mouth, nails, skin. Other sites occasionally involved		Before the age of 10 years
(ii)	Diffuse mucocutaneous candidosis	Unknown	Mouth, nails, skin and occasionally eyes, pharynx and larynx	Sporadic cases usually	Before the age of 5 years
(iii)	Candida–endocrinopathy syndrome	Autosomal recessive	Mouth, nails, skin. Larynx or vagina sometimes.	Hypoadrenocorticism, hypoparathyroidism. Occasionally diabetes mellitus or hypothyroidism.	By second decade

Median rhomboid glossitis

This is an elliptical area of papillary atrophy in the midline of the posterior third of the tongue. The lesion is now thought to represent an acquired form of oral candidosis, rather than a developmental anomaly as was originally maintained. Smoking and denture wearing are common local predisposing factors. The location of median rhomboid glossitis may be due to the fact that the posterior third of the tongue is the most frequently and most densely colonized intra-oral site for *C. albicans*.

Chronic mucocutaneous candidosis

Soon after birth, or in early childhood, the oral lesions invariably form the presenting feature, followed in most cases by skin involvement. The disorder is usually genetically determined and chronic mucocutaneous candidoses have been classified on the basis of their different modes of inheritance and the clinical features. In the endocrine candidosis syndrome there may be associated hypoparathyroidism or hypothyroidism. Immune unresponsiveness either specific for *Candida* antigens or sometimes other antigens or mitogens has been demonstrated by skin tests or by lymphocyte transformation in chronic mucocutaneous candidosis (see Chapter 11).

Immunological diagnosis

There is only an approximate correlation between the levels of serum or salivary antibody to *C. albicans* and the clinical status. Thus there is no significant differencf in the levels of candidal antibody in the serum and saliva of healthy oral carriers and non-carriers of the yeast. High antibody levels are usually found in chronic oral candidoses such as denture stomatitis. The overlapping between antibody levels in oral candidosis and in health invalidates their estimation for diagnostic purposes and smears, biopsies or imprint cultures (see below) are more convenient. Serological tests are invaluable, however, in disseminated candidosis. Matthews and colleagues have recently identified a *Candida* antigen of molecular weight 47 kilodaltons in the peripheral blood of patients with deep-seated candidosis such as candidal endocarditis. Patients subsequently developing antibody to this antigen tended to survive their disease. The test may prove to be of value both in diagnosis and for assessing the prognosis. The same antigen might possibly be used to vaccinate patients at risk.

Key laboratory tests

The diagnosis of thrush can usually be made on clinical grounds. It can be confirmed by a PAS-stained smear showing candidal hyphae, spores and polymorphs. Imprint cultures provide a sensitive means for isolating

Candida from the mouth and quantitating the density of organisms, which helps to distinguish oral infection from the carrier state. In candidal leukoplakia a biopsy is mandatory to assess the presence of epithelial dysplasia or carcinomatous change. A routine blood examination, including haemoglobin level, red cell values and film, is a suitable initial screening test for an underlying predisposing anaemia. A urine test for glucose is used to exclude diabetes mellitus.

SYPHILIS

General considerations

This sexually transmitted bacterial infection due to the spirochaete *Treponema pallidum* passes through primary, secondary and tertiary stages or may be acquired *in utero* (congenital or prenatal syphilis).

Immunological aspects of pathogenesis

In tertiary syphilis, small arteries become narrowed by a fibrous thickening of their walls (endarteritis obliterans). They are usually surrounded by a cuff of lymphocytes and plasma cells. The gumma is an area of coagulative necrosis, surrounded by a dense zone of fibrous tissue, and probably represents a delayed hypersensitivity reaction. The tissue necrosis could be a product of non-specific destruction caused by cytotoxic factor released by sensitized lymphocytes encountering tissue-bound treponemal antigens or mediated by specific cytotoxic lymphocytes.

Oral and systemic manifestations

The *primary* chancre develops as a painless, red papule after an incubation period varying between 2 and 6 weeks after the venereal infection. This papule soon develops a well-demarcated ulcer which lacks significant secondary bacterial infection. Chancres are usually located on the penis or vulva, but occasionally may be situated at extragenital sites such as the lip or tongue. There is a marked regional lymphadenopathy. Untreated, the chancre heals uneventfully, but 1–4 months later the signs and symptoms of *secondary* syphilis appear. The patient may feel generally unwell with a variety of maculopapular skin rashes and a generalized lymphadenopathy and mild pyrexia. The oral features include snail-track ulcers or grey mucous patches.

The *tertiary* stages of syphilis follow 3 or more years later. Leukoplakia of the tongue or a gumma, presenting as a painless, indolent, round or oval punched-out ulcer with a 'wash-leather' base are the characteristic oral manifestations. On the palate a gumma may cause perforation. Bones, liver and testes are the other sites of election. Other tertiary lesions include syphilitic aortitis, with sometimes an aortic aneurysm, and aortic valvular incompetence. In the nervous system, gummas may form in the brain or meninges and there may be cerebral ischaemia as a result of syphilitic arteritis. General paralysis of the insane and tabes dorsalis are other major forms of other neurosyphilis. A painless disorganization of joints, particularly of the knees, is known as Charcot's joint.

In *congenital* syphilis the fetus acquires infection from the mother via the placenta. The permanent maxillary incisors, and less often the mandibular incisors, are notched at their incisal edges and are barrel-shaped. The first permanent molars may have a rough, pitted occlusal surface with nodules replacing cusps (mulberry molars) or may be dome-shaped (Moon's molars).

The classic triad of congenital syphilis comprises an interstitial keratitis resulting in corneal opacity and blindness, mental retardation and nerve deafness. There may be ulcerated fissure (rhagades) radiating from the angles of the mouth. Gummas of the palate or nasal septum may be complicated by perforation.

Immunological diagnosis

The antibodies appearing in the blood, and in some circumstances in the cerebrospinal fluid (CSF), of patients contracting syphilis are of three types: non-specific, group anti-treponemal and specific anti-treponemal (Table 5.4).

Table 5.4 Diagnosis of syphilis before treatment

| | Dark-field microscopy of ulcerated lesions | Serology | | | |
| | | VDRL | TPHA | FTA–ABS | |
				IgG	IgM
Primary	+	+ or − (rising titre)	+ or −	+	+
Secondary	+	+	+	+	+
Tertiary – gumma neurosyphilis }	−	+	+	+	+
cardiovascular }	−	+ or −	+ or −	+	+
Congenital	+	+	+	+	+

Adapted from Csonka, 1983, with permission

Non-specific

The Wassermann reaction (WR) is a complement fixation test which detects a non-specific antibody that recognizes a phospholipid called cardiolipin present in normal tissues. A standardized antigen mixture of cardiolipin, cholesterol and lecithin are employed in the WR. The same antigen is used in the *Venereal Disease Reference Laboratory* (VDRL) test and *Kahn* tests, which are flocculation reactions monitoring a change from opalescence to flocculation (clumping). Biological false-positive (BFP) reactions due to this anti-lipoidal antibody occur in conditions unrelated to syphilis. Short-lived 'acute' BFP reactions occur occasionally in infections such as glandular fever or rubella. A positive reaction also occurs in the tropical infection yaws due to a related spirochaete *T. pertenue.*

Group anti-treponemal

Antigens are obtained from the commercial Reiter treponeme for the *Reiter complement fixation test.* Positive results will be obtained in other treponemal infections such as yaws or pinta.

Specific anti-treponemal antibodies

In a positive *treponemal immobilization test*, syphilitic serum immobilizes and then lyses *T. pallidum* in the presence of complement. It is also positive in yaws and pinta. For the modified *fluorescent treponemal antibody test* (FTA-ABS) organisms are incubated with the patient's serum, washed, and a fluorescent anti-human immunoglobulin is used to detect bound anti-treponemal antibody. The specificity of this indirect immunofluorescent test is increased by absorbing out group-specific antibodies from the patient's serum with the Reiter organism.

The highly specific *T. pallidum haemagglutination test* (TPHA) depends on the agglutination of tanned erythrocytes pretreated with a *T. pallidum* extract by absorbed patient's serum.

Key laboratory tests

In addition to the serological tests detailed above dark-field microscopy of unfixed fresh scrapings from the lesions in primary, secondary or congenital syphilis may detect the spirochaete with its characteristic 'spiral spring' movements.

The VDRL and the TPHA tests are usually sufficient for screening. If the results of these are equivocal, the FTA-ABS is a useful further investigation.

119

TUBERCULOSIS

General considerations

Tuberculosis of the oral cavity is uncommon. It is usually secondary to active pulmonary infection due to the human strain of the bacillus *Mycobacterium tuberculosis*. The incidence of tuberculosis is approximately twenty times higher in immigrants to Britain from those Asian countries where the disease remains endemic. Tuberculous cervical lymphadenitis due to the bovine strain is now encountered only in elderly people due to reactivation of bacilli, acquired by drinking contaminated milk many years previously. In children in Western industrialized countries, atypical or opportunist mycobacteria, such as *M. intracellulare* or *M. avium* cause a steady incidence of mycobacterial infection of cervical lymph nodes compared with that due to *M. tuberculosis* which is steadily declining. This is because the opportunist mycobacteria are not transmitted from other infected patients, as in a classical type of human tuberculosis, but are acquired from the environment, such as the soil in the case of *M. intracellulare*, or from animals, as in the case of *M. avium* from birds in poultry farms.

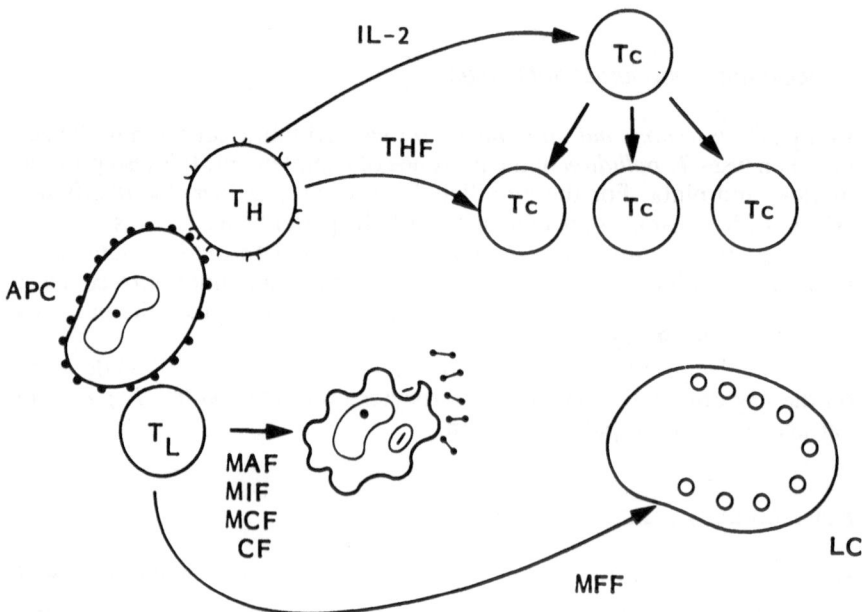

Figure 5.10 The tuberculous granuloma. Mycobacterial antigens recognized on the surface of antigen-presenting epithelioid histiocytes (APC), activate helper T lymphocytes (T_H) to secrete interleukin-2 and helper factor, THF inducing proliferation and activation respectively of cytotoxic T cells (Tc). Other lymphocytes (T_L) are stimulated to secrete macrophage migration inhibitory factor (MIF), macrophage chemotactic factor (MCF), macrophage activation factor (MAF) and cytotoxic factor (CF). Macrophage fusion factor (MFF) promotes giant cell formation (Langerhans cells, LC)

Immunological aspects of pathogenesis (Figure 5.10)

Tuberculosis is a granulomatous disorder, i.e. it causes a chronic inflammatory reaction in which macrophages predominate. A tuberculous focus characteristically has a central area of caseation necrosis surrounded by epithelioid macrophages. Some macrophages fuse, forming multi-nucleated giant cells with peripherally placed nuclei, often arranged in a horseshoe formation (Langerhans giant cells). Lymphocytes also form part of the infiltrate. The tubercle bacillus owes its virulence to its waxy outer envelope of mycolic acids and arabinogalactan, making it resistant to intracellular killing when ingested by polymorphs or macrophages. After phagocytosis the resulting phagosomes, containing the bacilli, do not fuse as usual with the lysosomes. The immune system has evolved ways of potentiating macrophages to overcome the mycobacteria. Mycobacterial antigens presented on the surface of antigen-presenting cells probably the epithelioid histiocytes, which are not themselves phagocytic, are recognized by helper T lymphocytes situated centrally in the lesion. These activated helper T cells in turn secrete helper factor and interleukin-2, which induce activation and proliferation respectively of cytotoxic T cells. These, in turn, also secrete lymphokines such as macrophage migration inhibitory factor (MIF) and a macrophage chemotactic factor, which intensify the cellular infiltrate. Another lymphokine, macrophage activating factor (MAF), possibly identical to gamma-interferon (IFN-γ) potentiates intracellular killing of the tubercle bacilli. Cytotoxic factor released from sensitized lymphocytes causes non-specific tissue destruction which could neatly account for the caseation necrosis. Macrophage fusion factor is released, promoting giant cell formation.

Systemic manifestations

Mycobacterium tuberculosis of human type most commonly causes pulmonary tuberculosis. Dissemination of bacilli by the blood stream may cause a widely dispersed form of the disease in which small tuberculous lesions develop on the pleura, pericardium, peritoneum, lungs, liver, spleen and other organs (acute miliary tuberculosis). This form of tuberculosis is less common in the Western world where extrapulmonary forms of tuberculosis tend to occur as chronic lesions in bone, joints and kidneys. Tuberculous meningitis also results from blood-stream spread.

Oral manifestations

Undermined painful ulcers, lined by pale granulation tissue, situated on the tongue or the mucosa of the lips and cheeks, are the typical oral manifestations. Periapical granulomas on non-vital teeth with the characteristic microscopic features of tuberculosis are an occasional incidental histological finding in patients with open pulmonary tuberculosis.

Immunological diagnosis

In the Mantoux skin test, immunity to tuberculin is tested by the intradermal injection of purified ⁿrotein derivative (PPD) an extract from *M. tuberculosis* cultures. In ᴜ positive test an indurated swelling appears after 48 hours, representing a delayed hypersensitivity (DTH) reaction due to local infiltration by Tdth lymphocytes and macrophages. Positive reactions signify active or healed tuberculosis, or follow successful vaccination. A negative result is useful diagnostically for excluding tuberculous infection. It now seems that a positive skin test with PPD combines two different immunological reactions. One is caused by macrophage activation, conferring protection (the Listerin-type reaction) and the second, necrotic Koch reaction, is an index of hypersensitivity possibly to a protein denatured in the manufacture of PPD, and is not related to protective immunity. New tuberculins, richer in species-specific antigens, are currently being evaluated.

A differential tuberculin skin test employs extracts of *M. tuberculosis* and *M. intracellulare*. It is useful diagnostically in children presenting with cervical lymphadenitis, in distinguishing infections due to the human type of *M. tuberculosis* and those due to opportunist mycobacteria.

Vaccination against tuberculosis

Intracutaneous injection of the attenuated organisms of Bacillus Calmette-Guérin protects 77% of recipients. Macrophage activation by T cells seems to be the likely mechanism of protection.

Key laboratory tests and other investigations

A biopsy of the oral lesions is mandatory and will reveal the cardinal histological changes (see the section on Pathogenesis).

The confirmatory tests include a tuberculin skin test (see the section on Immunological diagnosis) and a chest X-ray to exclude primary pulmonary disease is essential in all cases of oral tuberculosis. A swab from the oral lesions, the sputum (or in children, gastric washings) and early morning urine, are examined by microscopy of a Ziehl-Nielsen stained preparation for acid- and alcohol-fast bacilli. These specimens are also cultured on Löwenstein–Jensen selective medium, both to confirm the diagnosis and to subsequently establish the sensitivity of the bacilli to the standard antituberculous drugs.

FURTHER READING

Candida

Arendorf, T. M. and Walker, D. M. (1980). The prevalence and intra-oral distribution of *Candida albicans* in man. *Arch. Oral Biol.*, **25**, 1–10

Lehrer, R. I. (1978). Host defence mechanisms against disseminated candidiasis. p. 94. In: Severe candidal infections. Clinical perspectives, immune defence mechanisms and current concepts of therapy. *Ann. Intern. Med.*, **89**, 91

Matthews, R. C., Burnie, J. P. and Tabaqchali, S. (1984). Immunoblot analysis of the serological response in systemic candidosis. *Lancet*, **2**, 1415–18

Stiehm, E. R. (1978). Chronic mucocutaneous candidiasis: Clinical aspects. p. 96. In: Edwards, J. E. (moderator). Severe candidal infections. Clinical perspective, immune defence mechanisms and current concepts of therapy. *Ann. Intern. Med.*, **89**, 91

Valdimarsson, H., Higgs, J. M., Wells, R. S. *et al.* (1973). Immune abnormalities associated with chronic mucocutaneous candidiasis. *Cell. Immunol.*, **6**, 348

Herpes simplex virus

Adler, R. M., Glorioso, J. C., Cossman, J. *et al.* (1978). Possible role of Fc receptors on cells infected and transformed by herpes virus: escape from immune lysis. *Infect. Immun.*, **21**, 442

Mims, C. A. and White, D. O. (1984). *Viral Pathogenesis and Immunology.* pp. 87–134. (Oxford: Blackwell Scientific Publications)

Rola-Pleszczynski, M. and Lieu, H. (1983). Natural cytotoxic cell activity linked to time of recurrence of herpes labialis. *Clin. Exp. Immunol.*, **55**, 224

Sethi, K. K., Stroemann, I. and Brandis, H. (1980). Human T cell cultures from virus-sensitised donors can mediate virus-specific and HLA-restricted cell lysis. *Nature*, **286**, 718

Shillitoe, E. J., Wilton, J. M. E. and Lehner, T. (1978). Sequential change in T and B lymphocyte response to herpes simplex virus in man. *Scand. J. Immunol.*, **7**, 357

Syphilis

Csonka, G. W. (1983). Syphilis. In Weatherall, D. J. *et al.* (eds) *Oxford Textbook of Medicine.* Vol. 1. pp. 5.277–5.292. (Oxford: Oxford University Press)

Tuberculosis

Rook, G. A. W. and Stanford, J. L. (1979). The relevance of protection of three forms of delayed skin-tests response induced by *M. leprae* and other mycobacteria in mice. *Parasite Immunol.*, **1**, 111–23

Stanford, J. L. and Lema, A. E. (1983). The use of a sonicate preparation of *Mycobacterium tuberculosis* in the assessment of BCG. *Tubercle*, **64**, 275–82

6
Autoimmune Mucocutaneous Diseases and Diseases of Uncertain Aetiology

D. M. WILLIAMS and D. WRAY

INTRODUCTION

Although the immune system functions principally to protect an individual against an essentially hostile environment, there are circumstances when the effect of the system on the host is damaging. In addition there are a range of diseases in which the immune system is directed against the host. This concept of autoimmune disease was introduced to explain the mechanism of tissue damage in patients with thyroiditis, in whom destruction of the thyroid gland was associated with the production of autoantibodies against thyroglobulin. It is now known that normal individuals also produce 'autoantibodies' and that it is not merely their presence but their titre which determines whether organic disease occurs. Thus autoimmune diseases are characterized by significant levels of autoantibodies, which are primarily responsible for the clinical disease and result from a variety of stimuli and immunoregulatory events. Such diseases may be classified into organ-specific autoimmune disorders, such as thyroiditis in which a single organ is affected, or non-organ-specific disorders – diseases, for example rheumatoid arthritis and systemic lupus erythematosus, in which a number of organs and tissues are affected.

The diseases to be discussed in this chapter all have a strong immunological component to their aetiology, although the extent to which they are truly autoimmune is open to question. They are all well characterized clinically and pathologically and much is known of their aetiology. However, in most instances the precise nature of the antigen against which the immune system is directed is not fully established, nor is it always clear whether this antigenicity is the result of alteration or modification of a native structure, cross-reactivity with an exogenous antigen or the consequence of a primary change within the immune system.

Earlier autoimmune hypotheses proposed to explain the aetiology of recurrent aphthous stomatitis (RAS) and Behçet's syndrome have now largely been discarded. Nevertheless it is convenient to consider the immunology of the vesicular and bullous diseases and RAS in the same chapter. The collagen diseases will be considered elsewhere.

VESICULAR AND BULLOUS DISEASES

The diseases within this group present clinically as vesicles or larger bullae, which rupture more or less rapidly, producing ulcers. In addition to the oral mucosal lesions, there is skin involvement to a variable extent and ocular and genital lesions may also develop. The initial site within the mucosa at which the lesion develops characterizes the presentation of the disease and has an important bearing on the subsequent clinical course: pemphigus is characterized by degeneration within the prickle cell layer – acantholysis – leading to the formation of non-healing bullae and erosions; the other diseases in this group are associated with separation within the basement membrane zone. The common site of bulla formation in the latter group gives rise to similarities in clinical presentation and behaviour, and raises the possibility of a common approach to treatment.

Intraepithelial bullous disease – pemphigus vulgaris

General considerations

Pemphigus presents on the skin in essentially two forms: pemphigus vulgaris and pemphigus foliaceus, which can be separated on clinical grounds. Pemphigus foliaceus is characterized by high-level acantholysis, and pemphigus vulgaris by low-level separation, involving both skin and mucous membranes. It is with the latter form of the disease that this section is concerned.

Typically pemphigus vulgaris presents with superficial bullae affecting mucous membranes and skin. Over 50% of lesions begin within the mouth and may remain localized there for several months. This localization can lead to difficulties and delay in clinical diagnosis, but lesions eventually become generalized with extensive bulla formation, subsequent ulceration and little tendency towards healing.

Pathological features

By routine light microscopy, the characterizing feature of pemphigus is acantholysis with separation occurring immediately suprabasally. However, this is a late stage in the pathogenesis of the disease and ultrastructural examination at an earlier stage reveals dissolution of the intercellular cementing substance (ICS), or glycocalyx, followed by widening of

126

intercellular spaces. Subsequently there is condensation of the tonofilaments which insert into attachment plaques and, as separation progresses, desmosomes disappear In contrast to the sub-epithelial bullous diseases, these processes occur in the absence of inflammatory cells, although accumulations of eosinophils may rarely be present within the epithelium. Once acantholysis has become extensive, however, neutrophil accumulation occurs and, with subsequent ulceration, the inflammatory cell influx overwhelms the specific changes associated with the disease.

Immunological aspects of pathogenesis

Immunogenetic considerations – Studies have shown an increased prevalence of several HLA types, of which the most striking is HLA-DR4. Such HLA associations account for the earlier reports of unexpectedly high incidences of pemphigus in certain ethnic groups, most notably Arabs and Jews, in which there is a higher frequency of these HLA types.

Autoantibody studies – Pemphigus was the first skin disease in which both bound and circulating autoantibodies were identified. Bound auto-antibodies to ICS are detectable by direct immunofluorescence (IF) in perilesional skin and mucosa, and circulating autoantibodies are present in

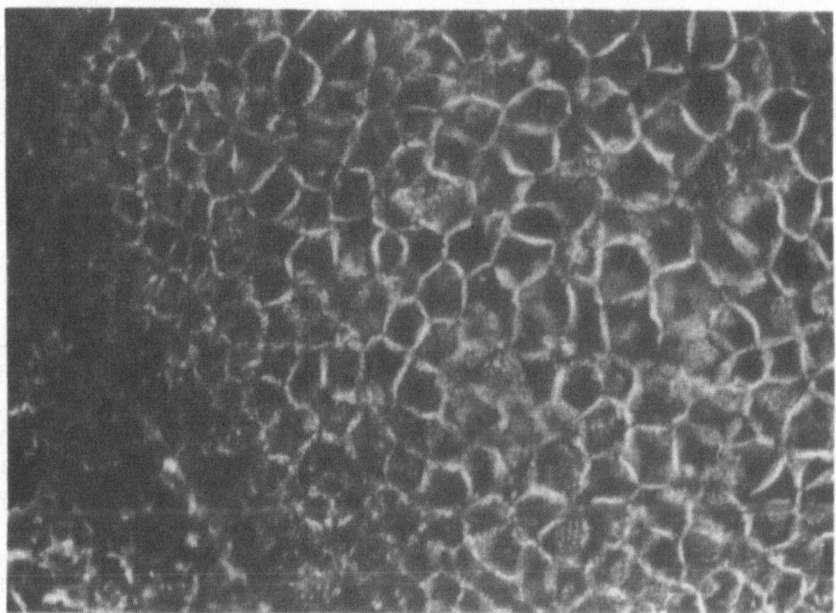

Figure 6.1 Pemphigus vulgaris – direct immunofluorescence. This photomicrograph shows a frozen section of mucosa, from a patient with pemphigus vulgaris, which has been reacted with anti-human IgG conjugated with fluorescein isothiocyanate and photographed in ultraviolet light. The diagnostic pattern of intercellular IgG binding in the prickle cell layer is evident

all patients with active disease. Titres usually, but not always, reflect the severity of the disease and may be used to monitor the response to treatment. The pattern of immunoglobulin (Ig) deposition revealed by direct IF in pemphigus vulgaris is striking, comprising cell membrane binding in the stratum spinosum (Figure 6.1). Binding in mucosa occurs most strongly in the immediately suprabasal layers, correlating well with the site of initial acantholysis. In more advanced lesions occasional cytoplasmic staining may be seen, probably reflecting non-specific absorption of reactants by lysed cells. IgG binding is consistently found; other Ig classes being present less frequently. The presence of complement binding appears to vary and is probably not of central pathogenic significance (see below).

Ultrastructural studies using the immunoperoxidase technique have confirmed the pattern of Ig localization observed by light microscopy. At the earliest stages of Ig binding to ICS there is no evidence of cell damage, indicating that Ig binding is the primary event in lesion development. The areas of strong binding observed on direct IF may represent areas of incipient acantholysis and result from binding of Ig to the convoluted cytoplasmic processes of keratinocytes which are still in contact with each other. The site to which Ig binds has been shown to correspond to the glycocalyx of the cell, even in advanced acantholysis. There is thus strong morphological evidence for the conclusion that the antigen in pemphigus vulgaris resides either within the ICS or on the surface of keratinocytes.

The observation that pemphigus serum binds strongly to normal mucosa strongly supports the view that the antigen is a normal component of skin and mucosa. The most recent studies have detected an immunoglobulin in the serum of patients with pemphigus which is specific for the desmosomes of stratified squamous epithelia. The pathogenic significance of these autoantibodies remains to be established, because desmosomal breakdown appears to be a late event in the acantholytic process. Nevertheless, autoantibody binding to desmosomes is likely to be a key event in lesion formation and further developments of this work are awaited with keen interest.

Experimental acantholysis and the nature of the pemphigus antigen – When injected into neonatal mice IgG fractions purified from serum of patients with pemphigus vulgaris can induce lesions which are clinically, histopathologically and immunologically similar to those of the disease in humans. Antibody binding can be induced in nude mice by passive transfer of IgG from patients with the disease, but detectable lesions occurred in only a small number of cases.

It is now clearly established that Ig production directed against an antigen, either in or closely related to the ICS, is important in the induction of acantholysis in pemphigus, but the nature of the antigen, or antigens, remains to be established. Dose-dependent acantholysis occurs when IgG from the serum of patients with pemphigus vulgaris is added to sections of normal skin. The phenomenon can be induced even when Fab fragments of IgG are used, thus indicating that complement activation is not necessary for acantholysis to occur. Complement may, however, have a role in the subsequent amplification of damage and the attraction of neutrophils and eosinophils to the area. It is necessary, therefore, to construct a mechanism for acantholysis which is independent of inflammatory cells and their products.

In vitro studies using primary keratinocyte culture have shown that pemphigus serum causes detachment of keratinocytes from their culture dishes, and that this can be blocked with proteinase inhibitors, although binding of pemphigus vulgaris serum is not affected. There is thus evidence that binding of pemphigus vulgaris serum to keratinocytes leads to the production or activation of proteinases which may act on the cell surface and result in acantholysis. Furthermore, this process is a reaction of intact, metabolically active cells and is not the result of cell damage. It has also been suggested that plasminogen activator (PA) may be the proteinase implicated in acantholysis; PA production results in the activation of plasminogen to plasmin which may be responsible for the loss of cell adhesion. Antibodies against a desmosomal protein may also be important in acantholysis, but the process by which binding leads to acantholysis is not yet established.

There has been a considerable amount of research into the precise location and nature of the antigen in pemphigus. However, further work is required to characterize the antigen fully and to determine whether it is part of the ICS, a receptor-like component of the plasma membrane or a component of desmosomes. The problems of identifying the antigen are compounded by the fact that it appears to be present only in low levels on epidermal keratinocytes, thus making it difficult to obtain in significant amounts for analysis.

Given the autoimmune nature of pemphigus and its known association with other autoimmune conditions (see below), it is possible that autoantibodies against a number of antigens are produced in pemphigus. It is thus possible that the clinical manifestations of the disease result from the sequential emergence of a range of different autoantibodies with different specificities. The differences in the location and distribution of the lesions in pemphigus vulgaris and foliaceus may well be a reflection of such antigenic differences.

Other disease associations – Pemphigus may be associated with other autoimmune diseases, the most frequent association being that of pemphigus foliaceus with thymoma and myasthenia gravis. Given the probable location of pemphigus antigen the latter association is particularly fascinating, because the antigen in myasthenia gravis is the membrane-located acetylcholine receptor of neuromuscular junctions. It is interesting in the light of developing understanding of lymphocyte–epithelial interactions to note that pemphigus antibodies have been reported to bind to Hassal's corpuscles in the thymus. Recognition that the thymus and squamous epithelia share cell surface and differentiation markers makes the association of pemphigus and thymoma still more tantalizing. There are also numerous reports of pemphigus developing in patients receiving long-term treatment with D-penicillamine for rheumatoid arthritis. It is probable that

129

such patients are already predisposed to autoantibody production against a range of tissues, but it is not certain whether penicillamine acts as a trigger or if all or part of the molecule functions as a hapten, becoming bound to the surface of keratinocytes.

Systemic manifestations

In pemphigus vulgaris both skin and oral lesions occur, although lesions may be restricted to one of these sites for several months before more generalized involvement occurs. Typically there is sudden onset of blisters which burst to form large, superficial, spreading erosions. The lesions show no tendency to heal and, with the continued formation of new lesions, extensive involvement of skin and mucosa results. Nikolski's sign (bulla formation on stroking the skin with light pressure) is an established clinical sign in pemphigus. However, it is not pathognomonic of the disease, because bulla formation in pemphigoid may be elicited in the same way.

Oral manifestations

In less severe forms of the disease, and during the early localized stage, presentation may be in the form of chronic erosions and ulcers in the oral mucosa alone. Failure to investigate the patient adequately at this stage may lead to the diagnosis being delayed until extensive spread of the lesions has occurred.

Diagnosis and laboratory investigation

Although the clinical presentation is characteristic in severe cases, laboratory examination is mandatory. Biopsy reveals characteristic suprabasal acantholysis, and direct immunofluorescence, performed on frozen sections of perilesional mucosa or skin, shows binding of immunoglobulin to the surface of prickle cells. Indirect immunofluorescence performed using serum from patients with active disease demonstrates the presence of circulating autoantibodies against the surface of prickle cells. Autoantibodies are usually present in high titre during active widespread disease, but disappear from the circulation as lesions respond to immunosuppressive therapy.

Treatment usually involves initial high-dose corticosteroid therapy, tapering the dose as lesions remit. In instances where lesions do not respond to corticosteroids, or where extremely high doses of the order of 300 mg per day are necessary to achieve remission, azathioprine may be used in conjunction with steroids.

Sub-epithelial bullous diseases

The range of conditions which present with sub-epithelial bulla formation is large and includes bullous lichen planus as well as bullous pemphigoid (BP), benign mucous membrane pemphigoid (BMMP), dermatitis herpetiformis (DH), and linear IgA bullous dermatosis (LABD). Erythema multiforme and epidermolysis bullosa acquisita (EBA) may also produce bullae within the mouth, further complicating the clinical picture. EBA is an acquired mechanobullous disease which should be differentiated from the hereditary forms of epidermolysis bullosa; linear IgG deposition in the basement membrane zone (BMZ) occurs, similar to that seen in BP, but recent studies using serum from patients with BP and EBA have shown the antigens in each case to be different, with sub-basal lamina separation in the latter. The overwhelming weight of recent evidence indicates that erythema multiforme is the consequence of an immune complex vasculitis, and we have confirmed the observation of others that complement is deposited in the walls of blood vessels in recent lesions. Erythema multiforme is discussed in Chapter 12 on Allergies.

It is with the first four conditions in this group that the remainder of this section is principally concerned. Clinical diagnosis in patients with these diseases is complicated by the fact that BMMP in particular may present with areas of desquamation and erosion of the attached gingiva in the absence of bullae. Because of the similarity in the site at which lesions develop, clinical differentiation of the diseases within this group is notoriously difficult and unreliable, placing a strong dependence on histopathological examination with emphasis on immunofluorescence. Before going on to consider these conditions in detail, lichen planus will be discussed.

Lichen planus

General considerations

Lichen planus may present in the mouth as a blistering condition or with desquamation of the gingivae, but more commonly it manifests as bilaterally symmetrical white patches or striae on the mucosa. These oral manifestations are discussed in more detail below. On the skin the disease, which is self-limiting, appears as a papular rash affecting the flexor surfaces. It is a relatively common condition, affecting predominantly the middle-aged and elderly.

The condition is not generally regarded as being pre-malignant, although up to 2% of patients with erosive lichen planus develop oral cancer during follow-up. Lichenoid drug eruptions, which closely resemble lichen planus, are precipitated by a number of drugs, including methyldopa and some anti-malarials. The relationship between 'true' lichen planus and such lichenoid reactions is unclear.

Pathological features

Histologically lichen planus is characterized by a dense, often band-like, connective tissue infiltrate of lymphocytes which hugs the epithelium. This is

131

associated with widening of the basement membrane zone and loss of the basal cell layer, a phenomenon referred to as liquefaction degeneration. In early lesions the infiltrate is limited to the tips of the rete pegs, but becomes more uniform as the lesion progresses.

Circular, eosinophilic cytoid or civatte bodies, which represent degenerate epithelial cells, are found in the lower epithelial layers. A saw-tooth irregularity of the rete pegs is described as a classical feature of lichen planus, but this is seen more commonly in the skin than in oral mucosa. More consistent features of the .disease are epithelial atrophy and hyperkeratosis, although the latter is not seen in erosive lichen planus. These features prompt the conclusion that the primary events in the disease are epithelial and that the inflammatory infiltrate is a secondary phenomenon. The histopathological features of the disease are remarkably similar to those seen in graft versus host disease.

Immunological aspects of pathogenesis

There is little evidence to support the view that lichen planus is an autoimmune disease, but immunological mechanisms are of major importance in the pathogenesis.

Among the early changes reported in lichen planus are the increases in the number of Langerhans cells in the epithelium, the expression of HLA-DR by keratinocytes and the accumulation of lymphocytes within the epithelium. The significance of the Langerhans cell changes requires considerable elucidation, but points to the possibility that these cells are functioning as antigen-presenting cells, interacting with the lymphocytic infiltrate. HLA-DR expression by keratinocytes also provides a possible mechanism by which an epithelial-associated antigen could be presented to the lymphocytic infiltrate.

The juxta-epithelial inflammatory infiltrate is composed of T lymphocytes, and recent studies have shown that the ratio of helper-inducer lymphocytes to suppressor-cytotoxic cells is higher in early lesions than later.

The nature of the antigen in lichen planus and the processes which initiate epithelial damage remain to be established. Furthermore, it is uncertain whether the expression of HLA-DR by keratinocytes is one of the primary events or whether this is 'switched-on' by gamma-interferon produced by the infiltrating lymphocytes. Nevertheless, a hypothetical model to explain the events in lichen planus can be constructed as follows:

1. An epithelial antigen, possibly drug-related or associated with local virus infection, is presented to lymphocytes in the connective tissue by Langerhans cells migrating from the epithelium.

2. Accumulating helper–inducer T cells in turn lead to the build-up of cytotoxic T cells, which effect keratinocyte damage.

3.   Interferon-induced HLA-DR expression by keratinocytes may then become important as one of the mechanisms responsible for the persistence of this damaging sequence of events, rather than as an initiating event.

Systemic manifestations

The principal systemic manifestation of lichen planus is cutaneous involvement which may precede, follow or occur simultaneously with oral lesions. The skin lesions are typically flat-topped violaceous papules several millimetres in diameter which last for up to 2 years, before resolving spontaneously. The lesions may be pruritic and occur most commonly, but not exclusively, on flexor surfaces and may be associated with white striae (Whickham's striae).

It has been suggested that there is a relationship between lichen planus and diabetes mellitus, with some patients suffering from both diseases. The issue remains equivocal. Reports that lichen planus is associated with stress, liver dysfunction and other abnormalities also await substantiation.

Oral manifestations

The commonest oral form of lichen planus is the reticular pattern with a lacework of white striae principally on the buccal mucosa. Lesions may also appear as white plaques, but these are usually associated with radiating peripheral white striae. Less commonly oral lichen planus may present in atrophic erosive and bullous forms and gives rise to desquamative gingivitis when the attached gingiva is involved. In contrast to the cutaneous lesions, which usually resolve spontaneously within 2 years, lesions of the oral mucosa persist.

Diagnosis and laboratory investigation

In its classical forms lichen planus is usually diagnosed on clinical grounds and routine histopathological examination is confirmatory. However, the erosive and bullous forms of the disease may present difficulties in clinical diagnosis and routine microscopy often fails to discriminate lichen planus from the other vesicular and bullous diseases. In such instances direct immunofluorescence is helpful in establishing the diagnosis. Direct immunofluorescence may also help in differentiating lichen planus from lupus erythematosus.

Bullous pemphigoid and benign mucous membrane (cicatricial) pemphigoid

General considerations

BP and BMMP share many common features and have been regarded in the past as being part of a continuous spectrum of disease, although recent studies indicate that there is a subtle difference in antigen location in the two diseases. BP is a relatively benign disease lasting up to 5 or 6 years, during which period there may be remissions and recurrences. Bulla formation on the skin is characteristic and oral lesions occur in up to 30% of cases.

BMMP usually presents in the sixth and seventh decades and affects the mouth in most cases, less commonly the eyes and occasionally other mucosal surfaces, including the nasopharynx, oesophagus and genitalia. Oral bullae, which may be blood-filled, ulcerate and tend to heal with scarring, leading to the term cicatricial pemphigoid, although scar formation does not appear to be universal. Eye involvement produces scarring of the conjunctiva and dry eye due to lacrimal gland duct involvement.

Pathological features

At the light microscope level the changes in BP and BMMP are fundamentally similar, with separation at the basement membrane in the presence of an inflammatory response of variable intensity. Much of the evidence for the importance of particular pathogenic mechanisms comes from studies of BP, and caution should be exercised in extrapolating these findings to include BMMP. Two types of lesions are described in BP, appearing respectively in inflamed and non-inflamed skin. Leukocytes are involved in lesion development in both forms, but are more numerous in the inflamed lesions, with progressive accumulation of eosinophils in the upper dermis. The inflammatory response begins in apparently normal skin or mucosa with the accumulation of neutrophils and eosinophils in the BMZ. Ultrastructural studies have shown contact between leukocytes and BMZ components in both lesion types, but there is relatively mild anchoring fibril disruption and separation at the level of the lamina lucida in infiltrate-poor lesions, in contrast to the extensive damage seen in infiltrate-rich lesions. The demonstration of the membrane attack complex of complement at the BMZ suggests a possible mechanism for bulla formation in infiltrate-poor lesions. It is likely that a fundamentally similar series of events occurs in BMMP.

Immunological aspects of pathogenesis

Immunogenetic considerations – There is somewhat equivocal evidence for the existence of a genetic predisposition to BMMP, and a study showing a 44.4% frequency of HLA-B12 has not been confirmed. The matter requires further investigation and it should be noted that the reported frequency is insufficient to indicate a direct relationship between HLA-B12 and BMMP.

Immunopathological studies – Both BP and BMMP are characterized on direct immunofluorescence by linear binding of Ig with or without complement components, in the BMZ of perilesional skin and mucosa. In some instances, where complement components are demonstrable in the absence of Ig, failure to demonstrate the latter probably reflects methodological sensitivity rather than true absence. IgG is almost always present in BP, with a much lower incidence of IgA and IgM. In BMMP, however, although IgG is commonly present the frequency of IgA is much higher and approaches 50%. Circulating antibodies against BMZ are found in 70% or more of patients with BP although the titre does not reflect disease severity. In BMMP, by contrast, circulating BMZ antibodies are only found occasionally. This low incidence has been variously attributed to overspill into the circulation of Ig produced within the lesion or insensitivity of the detection system coupled with low circulating BMZ antibody levels. The issue is currently unresolved and awaits clarification.

Ultrastructural immunocytochemistry has been applied to the study of BP and BMMP, showing localization of Ig to the lamina lucida in both instances, and until recently it was assumed that the site of binding was identical in the two diseases. However this view has recently been challenged, because in BMMP Ig binding is present in the base of the blister but in BP binding is present in the roof. It has thus been proposed that the BMMP antigen is a component of the lower lamina lucida, although there is currently no indication of its nature.

The nature of the antigen in bullous pemphigoid – Although virtually nothing is known of the nature of the antigen in BMMP, recent studies have shed considerable light on the molecule involved in the antigen–antibody reaction which triggers lesion development in BP. The current area of uncertainty concerns the observation that, although the molecule has been demonstrated serologically in the lamina lucida in BP, there is accumulating evidence that it is synthesized by basal keratinocytes, where it is involved in hemidesmosome formation. Thus it can be hypothesized that BP antigen is not a normal lamina lucida component, and that its presence in the lamina lucida may be a consequence of cell damage. It is thus possible that the extracellular release of BP antigen, with subsequent antibody binding triggering bulla formation, is a secondary event in the pathogenesis of the disease. This is clearly an issue of fundamental importance which has not yet been addressed and requires further investigation.

To summarize these observations, a model for lesion development in BP can now be constructed, although it is far from certain that precisely the same sequence of events occurs in BMMP:

1. Binding of Ig to antigen within the lamina lucida is the earliest detectable event but the reason for the antigenicity of the binding site

is unclear. IgG deposition leads to complement activation with the production of factors chemotactic for neutrophils. C3a and C5a lead to mast cell degranulation with consequent generation of eosinophil chemotactic factors.

2. Release of enzymes and unstable oxygen intermediates from activated neutrophils and eosinophils leads to separation in the lamina lucida and subsequent damage to lamina densa and anchoring fibrils.

Systemic manifestations

The clinical presentations of BP and BMMP have already been alluded to. These are essentially diseases of the elderly and are uncommon below the age of 60 years. Females are affected twice as commonly as males.

BP is characterized by the presence on the skin of tense fluid-filled blisters which, because of their sub-epithelial location, persist longer than those in pemphigus. The blisters tend to collapse and heal after crusting.

Oral manifestations

Oral lesions in BP are transient and are not a significant feature of the disease. In contrast oral involvement is a major component of BMMP, which is characterized by the rapid formation of bullae which then burst quickly to leave extensive shallow erosions. These then usually heal within 7 to 10 days, but often with scarring. A characteristic of the disease is that lesions tend to recur at the same site. The other major clinical presentation of BMMP is as desquamative gingivitis, with fiery red erosions affecting the attached gingiva, but sparing edentulous areas.

In BMMP oesophageal involvement occurs in approximately 15% of patients, causing considerable discomfort, and where healing is accompanied by stricture formations dysphagia may result. Hoarseness may result from laryngeal involvement. The other aspect of BMMP of major clinical importance is ocular involvement. This may be severe, leading to blindness, and in a recent study 55% of patients with BMMP exhibited ocular stigmata of the disease. Symptomatic eye involvement was present in a much smaller proportion of patients, which raises the necessity for competent ophthalmological examination of all patients diagnosed as having BMMP.

Diagnosis and laboratory investigation

Because of the clinical similarities between BP, BMMP and the other sub-epithelial bullous diseases, biopsy with immunofluorescent examination of frozen sections of perilesional mucosa is mandatory. Direct immunofluorescence of clinically uninvolved skin and indirect immunofluorescence of serum are desirable. Separation of epithelium from the underlying connective tissue is seen on routine light microscopy and direct immunofluorescence reveals linear binding of Ig in the BMZ (Figure 6.2). In most patients with BMMP indirect immunofluorescence is negative, for reasons discussed above.

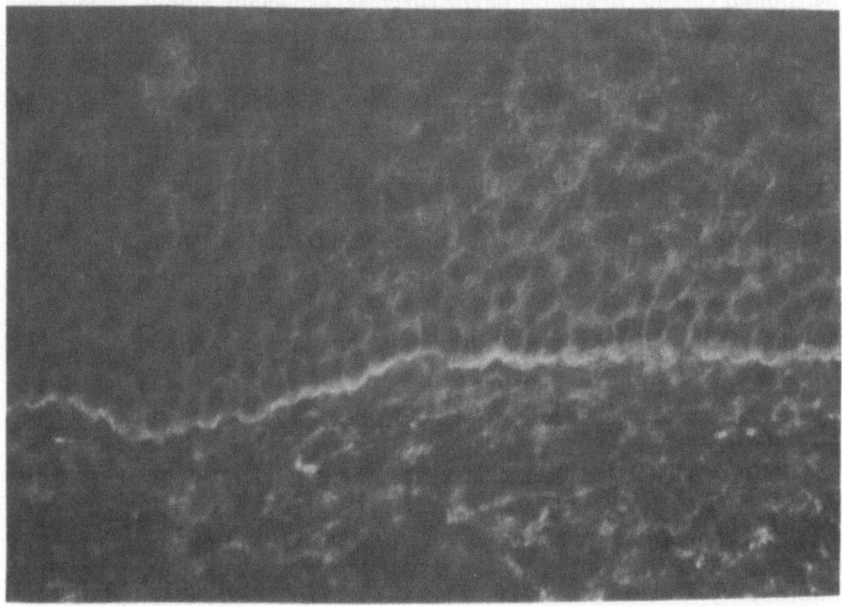

Figure 6.2 Benign mucous membrane pemphigoid – direct immunofluorescence. This photomicrograph shows a frozen section of mucosa from a patient with BMMP, which has been reacted with anti-human IgG conjugated with fluorescein. Linear binding of IgG can be seen at the BMZ

The variation in Ig class found at the BMZ has already been discussed, and was the subject of a recent study. From a series of 30 patients with BMMP, skin and mucosal biopsies together with serum samples were taken. Of the total group, 17 had active mucosal disease, with IgA in ten instances, and seven had Ig deposited at the BMZ in clinically uninvolved skin. A further patient with conjunctival lesions, but no active disease in the mouth, also had skin deposits of Ig and C3. No consistent relationship could be demonstrated between Ig classes deposited in mucosa and skin, and the significance of these differences is hard to assess. It may transpire that BMMP patients with IgG in skin constitute an overlap group with BP and those with IgA an overlap with linear IgA disease, to be discussed below. This issue is currently unresolved and requires further systematic examination, including the application of ultrastructural immunocyto-chemistry to permit more precise determination of the site of Ig binding.

Dermatitis herpetiformis

General considerations

Dermatitis herpetiformis (DH) is associated with gluten-sensitive enteropathy and is characterized by the presence of an intensely itchy papulovesicular eruption on an erythematous base. Lesions are usually distributed symmetrically on flexor surfaces, especially elbows, knees and buttocks, but oral lesions also occur. The clinical presentation is discussed below.

Pathological features

The typical pathological features in DH are well recognized, consisting initially of accumulations of neutrophils and eosinophils at the tips of connective tissue papillae. As lesions develop these microabscesses increase in size and become confluent, forming large, fluid-filled bullae at the level of the basement membrane.

Immunopathological aspects of pathogenesis

A number of immunogenetic studies have consistently shown an increased frequency of HLA-B8 and HLA-Dw3 both in patients with DH and those with coeliac disease, and it has recently been shown that HLA-DQw2 is also raised in both diseases. Both conditions are associated with gluten sensitive enteropathy but differ in that this is usually asymptomatic in DH. Furthermore, skin lesions occur in DH but not in coeliac disease. This leads to the suggestion that different genes play a role in the manifestation of the underlying disease in the two groups. Evidence for this view comes from a study which has shown an increase in HLA-DR2 associated with DH, but not coeliac disease.

Immunological features – One of the definitive characteristics of DH is the presence of granular IgA deposits near the basement membrane of clinically uninvolved skin. The majority of patients exhibit granular IgA binding at the tips of the dermal papillae, but in 10–15% a linear pattern is observed. Although debate continues in the literature, there is substantial justification for the separation of patients with a linear IgA pattern into a separate group, as discussed in the next section.

The pathogenesis of DH has been under intense investigation during the past two decades. The reason why IgA originating in the gut should bind in a granular distribution in the skin remains obscure and the antigen to which it binds is unknown. There is general consensus that gluten-associated small bowel damage is present in all patients and anti-gliadin antibodies (AGAs) are present in the serum in levels which correlate with the severity of gut disease. AGAs are of IgG class in all cases and IgA in approximately 50%,

138

but their precise association with the skin lesions remains unclear. It has been shown that wheat gliadin binds to reticulin-like fibres of human skin, leading to speculation that immune complexes composed of IgA and gliadin form in the gut and are carried to skin and mucosa, where they bind to reticulin fibres. However, attempts to isolate such IgA containing immune complexes have been unsuccessful. The alternative possibility that IgA deposition in the skin and mucosa might be secondary to gliadin deposition does not appear to have been fully investigated, nor is it certain that IgA binding is not the consequence of cross-reactivity involving gliadin and a component of skin and mucosa. Very recently, bound IgA has been isolated from the skin of patients with DH, although it has not yet been possible to establish the antigens to which it is bound. Nevertheless, this is a promising approach and the outcome of further studies is awaited with keen anticipation.

In summary, DH is triggered by gluten-sensitive enteropathy, to which there is a strong genetic predisposition, and is characterized by granular IgA deposition in connective tissue papillae of skin and mucosa. The ensuing accumulation of PMNs leads to sub-epithelial bulla formation. The mechanism by which IgA becomes localized on reticulin fibres in connective tissue awaits clarification and the antigen to which it binds is unknown.

Systemic manifestations

The main incidence of DH is between 20 and 55 years, and males are affected twice as frequently as females. DH takes its name from the skin lesions, which appear as herpes-like vesicles on an erythematous base. However, because they are intensely itchy, the lesions are often excoriated, leading to crusting.

Oral manifestations

Until recently oral lesions in DH were thought to be rare. However, oral involvement occurs in over 70% of the DH patients. Four different types of lesion can be distinguished: erythematous, pseudo-vesicular, purpuric and erosive. The determination of these categories is, however, subjective and does not permit DH to be differentiated reliably from the other sub-epithelial bullous diseases on the basis of the oral lesions. Thus, as with BMMP, pathological examination is important in establishing the definitive diagnosis.

Diagnosis and laboratory investigation

In patients who have DH, skin lesions are likely to be present in addition to oral lesions. Although diagnosis may be possible on clinical grounds, biopsy, with immunological investigation, is confirmatory.

The classical features of DH seen on routine biopsy of perilesional mucosa or skin comprise leukocyte microabscesses at the tips of connective tissue papillae. As described above, these accumulations are initially small but, as they enlarge, microabscesses in adjacent papillae become confluent, forming large vesicles. Once these burst, ulceration ensues and the diagnostic features are no longer recognizable.

Definitive diagnosis in DH depends on the demonstration, by direct immunofluorescence, of granular deposits of IgA beneath the BMZ in clinically normal skin and mucosa. Once lesion development begins, with neutrophil accumulation, this characteristic appearance is lost. Indirect immunofluorescence is negative, but in patients with active disease anti-gliadin antibodies are detectable in serum, reflecting the underlying enteropathy. Variably severe villous atrophy affecting the small bowel can be seen on jejunal biopsy.

Although patients with DH can be treated by strict adherence to a gluten-free diet, lesions are slow to respond and patient compliance is sometimes poor. Lesions respond more rapidly to sulphones, particularly dapsone, and this has now become the treatment of choice, although its mechanism of action is unknown.

Linear IgA bullous dermatosis (linear IgA disease)

General considerations

Linear IgA bullous dermatosis (LABD), or linear IgA disease is a recently defined skin disease characterized by spontaneous blistering and the presence of linear deposits of IgA in the BMZ of clinically uninvolved skin. Of the conditions discussed so far, LABD is the least well defined.

Pathological features

In LABD there is separation of epithelium from underlying connective tissue at the level of the basement membrane, producing appearances on routine microscopy which are not appreciably different from the appearances seen in BP, BMMP or DH.

Immunological aspects of pathogenesis

Immunogenetic considerations – It is possible that LABD as currently defined may include two separate entities. The reported 56% incidence of HLA-B8 in the patients with linear deposits of IgA may be interpreted as a reflection of unexpected grouping of patients with low HLA-B8 incidence and lamina lucida binding and high HLA-B8 incidence with sub-basal lamina binding. The origin of the IgA which binds in LABD is unclear and may differ in the two variants, but recent and as yet unsubstantiated evidence suggests that it comes from an extra-gut site, in contrast to DH.

Immunological features – One third of patients show IgG deposition in addition to linear IgA, but this does not appear to be associated with specific clinical features. However the value of such studies is somewhat limited because routine immunofluorescence does not permit precise localization of the site of antibody binding. Recent immunoelectron microscope studies of skin have shown two distinct patterns of reaction product deposition, to lamina lucida and sub-basal lamina region respectively. Further studies are necessary to clarify the relationship between the former pattern of binding and that seen in BMMP. However, the two different binding sites clearly raise the possibility that the IgA in each case is directed against a completely different antigenic determinant.

It is important to extend the current studies, relating findings to HLA type, the presence of anti-gliadin antibody and features of DH and BMMP respectively. In the long term, establishment of the antigenic determinants to which the IgA binds will enable the true nature of this disease to be established.

Systemic manifestations

Although it may present at any age from 12 years onwards, the peak age of onset is 45 years. The clinical presentation of LABD is variable, with some patients having features of DH and others BP. The majority of patients, however, have a disease which cannot be distinguished with certainty on clinical grounds alone.

In addition to skin involvement, there is a high incidence of cicatrizing conjunctivitis, with entropion and trichiasis. The rate of progress of eye involvement cannot be determined at this stage but, as with BMMP, there is a strong case for competent ophthalmologic examination of all patients suspected of having LABD.

Oral manifestations

Although no systematic study of the type, frequency and distribution of oral mucosal lesions has yet been published, it is recognized that these occur. The appearances seen include ulcers, erosions and bullae, which are no more specific than the skin lesions. Diagnosis thus rests on findings of pathological investigation.

Diagnosis and laboratory investigation

Routine histology does not permit differentiation of LABD from BMMP, and direct immunofluorescence of perilesional mucosa in both instances may reveal the presence of linear IgA binding in the BMZ. Thus, the demonstration of linear IgA binding in clinically uninvolved skin is necessary for the diagnosis of LABD. It is for this reason that direct immunofluorescence on punch biopsies of clinically normal forearm skin is advocated in the investigation of vesicular and bullous lesions affecting the oral mucosa.

The lesions of LABD show a good response to sulphones, in common with DH and BP. However, in contrast to the BMMP, lesions in LABD heal without scarring.

RECURRENT ORAL ULCERATION

Recurrent aphthous stomatitis (RAS) is the commonest oral mucosal disease and is characterized by the appearance of oral ulcers occurring singly or in crops, and affecting the non-keratinizing mucosa. The most striking clinical feature of RAS is that the lesions heal spontaneously, distinguishing them from most other immune related disorders and suggesting that fluctuating immunoregulatory influences are involved. Whereas RAS is confined to the oral mucosa, Behçet's syndrome (BS) is characterized, in addition to RAS, by genital ulcers, skin involvement and disorders of other systems: it may thus be regarded as the multi-system equivalent of the unifocal RAS. The aetiology of RAS and BS has not been fully established, but evidence is accumulating that the epithelial prickle cells are the target of immune damage. Thus the immunopathogenesis of these ulcers has features in common with the vesiculo-bullous disorders, although there is little good evidence that RAS and BS are autoimmune diseases.

Recurrent aphthous stomatitis

General considerations

RAS occurs in three distinct forms: minor, major and herpetiform. Minor aphthae are the commonest and are characterized by the occurrence of spontaneously healing, small (less than 1 cm) ulcers of the non-keratinizing oral mucosa. They occur singly or in crops of up to 20 ulcers which last from 4 to 21 days, before healing spontaneously without scarring. Major aphthae are also usually confined to the non-keratinizing mucosa but are larger (usually more than 1 cm), usually single and last for several weeks or months before healing with scar formation. Herpetiform ulcers are the least common form, and are so called because of their clinical similarity to herpetic gingivo-stomatitis. They are not due to viral infection, however, they are confined to the non-keratinizing mucosa, and are recurrent. Fifty to 200 ulcers, 1 to 2 mm in diameter, occur simultaneously on the oral mucosa and often become confluent before healing without scarring in 2–3 weeks.

Women are affected by RAS up to twice as often as men, indicating that hormonal influences are important, and the onset of ulcers is usually during the second decade. They may arise at any age, however, and are reported to occur in 20% of the population at some time.

Immunological aspects of pathogenesis

Immunogenetic considerations – RAS occurs more commonly in the first-degree relatives of patients than in the general population, which implies a

142

genetic component in their aetiology. Family studies have not shown a Mendelian inheritance pattern, but HLA typing of patients reveals an association between RAS and HLA A2 and Bw44 (relative risk 3.0 and 2.9 respectively).

Immunological features

The aetiology of recurrent aphthous stomatitis has evaded research workers for decades. Much of the immunopathogenesis, however, has been established. Data have been derived both from careful examination of tissue specimens and also from functional assays of peripheral immunocytes in these patients. Examination of lesional tissue specimens reveals that epithelial prickle cells are the initial targets of the mucosal destructive mechanisms. These prickle cells show initial degenerative changes which occur before the appearance of intra-epithelial immunocytes or inflammatory cells. Subsequently, macrophages can be seen phagocytosing these cells and recruiting T lymphocytes, which are probably cytotoxic, but the mechanisms which cause this cascade of events remain unclear. The epithelial prickle cells become coated with immunoglobulin, although this is probably an epiphenomenon, and simultaneously the subjacent lamina propria becomes infiltrated with lymphocytes and phagocytic cells. Initially this infiltrate is dominated by cells of the monocyte–macrophage series, until frank ulceration ensues, when neutrophils become most prevalent within the centre of the lesion. Accessory cells, such as mast cells and eosinophils, are seen in small numbers and amplify the immunological events. Monoclonal immunostaining of the lymphocytic infiltrate reveals an initial preponderance of inducer/helper T cells over suppressor/cytotoxic T cells. Once ulceration is established, however, this ratio is reversed and suppressor/cytotoxic T cells show a preponderance. This distribution of T cells subsets is reversed yet again as the ulcer enters a healing phase, implying that immunoregulation is important in dictating the clinical course of events.

In vitro studies – Functional studies of peripheral blood immunocytes assume lesional events are reflected systemically. Indeed, many studies have reported alterations in cellular and humoral responses, especially to bacterial and mucosal antigens. The existence of generalized systemic immune defects appears unlikely however because RAS usually occurs in healthy individuals. Notwithstanding these observations, it is significant that the relative number of circulating monocytes appears to be increased, in parallel with the severity of local events. A number of cytotoxicity mechanisms have been implicated in the pathogenesis of RAS, including complement-mediated cytotoxicity, antibody-dependent cellular cytotoxicity and natural killer cell activity. Circulating polymorphonuclear leukocytes, although metabolically intact, appear more adherent in RAS, but this is probably due to serum factors and is unlikely to be of central aetiological significance.

Systemic manifestations

As has already been stated, the majority of RAS patients are healthy, but a minority have associated disease which is often occult. Specifically, 20% of patients have an associated deficiency of iron, folic acid or vitamin B_{12} alone or in combination. In the majority of these patients the deficiency is latent, with no detectable changes in the peripheral blood, but careful investigation reveals further disease associations, which usually affect the gut and include gluten-sensitive enteropathy, Crohn's disease and pernicious anaemia. Correction of the underlying disease or replacement therapy is usually associated with resolution of the oral ulcers. Patients may also show evidence of food allergy, which is increased among non-atopic patients, and careful regulation of the diet may result in improvement of oral lesions. Oral ulcers may also arise secondary to mild trauma, and it seems probable that allergy and trauma exert early effects in the pathogenesis of ulceration, perhaps modulating the immune response through local histamine release. Hormonal influences, which are apparent in some women, and nutritional factors, may have effects both on the oral epithelium and the immune system. Interestingly, smoking appears to protect individuals from RAS.

Oral manifestations

The clinical appearances of the different types of RAS have been described above. Characterization of the oral lesions, however, is unhelpful in the management or investigation of these lesions. Onset in later life, lingual ulcers or the presence of other conditions, such as glossitis or angular cheilitis, are suggestive of an underlying nutritional disorder, but haematological investigation is still necessary to confirm and characterize the deficiency.

Diagnosis and treatment

RAS is diagnosed on the basis of its clinical presentation, and laboratory investigation is unhelpful. The occurrence of multiple-healing recurrent oral ulcers affecting the non-keratinized mucosa is the defining characteristic of RAS. Apart from a minority of instances, in which patients respond to replacement therapy or dietary manipulation, the treatment of RAS is empirical. Topical corticosteroids are usually helpful, and systemic therapy is only rarely justified.

Behçet's syndrome

General considerations

BS comprises the classical triad of oral and genital ulceration associated with iritis. In addition, a proportion of patients also exhibit cardiovascular, skeletal, cutaneous, neurological and gastrointestinal manifestations. Because the disease is cyclical in nature, investigation is difficult and the effect of treatment is hard to assess.

Immunological aspects of the pathogenesis

Immunogenetic considerations – recent studies of histocompatibility antigens in BS have been carried out and support the subdivision of BS into four subtypes. Thus, HLA B5 is related to ocular BS (relative risk 7.3), HLA B27 to the arthritic type (relative risk 12.1) and HLA B12 to the mucocutaneous type (relative risk 3.9). The neurological type shows no such association. Interestingly, RAS patients show an increased frequency of HLA-Bw44, a subtype of HLA B12, linking the condition with the mucocutaneous form of BS.

Immunological features

The immunological features of BS are broadly similar to those seen in RAS, although there are minor differences in the intra-epithelial cellular infiltrate. Polymorphonuclear leukocyte chemotaxis shows derangement in BS, with reduced spontaneous migration but enhanced chemotaxis. The principal differentiating feature from RAS appears to be the presence of immune complexes in BS. Some patients show increased levels of circulating IgG immune complexes, C9, acute phase proteins, factor B, and lysozyme. Although an aetiological link between BS and RAS seems probable, the immunopathogenesis of both conditions remains unclear.

Systemic manifestations

BS may be grouped into four types: ocular, arthritic, mucocutaneous and neurological, although a combination of these types may also be seen. Ocular involvement is seen most commonly in Japan and the Middle East. In Europe and the United States orogenital ulceration alone is more common. Fortunately, for prognostic purposes, progression from the orogenital type to more systemic involvement is rare. When there is ocular involvement, BS is associated with a significant mortality and morbidity.

Oral manifestations

The oral ulceration, which is a consistent feature of BS, is indistinguishable from RAS, and an aetiological link between the two disorders has long been suspected. Each of the forms of RAS has been described in BS.

The discrepancy in the incidence of the two diseases is consistent with the view that progression from RAS to BS is uncommon, although oral ulceration is usually the earliest sign of BS. Less than 3% of patients presenting with RAS are diagnosed as having BS.

Diagnosis

Absolute criteria for the diagnosis and classification of BS remain unclear. The consensus among clinicians is that two or more major criteria (oral, genital, ocular or mucocutaneous involvement) or a combination of major and minor criteria (vascular, neurological, skeletal or intestinal) constitute a positive diagnosis of BS. HLA typing is helpful in identifying the type of BS and its prognosis. A positive prick test (sterile pustule formation following intradermal injection of saline) is pathognomonic.

Treatment

Because BS is a rare disease, assessment of treatment modalities is difficult and therapy is usually empirical. Topical corticosteroids are effective for milder oral manifestations but systemic corticosteroids are the mainstay of treatment. Azathioprine may be a useful adjunct to steroid therapy and colchicine, in low dosage, is also effective in some patients. Aggressive therapy for oral lesions is justified, as these often precede ocular exacerbations in patients with ocular BS, and control of the oral lesions may prevent irreversible eye damage.

CONCLUSIONS

In the conditions which have been described in this chapter there are significant differences in the level of our understanding. With the vesicular and bullous diseases, all of which have an important immunological component, it is clear that the site of immunoglobulin deposition corresponds to the site of damage. However, the mechanisms of this damage are distinctly different in pemphigus, where Ig binding in the prickle cell layer to a still unknown antigen appears to initiate proteinase synthesis by keratinocytes, and those conditions with sub-epithelial bulla formation. In the latter group, which includes BMMP, BP, DH and LABD, a common sequence of events can be identified:

1.   Ig deposition in or near the basement membrane, associated with
      complement activation, leads to mast cell degranulation and the
      release of leukocyte chemotactic factors. This results in neutrophil
      and eosinophil accumulation.

2.   Release of enzymes, including proteinases and active oxygen
      intermediate metabolites, from inflammatory cells causes damage
      and degeneration within the components of the basement membrane
      and adjacent structures.

3.   Damage in the basement membrane zone leads to bulla formation,
      with separation of epithelium from the underlying connective tissue.

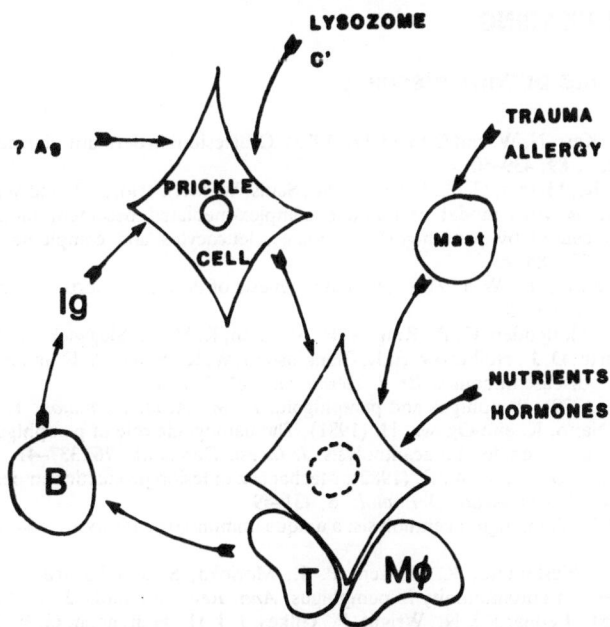

Figure 6.3 Hypothetical model of the early events in the immunopathogenesis of RAS. The epithelial prickle cell appears to be the target of immune damage. The initial events occur in the absence of immunocytes and may be mediated by complement (C') or lysozomal enzymes. The importance of cell surface antigenic alterations due to exogenous (infective) or endogenous (immunogenetic) factors remain unclear. Subsequent to initial prickle cell damage macrophages (Mφ) and lymphocytes (T) are recruited which indicate a cascade of humoral and cellular events culminating in oral epithelial destruction and frank ulceration. Initiating factors, such as trauma and allergy, may exert their effect via histamine release which both amplifies the immune response and is immunoregulatory. Haematinics and hormones may influence the oral epithelium *per se*, or may act upon the immune response

Thus the consequences of Ig deposition are now reasonably well
understood, although the mechanism of leukocyte accumulation when IgA
alone is present is unclear. The major areas which require research are to

establish the antigens in the different conditions, to obtain a better understanding of the factors which lead to Ig deposition and the initiation of bulla formation, about which remarkably little is yet known.

The aetiology of RAS and BS remains elusive. Much is known of the pathogenic mechanisms involved in the ulcerative process, however, and these have been summarized in Figure 6.3. As is the case with the vesiculo-bullous disorders, identifying the initial changes which stimulate the immune response is crucial to the understanding of the pathogenesis.

The elucidation of these points will prove to be a fascinating and taxing challenge, and will provide a better understanding of the role of immunological mechanisms in disease processes in general.

FURTHER READING

Vesicular and bullous diseases

Fraser, N. G., Kerr, N. W. and Donald, D. (1973). Oral lesions in dermatitis herpetiformis. *Br. J. Dermatol.*, **89**, 439–50

Gammon, W. R., Merritt, C. C., Lewis, D. M., Sams, W. M., Carlo, J. R. and Wheeler, C. E. (1982). An in vitro model of immune complex-mediated basement membrane zone separation caused by pemphigoid antibodies, leucocytes and complement. *J. Invest. Dermatol.*, **78**, 285–90

Katz, S. I. and Strober, W. (1978). The pathogenesis of dermatitis herpetiformis. *J. Invest. Dermatol.*, **70**, 63–75

Leonard, J. N., Haffenden, G. P., Ring, N. P., McMinn, R. M. H., Sidgwick, A., Mowbray, J. F., Unsworth, D. J., Holborow, E. J., Blenkinsopp, W. K., Sirain, A. F. and Fry, L. (1982). Linear IgA disease in adults. *Br. J. Dermatol.*, **107**, 301–16

Lever, W. F. (1979). Pemphigus and pemphigoid. *J. Am. Acad. Dermatol.*, **1**, 2–31

Morioka, S., Naito, K. and Ogawa, H. (1981). The pathogenic role of pemphigus antibodies and proteinase in epidermal acantholysis. *J. Invest. Dermatol.*, **76**, 337–41

Sams, W. M. and Gammon, W. R. (1982). Mechanism of lesion production in pemphigus and pemphigoid. *J. Am. Acad. Dermatol.*, **6**, 431–49

Schiltz, J. (1980). Pemphigus acantholysis: a unique immunologic injury. *J. Invest. Dermatol.*, **74**, 359–62

Singer, K. H., Hashimoto, K., Jensen, P. J., Morioka, S. and Lazarus, G. S. (1985). Pathogenesis of autoimmunity in pemphigus. *Ann. Rev. Immunol.*, **3**, 87–108

Williams, D. M., Leonard, J. N., Wright, P., Gilkes, J. J. H., Haffenden, G. P., McMinn, R. M. H. and Fry, L. (1984). Benign mucous membrane (cicatricial) pemphigoid revisited: a clinical and immunological re-appraisal. *Br. Dent. J.*, **157**, 313–16

Recurrent aphthous stomatitis

Gadol, N., Greenspan, J. S., Hoover, C. I. and Olson, J. A. (1985). Leukocyte migration inhibition in recurrent aphthous ulceration. *J. Oral Pathol.*, **14**, 121–32

Wray, D. (1984). Aphthous ulceration. *J. R. Soc. Med.*, **77**, 1–3

Behçet's syndrome

Lehner, T. and Barnes, C. G. (1979). *Behcet's Syndrome.* (London: Academic Press)

7
Connective Tissue Diseases with Oral Manifestations

K. W. LEE

INTRODUCTION

Included under the heading of connective tissue diseases is a group of heterogeneous conditions of unknown aetiology. Although the connective tissues are chiefly affected, it is not clear if collagen is the principal target tissue involved. Immunological phenomena abound, involving mainly the production of autoantibodies. Patients with one form of connective tissue disease may develop other forms. Some animals develop spontaneous disease; for example, the New Zealand black/white (NZ B/W) mouse develops systemic lupus erythematosus and Sjögren's syndrome-like lesions. Significant associations with the major histocompatibility genes are found in several diseases.

RHEUMATOID ARTHRITIS AND VARIANTS

General considerations

Twenty years ago, in a classical paper on 'Arthritis of the mandibular joint', it was stated that the aetiology of rheumatoid arthritis (RA) was still obscure, but that there was increasing evidence to show that the disease may come within the classification of so-called 'collagen diseases'. Current views have altered but little, but a number of genetically determined antigens may impart a genetic susceptibility to an unidentified environmental factor, such as a virus, that initiates the disease process. Classically, middle-aged women are predominantly affected, with the sex ratio of 3 : 1 in favour of women. The diagnostic criteria as laid down by the American Rheumatoid Association are still valid and these are:

1. morning stiffness;
2. pain on motion or tenderness in at least one joint;
3. swelling of at least one joint due to thickening of the soft tissue or effusion;
4. swelling of at least one other joint with an interval of not less than 3 months between the two events;
5. symmetrical joint swelling;
6. subcutaneous nodules over bony prominences or in the vicinity of joints;
7. increased radiolucency in the vicinity of the affected joints and erosions of the bone at the margins of the articular cartilages;
8. positive tests for the presence of rheumatoid factor.

If seven of these criteria are present, it is described as classical RA; if five are present, RA is definite; and if only three are present, it is probable. The wrists and metacarpophalangeal joints are usually the first to be affected, followed by the metatarsophalangeal joint. Larger joints such as the ankles, knees and elbows may be involved later, and may result in the patient becoming crippled.

It is difficult to know how often the temporomandibular joint is involved. Early studies suggested that as many as 50% of all cases of RA may involve the mandibular joint. More recent studies suggest a figure of less than 10%. In one study 53 patients with RA were investigated, and it was found that none showed clinical evidence of involvement of the temporomandibular joint. Of these patients, however, 43% gave a history of symptoms related to the temporomandibular joint at some time during the course of the disease. The changes that are seen in the joint are as follows; the synovial tissues of the lower joint compartment appear to be first affected and the lesion spreads from here to the articular surface of the condyle. Vascular granulation tissue called pannus diffusely infiltrated with inflammatory cells is formed, and the articular surface of the condyle undergoes resorption by osteoclasts, resulting in destruction of the subchondral bone with the formation of small adhesions between the articulating surface of the disc and the condyle. Fibrous ankylosis appears to be the end-result in most cases.

Immunological diagnosis

Autoantibodies known as rheumatoid factor (RF) with anti-IgG specificity are classically detected in sera of patients. The latex particle agglutination test utilizing human IgG to coat particles of latex is the test most widely used. This detects antibodies of the IgM class. Another test that is used is the sensitized sheep red cell test (Rose-Waaler test) where sheep red blood cells are coated with rabbit antibody against sheep red blood cells. The sensitized sheep cells will then agglutinate in the presence of RF.

Autoantibody of the IgG class can also be detected, but only by means of radioimmunoassay methods. The distribution of titres of RF is a continuous variable and a minority of patients with undoubted rheumatoid disease remain persistently seronegative. On the other hand, some non-rheumatoid conditions including leishmaniasis, infectious mononucleosis, some lung and liver diseases and dys- and paraproteinaemias may give rise to positive latex tests.

It has been shown that the synovial membrane in RA has many of the characteristics of a hyperactive immunologically stimulated lymphoid organ. Large, very strongly HLA-DR positive macrophage-like inter-digitating cells form close contacts with $OKT4^+$ (helper/inducer type-T cells) while the $OKT8^+$ population (T cells of the suppressor/cytotoxic type) is scanty (T4 : T8 = 9 : 1). These large interdigitating cells and $OKT4^+$ cells may be mutually stimulating, and in the absence of efficient suppression may lead to the activation of B lymphocytes to oligoclonal and polyclonal immunoglobulin synthesis.

Subcutaneous nodules over bony prominences, or in the vicinity of joints, are the commonest extra-articular signs of the disease. They may produce ulceration of the skin and erode underlying bone. They are thought to result from the depositions of immune complexes in the affected tissues with consequent vasculitis. Less frequently these nodules have been found on the pericardium, heart valves, pleura and lung, and in the sclera of the eye. Autoantibody levels are significantly higher in patients with nodules of vasculitis and the presence of raised rheumatoid factor levels points to a poor prognosis in RA.

Patients with RA may exhibit autoantibodies other than RF. Anti-DNA antibodies are seldom present except in so-called 'overlap' syndromes with features of both systemic lupus erythematosus and RA. Approximately 14% of males and 25% of females exhibit an antinuclear antibody (ANA) at serum levels at or above 25 IU/ml. Other autoantibodies described in rheumatoid patients include anti-collagen antibodies, anti-perinuclear factors, anti-keratin antibodies, anti-salivary duct antibodies, and anti-vimentin antibodies. The aetiological relevance of these autoantibodies remains to be established. Finally in RA there are significant associations in certain of the HLA tissue types; in particular HLA-D4 and HLA-DR4 have been demonstrated. There is also a significant decrease in the frequency of HLA-DR2.

The erythrocyte sedimentation rate, C-reactive protein levels and plasma viscosity are other useful laboratory tests in the diagnosis of RA. In particular the levels of C-reactive protein reflect the patient's clinical state more faithfully than the erythrocyte sedimentation rate.

FELTY'S SYNDROME

This is a combination of neutropenia and splenomegaly in a patient with RA. The neutropenia predisposes to recurrent infections which may prove fatal. Non-articular rheumatoid features are common. The patients are usually strongly positive by the latex test. The incidence of ANA is 50–60%, usually with specificity for granulocyte nuclei.

MIXED CONNECTIVE TISSUE DISEASE

This term has been used to describe a group of RA patients who also present with features of systemic lupus erythematosus, scleroderma and poly-myositis. The patients exhibit an antibody giving a 'speckled' pattern of ANA staining by immunofluorescence and an antibody specifically directed against ribonucleoprotein (RNP). The claim that the anti-RNP antibodies are present only in patients with mixed connective tissue disease has not been substantiated by later studies.

JUVENILE CHRONIC POLYARTHRITIS (juvenile rheumatoid arthritis)

This is a form of arthritis which affects children below 16 years, with pain, swelling and limitation of movement. The histopathology of the joint tissues is similar to RA. The condition is heterogeneous, and several subgroups are described based upon mode of onset.

Although certain abnormalities of immunoglobulin, complement and cellular immunity are compatible with the diagnosis of juvenile RA, no specific immunological test is available.

SYSTEMIC LUPUS ERYTHEMATOSUS

General considerations

Lupus erythematosus (red wolf) takes its name from the facial rash which has a butterfly distribution in these patients. In the United States one female in 500 is affected, and the female–male ratio is 10 : 1. It is particularly common in the Far East. Systemic lupus erythematosus (SLE) although affecting internal organs, generally produces a mild rash or flush on the face. Discoid lupus erythematosus (DLE), however, usually causes a much more pronounced, sometimes scarring rash in the face, and may result in severe hair loss and scarring of the scalp. About 5% of patients with DLE develop the systemic form of the disease. SLE affects skin, joints, blood vessels, heart, lungs, brain and kidneys, and signs and symptoms may include fever, malaise, skin rash, vascular inflammation, arthritis, pleurisy, pericarditis and glomerulonephritis. It is widely accepted that they are the result of the formation and deposition of immune complexes in the tissues.

Oral manifestations

Oral ulceration may be a presenting feature of SLE. The lesions present as erythematous areas with superficial ulcerations but no keratinization of the oral mucosa. Patients with DLE may similarly present with oral lesions. Sometimes these precede the appearance of skin lesions; at other times they

152

appear subsequently. The oral lesions of DLE may appear on the vermilion border of the lip and on the buccal mucosa. The lesions are classically described as areas of central erythema with white spots approximately 0.5 mm in diameter and a 2–5 mm wide border of white striae radiating from the centre. When transformation from the discoid into the systemic form occurs, ulceration may appear in these lesions. In addition the alveolar process and the gingiva become involved. The difficulty in distinguishing oral lesions of lupus erythematosus from lichen planus and leukoplakia is well recognized. The central areas of erythema and white spots resemble speckled leukoplakia, and the radiating border of white striae resembles Wickham's striae in lichen planus; even histological examination may not completely resolve the difficulty.

It has been stated that a diagnosis of oral lupus erythematosus, either in the absence of skin lesions or on the basis of oral lesions alone, should not be attempted. More recent views, however, suggest that provided there is at least one mucosal lesion clinically characterized by a central atrophic area with small white dots surrounded by a border with parallel white striae, it may be possible to make the clinical diagnosis.

The World Health Organization listed the following criteria for the histological diagnosis of oral DLE:

1. hyperorthokeratosis with keratotic plugs;
2. atrophy of the rete processes;
3. 'liquefaction degeneration' of the basal layer;
4. a band-like infiltration of lymphocytes in the lamina propria;
5. PAS-positive deposits juxta-epithelially, which resemble a thickening of the basement membrane.

Some authors evaluated these criteria and found that they were not sufficiently clear-cut for distinction in particular from lichen planus. They suggested further histological criteria which may be characteristic of the disease. These were multinucleated epithelial giant cells with three or more nuclei and the presence of epithelial islands in the connective tissue.

Immunological diagnosis

Antinuclear antibodies

The immunofluorescent antinuclear test is the most widely used test for SLE. It is positive in almost 99% of SLE patients though it may be negative in patients with DLE. The test has replaced the older LE cell test, as the latter is time-consuming and less sensitive.

It is not, however, diagnostic for SLE, as positive tests are occasionally seen in other non-lupus conditions. It has particular importance as a screening test, as a negative test virtually excludes lupus.

Anti-DNA antibodies

Anti-native (ds) antibodies are the most specific of antibodies in the diagnosis of SLE as they occur in 80% of patients and they fluctuate with disease activity. The DNA-binding test known as the Farr radio-immunoassay is the most useful diagnostic test at present. Anti-denatured (ss) antibodies are complement fixing, and generate a type III hypersensitivity reaction. Antigen–antibody complexes are detected in renal lesions in patients with glomerulonephritis. Patients with extensive involvement of skin, kidney and central nervous system show reduced levels of complement in their sera. The finding of low complement levels in the blood is indirect evidence of the presence of circulating immune complexes.

Other laboratory tests

Haematological examination may reveal the presence of an anaemia and thrombocytopenia purpura. The erythrocyte sedimentation rate may rise well above 100 mm per hour and gives a general guide to disease activity.

Kidney function tests

Urinalysis may reveal albuminuria and the presence of red blood cells, granular and hyaline casts. Blood levels of urea and creatinine also help to determine if filtration impairment is present.

SJÖGREN'S SYNDROME

General considerations

Sjögren's syndrome is defined by the presence of at least two of the following criteria:

1. keratoconjunctivitis sicca;
2. xerostomia;
3. another well-defined chronic inflammatory connective tissue disease.

Sjögren's syndrome is classified as primary when only the first two criteria are fulfilled and as secondary when the third is present. Primary Sjögren's is also referred to as the sicca syndrome. RA is the connective tissue disease most frequently associated with Sjögren's syndrome, but the syndrome may also be found in patients with SLE, progressive systemic sclerosis, mixed connective tissue disease, polymyositis and other chronic inflammatory connective tissue diseases.

   Although the true prevalence of Sjögren's syndrome is unknown, it is the most common connective tissue disease after RA. About half of the cases are primary and 25–50% of RA patients fulfil the criteria required for secondary Sjögren's syndrome. The female/male ratio is 9 : 1 with an age peak between 40 and 60 years. Secretory glands other than the lacrimal and salivary glands may be affected, with a resulting dry skin, larynx, bronchi, lungs, gastrointestinal tract, liver and pancreas. The patient may experience universal tiredness, fever, arthralgia and a diffuse myalgia. The kidney is affected in 15–20% of cases.

Oral manifestations

The salivary glands and lacrimal glands may be enlarged and show marked infiltration by lymphoid cells with epithelial islands called epimyoepithelial islands. These lesions used to be called benign lympho-epithelial lesions. However, it has been shown that the relative risk of patients with Sjögren's syndrome developing a lymphoproliferative malignancy is estimated to be 44 times that of the general population and a decrease of serum IgM level may accompany or precede malignancy. The dry mouth predisposes to rampant dental caries and candidiasis.

Diagnosis of Sjögren's syndrome

The diagnosis of keratoconjunctivitis sicca is made by demonstrating diminished lacrimation by the use of the Schirmer tear test and the finding of filamentary or punctate keratitis on slit lamp examination of the cornea after the instillation of rose bengal dye into the conjunctival sac.

Salivary flow rate estimation

Ninety per cent of patients with Sjögren's syndrome have flow rate values below the normal range. A standardized 10-min, bilateral stimulated parotid flow rate is measured. Both left and right flow rates are determined and averaged: 4 ml/10 min is used as the low range of normal flow.

Hydrostatic sialography

A water-soluble contrast medium is introduced into the salivary duct system at a constant pressure.

Salivary scintiscanning

^{99m}Tc pertechnetate is used as a scanning agent. Uptake by the salivary glands is reduced in patients with Sjögren's syndrome.

Labial gland biopsy

The original technique involved the removal of an ellipse of labial mucosa including underlying mucous glands and examination for foci of lymphocytes. A 'focus' is defined as consisting of an aggregate of 50 or more lymphocytes, usually with a few plasma cells placed peripherally, adjacent to and apparently replacing gland acini.

More recently a modified technique, using a 1.5–2.0 cm linear incision, parallel to the vermilion border and lateral to the midline has been recommended. The mucous gland lobules are removed by blunt dissection without removing any surface mucosa. At least five gland lobules should be removed to take into account the variability in appearance that may be found in the lobules. The presence or absence of 'focal' cell infiltration is assessed with a grading system ranging from 0 to 4. Grade 0 represents a labial salivary gland which is free of round cell infiltration and Grade 4 denotes the presence of more than one focus of 50 or more round cells per 4 mm^2 of section.

Immunological diagnosis

There is a marked tendency to hypergammaglobulinaemia and some patients develop a hyperviscosity syndrome, owing to the presence of cryoglobulins or circulating complexes. An organ-specific anti-salivary duct antibody has been described in 25% of patients with primary Sjögren's syndrome, in 69% with RA and Sjögren's syndrome, and in 26% with RA alone. Three other non-organ-specific antibodies to small nuclear ribonucleoproteins have been described. They are named anti-SS-A, anti-SS-B and anti-SS-C. It was originally suggested that anti-SS-A and anti-SS-B occurred exclusively in patients with primary Sjögren's syndrome, while anti-SS-C occurred predominantly in RA patients with or without Sjögren's syndrome, but these results have not been borne out in later studies.

There is also a striking association between primary Sjögren's syndrome and HLA phenotype. In the primary disease the frequency of HLA-A1, B8, and DR3 is 88%, 94% and 75% respectively, whereas in secondary Sjögren's syndrome the frequency is 38%, 29% and 14% respectively. This confirms the strong link between primary Sjögren's syndrome and HLA-B8 and DR3.

PROGRESSIVE SYSTEMIC SCLEROSIS (SCLERODERMA)

General considerations

This is a multi-system disorder in which there is a progressive deposition of collagen in the skin and subcutaneous tissue and fibrosis of many organs including the heart, lungs, gastrointestinal tract and kidney. A subset of generalized scleroderma, consisting of calcinosis cutis, Raynaud's phenomenon, oesophageal dysmobility, sclerodactyly and telangiectasia is known by its acronym as the CREST syndrome. This usually has a better prognosis than progressive systemic sclerosis.

The disease may begin in children, or in young adults, and females are affected twice as frequently as males. It usually begins on the face, hands or trunk. In more than half of the cases, Raynaud's phenomenon heralds the onset of the disease. Neuralgia or paresthesia may occur and there may be arthritis or vague joint pain. The skin becomes hardened and atrophic and cannot be wrinkled because of fixation to the deeper tissues.

Oral manifestations

The localized form of the disease, commonly termed morphea, presents as well-defined cutaneous patches which are white or yellowish and are surrounded by a violaceous halo. Occasionally the lesions occur as linear bands or ribbons on the face, and may be associated with facial hemiatrophy. Oral tissues, in particular the tongue and soft palate, may be involved in progressive systemic sclerosis. Limitation of mouth opening may be found in 80% of patients. The disease may thus resemble oral submucous fibrosis, a condition of unknown aetiology which results in the development of fibrous bands within the cheeks. The latter, however, appears to be confined to Indians and inhabitants of South-East Asia, and appears to be closely related to the habit of betel-nut chewing.

A radiological feature of oral interest is the extreme widening of the periodontal ligament. This is due to an increase of collagen and oxytalan fibres as well as hyalinization and sclerosis of collagen. Bone resorption of the angle of the mandibular ramus, the mandibular condyle, and of the coronoid process has also been reported.

Immunological diagnosis

Antinuclear antibodies are frequently found in these patients and they may exhibit several staining patterns of cell nuclei or nucleoli, including an anti-centromere antibody and another antibody which is reactive with a liver cell nuclear protein (Sci-70).

POLYMYOSITIS AND DERMATOMYOSITIS

General considerations

This is a heterogeneous group of conditions characterized by the presence of muscle weakness. When skin lesions are also present it is known as dermatomyositis. Some patients have a coexistent neoplasm, and there may be associated features of other connective tissue disorders. Listed below are the criteria for diagnosis:

157

1.   objective evidence of symmetrical weakness of proximal muscle groups;

2.   systemic or local evidence of necrosis of skeletal muscle;

3.   systemic or local evidence of inflammatory disease.

Most cases occur in the fifth or sixth decade and the male/female ratio is approximately 1 : 2.

The predominant clinical feature is symmetrical sustained weakness of proximal muscle groups. The facial and extraocular muscles are, however, spared. Weakness is much more apparent than wasting. When the skin is involved, lesions are also seen on the facial skin. These include:

1.   a dusky erythema of the face and oedema; the 'heliotrope' rash (a dusky, lilac colour of the upper eyelids) is pathognomonic;

2.   periungual erythema and haemorrhage;

3.   erythema over extensive surfaces such as the posterior neck, elbows, knuckles, knees and ankles.

Some patients may have a concomitant malignant tumour, and a diligent search should be made for it in a patient who develops the disease as an adult.

Oral manifestations

Diffuse stomatitis and pharyngitis are extremely common, as well as telangiectatic lesions on the vermilion border and cheeks. Involvement of the muscles of the jaws, tongue and pharynx may pose problems in eating and phonation.

Immunological diagnosis

Antibodies to extractable nuclear antigens have been described in some patients. The presence of antinuclear antibody, rheumatoid factor and hypergammaglobulinaemia probably reflects the association with diseases such as SLE and RA.

Other laboratory tests

An elevated erythrocyte sedimentation rate and a mild anaemia are very common. Myoglobinaemia and myoglobinuria are often seen. An elevated serum creatine kinase or an increase in urine creatine concentration is important evidence of skeletal muscle necrosis.

FURTHER READING

Blackwood, H. J. J. (1963). Arthritis of the mandibular joint. *Br. Dent. J.*, **115**, 317–26

Fye, K. K. and Sack, K. E. (1984). Rheumatic diseases. In Stites, D. P., Stobo, J. D., Fudenberg, H. H. and Wells, J. V. (eds) *Basic and Clinical Immunology*. 5th edition. pp. 423–41. (Los Altos: Lange)

Glynn, L. E. (1976). Rheumatoid arthritis. In Cohen, B. and Kramer, I. R. H. (eds). *Scientific Foundations of Dentistry*. pp. 616–20. (London: William Heinemann)

Holborow, E. J. and Swannell, A. J. (1983). The connective tissue diseases. In Holborow, E. J. and Reeves, W. G. (eds) *Immunology in Medicine*. pp. 246–73. (London: Grune & Stratton)

Janossy, G., Panayi, G., Duke, O., Bofill, M., Poulter, L. W. and Goldstein, G. (1981). Rheumatoid arthritis: a disease of T lymphocyte/macrophage immuno-regulation. *Lancet*, **2**, 839–42

Manthorpe, R., Frost-Larsen, K., Isager, H. and Prause, J. U. (1981). Sjögren's syndrome: a review. *Allergy*, **36**, 139–53

Motsopoulos, H. M. (1980). Sjögren's syndrome. *Curr. Iss. Am. Intern. Med.*, **92**, 212–26

Pindborg, J. J. (1980). *Oral Cancer and Precancer*. (Bristol: John Wright & Sons)

Schiødt, M. and Pindborg, J. J. (1984). Oral discoid lupus erythematosus. I. The validity of previous histopathologic diagnostic criteria. *Oral Surg.*, **57**, 46–51

8
Granulomatous and other Systemic Diseases with Oral Manifestations

M. M. FERGUSON and E. E. MacFADYEN

OROFACIAL GRANULOMATOSIS

Orofacial granulomatosis is a chronic, non-caseating granulomatous disorder involving the tissues of the mouth and face. Although this condition can exist as a localized entity it may also represent the oral manifestations of Crohn's disease or sarcoidosis.

Localized orofacial granulomatosis

General considerations

An association between episodes of seventh nerve palsy and transient facial oedema has been recognized in the literature for over a century, but is most commonly referred to as the 'Melkersson–Rosenthal syndrome' when there is associated fissuring of the tongue. An alternative title which was adopted for swelling of the lips and face, due to granulomatous infiltrate, was 'cheilitis granulomatosa of Miescher'. These are now known to be the same entity and also include the 'Melkersson–Rossolimo syndrome'. However, in an attempt to overcome confusion with multiple eponyms, as well as take cognizance of a similar oral presentation in some cases of Crohn's disease and sarcoidosis, the term 'orofacial granulomatosis' was proposed.

Immunological aspects of pathogenesis

The aetiology of orofacial granulomatosis, in the absence of Crohn's disease or sarcoidosis, has been unclear, although there are a number of reported cases where parents or siblings are also affected; however this is relatively uncommon. No studies appear to have been undertaken either to associate the localized form of orofacial granulomatosis with specific histo-compatibility lymphocyte A (HLA) types or to detect abnormalities in parameters of the immune response. An analysis of one substantial group of patients revealed that about 60% of the group were clinically atopic with a history of infantile eczema, hay fever or asthma. This is significantly greater than the 10–15% of atopy in the general population and so raised the possibility of a defect in cell-mediated immunity.

Recent work indicates that an aetiological factor in a significant number of individuals is an intolerance to foods, flavourings or other agents placed in or near the mouth. Some patients, by correlating episodes of orofacial swelling with recent dietary experience, have been able to identify provoking foods, but a more productive approach has been the use of a very low allergen diet. This consists of starting a diet comprising lamb, pears, apples, rice and water, together with a synthetic supplement – Peptisorbon (Phrimmer & Co.) or Vivonex (Norwich Eaton Ltd. – to maintain an adequate nutritional balance and provide energy requirements. After 2 weeks of this regime new foods are introduced every third day until a comprehensive diet is established. In the event of such a food precipitating an episode of orofacial swelling this and other members of the same family (e.g. solanacea) are then avoided until completion of the reintroduction phase. At this time the suspected foods are again used as a challenge and if positive they are subsequently eliminated from the diet. During such procedures it is important for the clinician to work in close co-operation with a dietician, not only to maintain an adequate diet but also to arrange appropriate counselling and encouragement for the patient.

There is some evidence to suggest that in a number of orofacial granulomatosis patients there may be a form of hypersensitivity to certain micro-organisms, but this requires further substantiation. However, such a reaction is not inconsistent with the other individuals showing food intolerances; there is considerable overlap between microbial products and materials from plants. In some cases the responsible molecule has been identified as an electrophilic agent, e.g. cinnamaldehyde, which will have the capacity to combine with basic proteins, forming a hapten, whereas in others it is more probably a foreign peptide or protein.

The elucidation of the role of food intolerance as the precipitating factor in orofacial granulomatosis has allowed for the development of a rational approach to treatment for a number of these patients. Identification of further environmental agents as allergens should enable the extension of this approach.

Systemic manifestations

In the localized form of orofacial granulomatosis it is unusual to encounter any other systemic manifestations except neurological changes. A few patients have commented on a general malaise or joint pains in association with their facial swelling, which suggests the presence of circulating immune complexes. The commonest neurological disorder is seventh nerve paralysis. This usually precedes the orofacial swelling, is transient and may occur several times on either side. Less than half the patients with orofacial granulomatosis have experienced facial palsy which, it has been suggested, is due to ischaemia as the nerve traverses the facial canal. In addition, an upper motor neurone lesion of this nerve has also been reported and, less frequently, there may be involvement of the oculomotor, the trigeminal or the glossopharyngeal nerve. Changes in the central nervous system have been documented, with abnormalities in the EEG pattern and deterioration of the intellect. A further problem is psychologically coping with the facial disfigurement, and this may lead to anxiety and depression.

Oral manifestations

The clinical features include swelling of the lips, facial swelling, mucosal thickening, oral ulceration, hyperplasia of the gingivae, mucosal tags and angular cheilitis (Figures 8.1–8.3). Fissuring of the tongue is not particularly common and is perhaps not even a significant feature in this condition any more than is geographic tongue.

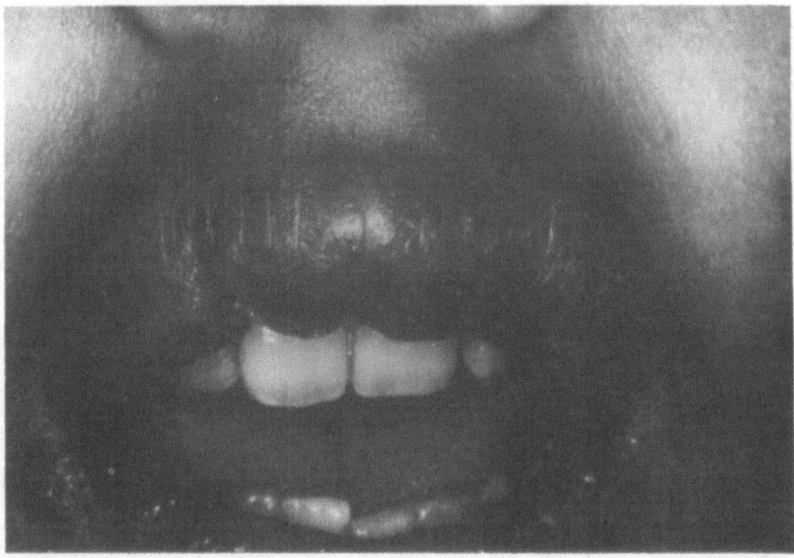

Figure 8.1 Case of orofacial granulomatosis associated with Crohn's disease of the bowel. This case demonstrates prominent lip swelling with vertical fissuring and crusted angular cheilitis

The labial swelling may involve both lips but it is somewhat more common to have this confined to one lip: the upper and lower lips are involved with equal frequency. In a few cases there is asymmetry with only a portion of the lip being affected. The swelling may fluctuate in magnitude or remain

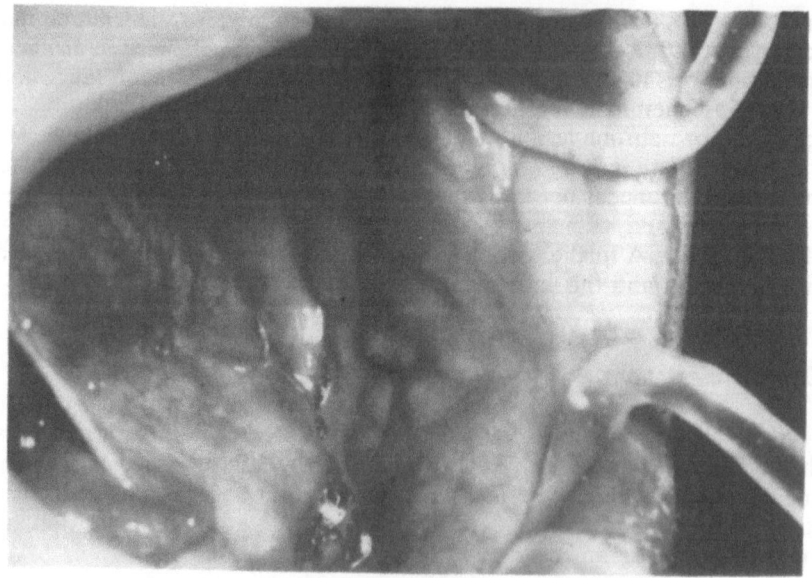

Figure 8.2 Localized orofacial granulomatosis where the thickened buccal mucosa has assumed a lobulated appearance

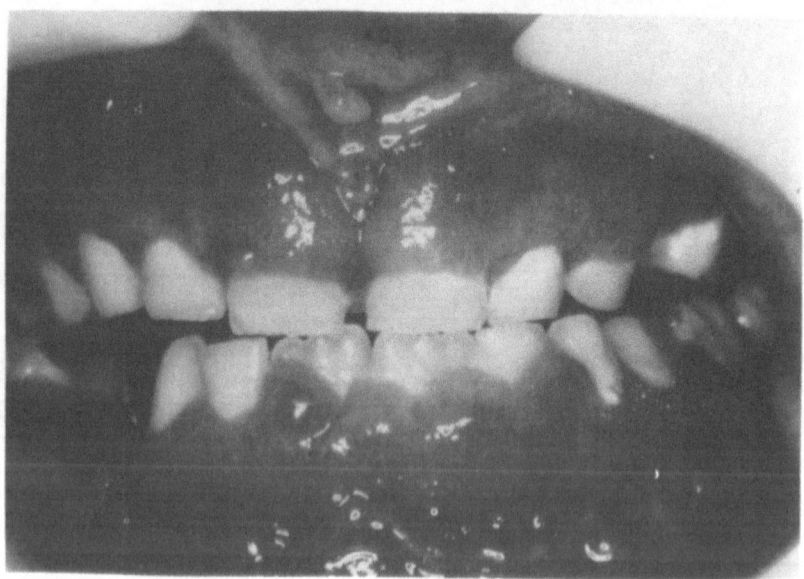

Figure 8.3 Gingival involvement in orofacial granulomatosis with granular changes extending from the attached mucosa to the sulcus. Hyperplastic tissue is evident in the lower sulcus

164

relatively constant with tense tissue causing discomfort or even paraesthesia, which is presumably a consequence of pressure on the sensory nerves. When the lips are enlarged and tense, their colour and that of the surrounding skin may develop a deep red or cyanosed appearance. Splits sometimes occur with the formation of vertical fissuring; these subsequently become infected with a range of micro-organisms such as *Candida albicans* and *Staphylococcus aureus*, leading to further inflammation. Angular cheilitis does not always appear to be related to mechanical distortion of the lips and tends to assume a crusted, eczematous appearance rather than prominent fissuring.

Swelling of the face is usually confined to the lower half, although there are a few documented cases where the eyelids and nose were similarly affected. This swelling can be bilateral or unilateral, and like the lips may be variable or constant. The overlying skin colour varies from normal to being erythematous.

Although the buccal and labial mucosa is most frequently involved with tense thickening and erythema any region of the oral mucosa can be affected; the pharynx, larynx and upper oesophagus do not appear to be thickened in the localized form of orofacial granulomatosis. The labial mucosa usually is abnormal in association with enlargement of the lips and may either be diffusely swollen or else assume a lobulated or cobblestone appearance. Thickening of the buccal mucosa results in the formation of folds or lobules; this prominent, swollen mucosa may be traumatized by the occlusion and become accentuated along the occlusal line; on other occasions this results in traumatic ulceration. Enlargement of part of the tongue may lead to similar damage or else the distorted tissue presses against the teeth leading to a scalloped or indented appearance around the lateral margins. Oedema of the floor of the mouth is uncomfortable and leads to difficulty with speech and swallowing.

A hyperplastic gingivitis can develop and in some individuals this is apparently the only manifestation of the disorder. It may be extensive, although more commonly the hyperplasia is patchy in distribution with the anterior gingivae being especially vulnerable. The gingivitis extends from the free gingival margin to involve the reflected mucosa. The surface may be smooth and shiny red or develop a granular appearance throughout.

Discrete tags may develop in any part of the mucosa either as small, isolated lesions or assuming a linear form in the sulcus. This looks similar to denture-induced hyperplasia, albeit the patients are fully dentate. The form of mucosal ulceration varies considerably, from very superficial ulcers to deep, persistent lesions. A number of these patients appear to have ulcers identical to recurrent aphthae and perhaps this is not unexpected as a coincidental finding since aphthae are so common in the general population. Enlargement of the cervical lymph nodes is not a frequent finding. In such cases where granulomata are present in the nodes then the diagnosis of sarcoidosis or even tuberculosis must be considered.

Immunological diagnosis

No diagnostic immunological test has been described in the localized form of orofacial granulomatosis, with the exception of the employment of patch testing on the skin using potential allergens.

Laboratory tests

The single investigative procedure in patients with this disorder is the biopsy. Histopathological features which characterize orofacial granulomatosis are non-caseating granulomata, a chronic inflammatory infiltrate, oedema and lymphatic dilatation. However, these granulomata may be sparsely distributed through the tissue and are more likely to be found when the biopsy is relatively large and includes some underlying skeletal muscle. The histology of the localized form of orofacial granulomatosis is indistinguishable from that of either Crohn's disease or sarcoidosis.

Crohn's disease (regional enteritis, granulomatous colitis)

General considerations

Crohn's disease is a chronic granulomatous disorder which may affect any part of the alimentary tract, although it has a particular predilection for the terminal ileum and colon. Any age group can be involved but it has its peak incidence in the second and third decades. In addition to its gastrointestinal lesions, up to 20% of patients with Crohn's disease may have lesions directly affecting other tissues in the body.

Immunological aspects

No specific aetiology has been identified for Crohn's disease. There is a hereditary pattern for some individuals. Patients and their first-degree relatives also have been noted to have a high incidence of atopy. This, like the local form of orofacial granulomatosis, is suggestive of defective cell-mediated immunity: lymphocyte transformation tests to PHA and PPD are often subnormal. Likewise there can be decreased skin reactions after intradermal injection of tuberculin and reduced responsiveness in contact hypersensitivity against dinitrochlorobenzene (DNCB). In Crohn's disease the highest number of granulomata are found in those patients with HLA-B8, a haplotype also associated with abnormal immune responsiveness.

Despite the increased incidence of atopy in patients with Crohn's disease, there is no evidence to indicate that the alimentary lesions represent an immediate hypersensitivity reaction. Serum levels of total IgE have not been found to be elevated and there is probably no increase in the number of mucosal IgE-bearing plasma cells or mast cells. However, there has been the suggestion of basophil and IgE participation in the affected tissue but this requires confirmation.

An increased number of IgM and IgA containing plasma cells have been observed in the non-involved oral mucosa of patients with alimentary Crohn's disease and whole saliva levels of IgG, IgA and IgM were also found to be elevated. Plasma cells and B lymphocytes are increased in the lamina propria of affected intestine and the number of IgA-bearing cells is disproportionately increased. Circulating antibodies to colonic epithelium of the IgG, IgA or IgM class have been reported in Crohn's patients. The antigen to which these are directed is a lipopolysaccharide located in the colonic epithelial goblet cells, but these specific autoantibodies have not been demonstrated at the tissue level. The significance of these circulating immunoglobulins is unclear and it has been impossible so far to demonstrate any cytotoxic effect of the anti-colonic epithelium immunoglobulin for human fetal colon cells in culture even in the presence of complement.

Evidence for immune complex reactions has been sought in Crohn's disease as this would be consistent with several of the associated extra-intestinal lesions. Tissue deposition of certain immune complexes will activate the components of complement and result in an inflammatory response. The nature of this depends both on complex size and ratio of antigen to antibody: one study reports the induction of a granulomatous reaction with complexes at equivalence, whereas those found in the presence of excess antigen led to an Arthus-type reaction.

In patients with Crohn's disease there is no impairment of pokeweed-stimulated lymphocyte transformation (a B-cell activator) but the responses to PHA or to mixed lymphocyte culture are impaired. A decrease in the number of circulating T lymphocytes has also been reported.

Lymphocytes from patients with Crohn's disease exhibit cytotoxicity towards colonic epithelial cells in culture and this can be blocked with polysaccharides from certain strains of *E. coli*. It has been suggested that these coliforms share an antigen with colon cells, but whether this is an aetiological factor or a consequence of mucosal damage and altered permeability to bacterial antigens remains to be established. There is also some evidence to implicate a transmissible agent in Crohn's, although this appears to have been better substantiated in cases of sarcoidosis.

A further possibility in the pathogenesis of Crohn's disease is the action of antibody-dependent K lymphocytes: the Fc receptors of these K lymphocytes are capable of binding to the antibody moiety of antigen–antibody complexes. Lymphoid cells obtained from normal, healthy human intestine exert no antibody-dependent cytotoxicity, whereas immuno-fluorescent studies of tissue from individuals with Crohn's disease have demonstrated inflammatory cells which might bear Fc receptors as they bind aggregated IgG.

Recently it has been found that a number of patients with Crohn's disease of bowel respond favourably to a very low allergen diet and that specific foods provoke symptoms. When these items are avoided it has been possible to withdraw steroids, which indicates that food intolerance is an aetiological factor, at least in some patients with Crohn's disease, as it is in the localized form of orofacial granulomatosis. Again the evidence to implicate micro-organisms in Crohn's disease does not exclude the dietary hypersensitivity theory.

Systemic manifestations

In Crohn's disease there is a characteristic inflammatory and granulomatous infiltrate in the bowel wall. Lesions are most commonly found in the terminal ileum but involvement of colon is also frequent. Skip lesions characterize Crohn's disease where there is patchy bowel involvement and the granulomatous lesions may occur anywhere in the alimentary canal. These give rise to abdominal pain, loose stools or constipation, fever and anorexia. Malabsorption is common and leads to the classical features of nutritional deficiency. Bowel perforation, acute obstruction, melaena or cutaneous fistulae may also develop.

Extraintestinal complications of Crohn's disease include arthritis, ankylosing spondylitis, sacroileitis, cutaneous granulomata, pyoderma gangrenosum, erythema nodosum, conjunctivitis, iridocyclitis, blepharitis and retrobulbar neuritis. Liver abnormalities and nodular pancreatitis have also been reported.

Oral manifestations

Oral manifestations of Crohn's disease are identical to those present in patients with localized orofacial granulomatosis, although there may be additional involvement of the pharyngeal mucosa, epiglottis and oesophagus with swelling and ulceration. As deficiencies of iron, folate, vitamin B_{12} and other B vitamins may develop these patients occasionally present with atrophic glossitis, angular cheilitis and ulceration of the oral mucosa.

Immunological diagnosis

There is no specific immunological diagnosis for Crohn's disease. The diagnosis is based firmly upon history and clinical examination. Markers of active tissue inflammation are elevation of erythrocyte sedimentation rate, C-reactive protein and α-globulin levels. Contrast radiography, with large and small bowel enemas, may reveal irregular narrowing, nodularity, ulcers and fistulae. Proctoscopy and colonoscopy are performed to show cobblestoning, ulceration and inflammation. Biopsies of colon and rectal mucosa are also performed to examine for the presence of the characteristic granulomata. Gastro-duodenoscopy and jejunal biopsy are used to reveal lesions in the upper intestine. Scanning for accumulation of ^{111}In-labelled leukocytes has been used to detect inflammatory changes in bowel loops. Tests of intestinal function (such as xylose absorption, faecal fat, and Schilling tests) have a lesser part to play in the diagnosis of Crohn's disease, although faecal [51]Co excretion has been employed to differentiate between inflammatory bowel disease and irritable bowel syndrome.

Sarcoidosis

General considerations

Sarcoidosis is a multisystem, granulomatous disorder of undetermined aetiology and may affect individuals of any age, although its peak occurrence is between the second and fourth decades. Females have a somewhat higher incidence and it has been found to develop more frequently in Negroes. In a small number of cases more than one individual in a family is involved, to an extent that this is more than could be expected by chance. Likewise there is some evidence to suggest a familial association between sarcoidosis and Crohn's disease.

Immunological aspects

A number of studies of HLA antigens have been performed in sarcoidosis in view of the evidence that genetic factors might influence susceptibility. In general, a higher frequency of HLA-B7 has been found in pulmonary sarcoidosis but in other areas greater numbers of HLA-B5 and HLA-A9 have been noted. There is further evidence to link HLA types with particular clinical manifestations; for example, B8 has been associated with arthropathy. The haplotype HLA-A1, B8 and DR3 occur in linkage disequilibrium, and this has also been associated with abnormal immune responsiveness.

Like Crohn's disease, cutaneous sensitization to DNCB has been found to be reduced in sarcoid patients, as has the reaction to tuberculin, mumps virus, *Candida* antigen and pertussis antigen. However, there does not appear to be a defective humoral response: serum IgE levels overall are higher than in controls and a number of studies have also found an increase in α-globulins with a slight reduction in albumin. Levels of IgM, IgA and IgG tend to be raised but no change has been recorded in IgE. Using latex fixation tests for rheumatoid factor, there is an increased number of positives in sarcoidosis but there is no change in the incidence of antinuclear factor. In acute cases of sarcoidosis, immune complexes have been found and these have been associated with disturbances of serum complement levels. Immune complexes of the size detected have been shown to be pathogenic in animals.

During the active phase of sarcoidosis the number of circulating T lymphocytes is reduced and a proportion of the lymphocytes have an atypical morphology, resembling those found in some acute viral diseases. Lymphocyte transformation tests have shown a decreased stimulation in sarcoid patients, with PHA, PPD and Con-A. These depressed responses have been attributed to some extent to a suppressor effect from monocytes, possibly related to their prostaglandin synthesis.

A range of hypotheses has been advanced regarding the aetiology of sarcoidosis. Pine pollen and beryllium have both been considered as possible non-infective causal agents, but current opinion does not support this. The similarity in the granulomatous appearance in histology of sarcoidosis and tuberculosis prompted earlier workers to search for a form of mycobacterium; epidemiological surveys of sarcoid patients suggested either a previous high contact rate with tuberculosis or else a greater incidence of sarcoidosis and tuberculosis in siblings. A series of experiments has been performed where tissues from sarcoid tissue homogenates were injected into footpads of mice and granulomata subsequently formed. Irradiation, autoclaving or prolonged storage of the homogenates at −20 °C inactivated this ability to produce granulomata, which is indicative of a transmissible agent. Further, although the human sarcoid tissue from which the tissue homogenates had been prepared was devoid of mycobacteria, acid-fast bacilli were found subsequently in the murine tissues. Pooled homogenates from the recipient mouse lungs and spleens grew myco-bacteria, having the characteristics of human *M. tuberculosis*, on Lowenstein–Jensen medium. The homogenates from the sarcoid tissue could also be passed through a 0.2 μm filter and still retain potency. Therefore such an agent would either require to be the size of a virus or be capable of being deformed sufficiently to pass through the filter. A protoplast or L-form tubercle bacillus may have this capacity and be the transmissible agent, at least in some patients with sarcoidosis. However, definitive identification of this agent remains to be established.

Systemic manifestations

Sarcoidosis can involve most organs of the body wherein impairment of function results from active granulomatous disease as well as secondary fibrosis. Non-specific presenting features are fever, weight loss and fatigue. An important early manifestation of sarcoidosis is bilateral hilar lymph node enlargement often accompanied by erythema nodosum; most of these patients have associated joint pains with the larger joints being most commonly affected. Symptoms related to the bilateral hilar node enlargement are variable and may include dyspnoea, chest pain and an unproductive cough. There may also be widespread granulomatous involvement of lung resulting in pulmonary fibrosis, often with exacerbation of secondary bacterial infections.

The skin lesions of sarcoidosis are lupus pernio, nodular infiltrations, plaques, subcutaneous nodules and infiltrations of old scars. Splenomegaly and enlargement of lymph nodes are frequent findings and the cervical groups of nodes are most involved, followed by those of the axilla. Ocular sarcoid lesions are uveitis, conjunctival granuloma, band keratopathy, episcleritis, dacryostenosis and fundal changes as well as enlargement of the lacrimal glands with reduced tear production. The kidneys may be affected directly by granulomata, as can the remainder of the genitourinary system or, more commonly, nephropathy results from hypercalcaemia.

The central and peripheral nervous systems may be involved. Granulomatous infiltration of the meninges at the base of the brain and adjacent hypothalamus may lead to neuroendocrine and visual disturbances. Neuropathies which occur tend to be variable and remittent. The seventh cranial nerve is most frequently involved with a transient lower motor neurone palsy. If the lesion is above the level of the chorda tympani, then a taste disturbance may accompany the palsy. Rarely an upper motor neurone palsy of the facial nerve results from a deposit in the brain, and is usually part of a hemiplegia. Most of the remaining cranial nerves can become involved; when the trigeminal nerve is affected it is more often in its sensory functions, and lesions in the glossopharyngeal and vagal nerves result in dysphagia due to paralysis of the pharyngeal and palatal muscles.

A number of sarcoid patients develop lesions in the nasal mucosa, especially of the inferior turbinates and adjacent septum, but granulomata may also occur in the nasal sinuses, pharynx, epiglottis and larynx. Granulomata may be present in the oesophagus, stomach, small intestine, appendix and colon; in these sites they are often asymptomatic and difficulty can arise in differentiating sarcoidosis from Crohn's disease.

Oral manifestations

Sarcoidosis may present as orofacial granulomatosis, the oral lesion being indistinguishable from those of the localized form of orofacial granulomatosis or Crohn's disease. Granulomatous infiltration of the salivary glands is another oral manifestation of sarcoidosis with enlargement of the parotid glands being a prominent feature. However, all of the salivary glands may be infiltrated and this leads to xerostomia. Such patients experience a persistent dry feeling which may also cause a burning sensation of the mucosa. Speech and mastication are difficult and their diet may require to be modified accordingly. As in any group of patients with prolonged xerostomia, dental caries and periodontal disease become a problem and require an active programme of preventive therapy.

Immunological diagnosis

A number of tests may contribute to the diagnosis of sarcoidosis. In active disease an increase in the serum α-globulins and a diminution in albumin may be found. Tuberculin tests as well as other delayed skin reactions can be depressed, and a negative Mantoux test supports the diagnosis of sarcoidosis, although a positive reaction is still compatible with it.

The Kveim reaction is a standard diagnostic test for sarcoidosis and gives the highest proportion of positive reactions in the early, active phases of the disorder. Essentially this test consists of injecting a homogenate of spleen, removed from a sarcoid patient, intradermally then biopsying the area about 6 weeks later and examining this for the development of granulomata. It is critical that, for the Kveim test, a properly validated suspension be used.

Laboratory tests

Biopsy of affected tissue is an important step in the diagnosis of sarcoidosis and this is usually taken from lymph nodes, skin, liver, bronchial mucosa, lung, skeletal muscle, conjunctiva, spleen or minor salivary glands.

Other useful diagnostic procedures are measurement of serum calcium for evidence of hypercalcaemia and serum levels of angiotensin-1-converting enzyme, adenosine deaminase and lysozyme; these three enzymes are produced by macrophages and epithelioid cells in the granulomata and hence are raised in active stages of sarcoidosis.

Scintiscanning with gallium may reveal active sarcoidosis, and both computerized tomography and NMR scanning have been used to detect cranial and pulmonary lesions. Routine chest radiographs alone may miss cases of respiratory involvement and therefore they should be augmented by pulmonary function tests.

ULCERATIVE COLITIS

General considerations

Ulcerative colitis is an inflammatory disorder affecting the mucosa of the rectum and colon. It is characterized histologically by ulceration of the mucosa, the presence of a purulent exudate together with blood on the epithelial surface, small abscesses around the crypts and an inflammatory infiltrate in the mucosa and submucosa. The abnormal mucosal reaction stops abruptly at its proximal extent in the colon and mesenteric lymph nodes are not involved.

Immunological aspects

One of the earlier theories of the aetiology of ulcerative colitis was that it represented an immediate hypersensitivity reaction to dietary proteins of which cows' milk antigens were most commonly implicated. However, this theory has not been substantiated.

Patients with ulcerative colitis have a higher incidence of atopy and an increased number of IgE-containing plasma cells have been reported in the affected colonic mucosa. Tissue mast cells appear to be increased and a greater number of circulating eosinophils have been reported during active phases of the disease. The further suggestion has been made that basophils may similarly be implicated in the reaction.

Immunoglobulins, of the IgA, IgG and IgM classes directed towards colonic epithelium, have been described in patients with ulcerative colitis but these have not been found to be cytotoxic towards the colon epithelial cells in culture, even with the addition of complement. It is thought that these antibodies probably do not play a significant role in the pathogenesis of the condition. Similar antibodies to colon epithelium have been raised in rabbits and no inflammatory changes developed in the colon: both enterobacteria and colonic antigen have been employed to induce antibodies.

Immune complex-mediated tissue damage is another possible mechanism of inducing mucosal inflammation as well as the extraintestinal manifestations of the disease. There is increased catabolism of C1q and C3, with fibrin, IgG, C1q and C3 having been demonstrated on the basement membrane of rectal biopsies taken from patients with ulcerative colitis. This is consistent with local deposition of immune complexes, although further studies are still necessary to establish a role for these complexes in the pathogenesis.

Lymphocyte toxins of the IgM class have been found in over 25% of patients with ulcerative colitis as well as in their first-degree relatives. The significance of these cytotoxic antibodies to lymphocytes is unclear and they have also been detected in a number of other disorders. As in Crohn's disease, lymphocytes from patients with ulcerative colitis have been found to be cytotoxic to human adult and fetal colon epithelial cells in tissue culture. This cytotoxic action was shown to be affected by a soluble factor released from the lymphocytes, namely a lymphotoxin. The cytotoxic potential could be conferred upon normal lymphocytes from healthy individuals by incubating either with the IgM fraction from ulcerative colitis patients or a crude extract of *E. coli*. The cytotoxic property of patients' lymphocytes, together with the ability of their serum to confer a similar cytotoxic reaction on normal lymphocytes, disappeared about a week following resection of the diseased colon. An *in vivo* study supported the *in vitro* findings where a leukocyte suspension prepared from ulcerative colitis patients was injected into healthy rectal mucosa and provoked a local inflammatory reaction.

Experimental models of ulcerative colitis have been developed in guinea pigs and rabbits. By employing DNCB sensitization in the guinea pig, an inflammatory reaction can be produced in the mucosa which shows similar histology to ulcerative colitis in humans. In addition, the same changes can then be induced in other guinea pigs by passage of lymphocytes from the first sensitized animals. Rabbits were given a diluted formalin solution per rectum following immunization with an antigen common to the enterobacteria, i.e. Kunin antigen. Then following intravenous injection of soluble immune complexes a chronic colitis appeared, suggesting that ulcerative colitis may develop in individuals who initially become sensitized to antigens from the colonic bacteria and then suffer an acute colonic infection.

Systemic manifestations

The intestinal features of ulcerative colitis are abdominal pain, weight loss and the frequent passage of liquid stools containing blood and pus. These symptoms are variable, with some individuals experiencing minimal direct colonic problems and even having constipation interspersed with bouts of diarrhoea. Severe cases with involvement of the entire colon present with very severe changes in the form of an acute fulminating colitis. Fatty infiltration of the liver appears in some cases and this may be related to a pericholangitis. Extraintestinal lesions include a monoarticular arthritis of large joints, polyarthritis of peripheral joints and ankylosing spondylitis. Pyoderma gangrenosum and erythema nodosum may appear in the skin, although the latter occurs more frequently in association with Crohn's disease. Ocular manifestations may also appear and include conjunctivitis, uveitis and episcleritis.

Oral manifestations

Nutritional deficiencies can occur consequent to malabsorption, and therefore the relatively non-specific features of atrophic glossitis, angular cheilitis and mucosal ulceration sometimes develop. Ulcers of the aphthous pattern may arise in patients with associated active disease but a more characteristic oral manifestation is pyostomatitis vegetans. In this latter condition the mucosa becomes erythematous and may form papillary folds and grooves, which impart a pebbly appearance. Numerous, small yellow pustules develop on the surface and as they become ulcerated tend to coalesce forming irregular linear lesions reminiscent of snail-track ulcers. Although any region of the oral mucosa may become involved, the most frequently affected sites are the labial mucosa, buccal mucosa, the palate and labial and buccal aspects of the gingivae. Equivalent oral lesions to cutaneous pyoderma gangrenosum have been described in a few patients with ulcerative colitis. Large irregular-shaped ulcers develop which can be very persistent. The deep base is covered in a yellow/grey slough and the mucosal margins assume a rolled form.

Immunological diagnosis

No specific immunological tests have been adopted in the diagnosis of ulcerative colitis. The diagnosis is confirmed by sigmoidoscopy or colonoscopy and a rectal biopsy. Barium enema also shows the characteristic changes in the colon.

COELIAC DISEASE (Gluten-induced enteropathy)

General considerations

Coeliac disease is a disorder of the jejunum characterized by an intolerance to gluten which results in malabsorption. This condition affects women more commonly, and tends to show a hereditary pattern suggestive of an autosomal dominant condition but with incomplete penetrance. Striking geographical differences exist and it has a particular association with haplotype HLA-DRW3 as well as a secondary association with HLA-B8.

174

Immunological aspects

The aetiology of coeliac disease appears to be an intolerance of gluten, a protein present in wheat, barley and rye. Fractionation of gluten indicates that the toxic component is α-gliaden which has a molecular weight of about 18 000. Omission of gluten from the diet results in a complete remission but the mechanism whereby the gluten causes the damage to the small intestine is unclear. A specific reaction to α-gliaden or a deficiency to a proteolytic enzyme in the jejunal mucosa have both been proposed.

Although there is an increased number of IgM-containing plasma cells in the involved jejunal mucosa, the plasma level of IgM is often decreased. The IgA plasma level is commonly increased, and both IgA and IgM concentrations tend to be elevated in the intestinal secretions.

Circulating antibodies directed towards a number of food antigens may be detected and probably are a consequence of an inflamed and ulcerated, leaky intestine. However, antibodies directed specifically towards α-gliaden also develop in a number of patients with active disease. Another immunoglobulin has been described in coeliac patients which is an IgA directed to reticulin fibres. The specificity is not absolute for coeliac disease as it has also been described in association with Crohn's disease and Sjögren's syndrome. There is some evidence suggesting that since α-gliadin shows a particular affinity for reticulin fibres then the reticulin antibody which has been demonstrated really represents gliaden–antigliaden immune complexes. Circulating immune complexes have been demonstrated in coeliac disease and those associated with IgG appear to bear a relationship to disease activity. The antigen component of these high-weight immune complexes remains to be identified.

The absolute lymphocyte count and the T lymphocyte count are reduced in cases of untreated coeliac disease and these are restored to a normal level following the institution of a gluten-free diet. Lymphocyte transformation tests, using PHA, Con-A and pokeweed as mitogens, are reduced in untreated cases. A cellular hypersensitivity has been demonstrated to α-gliadin using both lymphocyte transformation and the leukocyte migration inhibition assay.

Systemic manifestations

Clinical features of coeliac disease are diarrhoea, weight loss, malaise, steatorrhoea, abdominal distension and evidence of nutritional deficiency – especially anaemia. Metabolic bone disease may also be a feature with demineralization leading to compression fractures. Intestinal lymphomata occur more frequently in patients with coeliac disease.

Oral manifestations

There are no specific oral manifestations of coeliac disease but deficiencies of folic acid and iron are common features. As such, patients present with atrophic glossitis and angular cheilitis. Non-specific mucosal ulceration may be a feature and in a few individuals recurrent aphthae develop. These would appear to be indistinguishable from other cases of recurrent aphthae but represent an aetiological factor in under 5% of patients being referred to specialist clinics with this form of recurrent ulceration.

Immunological diagnosis

The immunological features which are used diagnostically for coeliac disease are the presence of circulating antibodies to α-gliadin and reticulin. The definitive diagnosis is established by the appearance of sub-total villous atrophy in a jejunal biopsy. Serum levels of folate and ferritin are commonly decreased and this tends to be reflected in anaemias.

HYPOADRENOCORTICALISM (ADDISON'S DISEASE)

General considerations

Hypoadrenocorticalism is a fairly rare condition associated with the progressive destruction of all layers of the adrenal cortex. The most frequent cause of primary hypoadrenocorticalism in the past was probably tuberculous infiltration; this is now more commonly attributed to an autoimmune disorder. Even less commonly, the adrenal cortex is destroyed by amyloid disease, protozoal or fungal infestation. The general manifestations of the condition are related to insufficient secretion of glucocorticoids and mineralocorticoids.

Immunological aspects

Hypoadrenocorticalism may exist on its own or in association with other disorders, namely autoimmune thyroiditis, diabetes mellitus, hypoparathyroidism and pernicious anaemia. No clear genetic pattern has been established although some families do show a predisposition. The Type II form is strongly associated with HLA-DR3, but no association has been found in the Type I form.

Two patterns of hypoadrenocorticalism have emerged. In Type I, which occurs in children and young adults, there is a sequence of presentation, starting with chronic mucocutaneous candidiasis, then hypoparathyroidism and finally Addison's disease; less frequently, hypogonadism, vitiligo, pernicious anaemia, chronic active hepatitis and malabsorption syndrome may also occur. Type II usually develops in middle age and shows no set order of disorders: it occurs in association with hypothyroidism, pernicious anaemia and juvenile onset (insulin-dependent) diabetes mellitus.

Approximately 70% of patients with autoimmune hypoadrenocorticalism have circulating antibodies directed to the microsomes of cortical cells. Other antibodies encountered are to thyroid microsomes, parietal cells, steroid-producing cells of the gonads, and pancreatic islet cells.

Some patients with hypoadrenocorticalism have been shown to have a cell-mediated reaction to adrenal cortical tissue, based on the leukocyte migration inhibition assay. However, the antigenic material in this case was apparently the mitochondrial fraction, which is in contrast to the microsomal fraction which reacts with the circulating immunoglobulin. Chronic mucocutaneous candidiasis has been associated with various defects of the cellular response, as well as IgA deficiency.

Systemic manifestations

The onset of hypoadrenocorticalism is usually insidious, with progressive weakness, anorexia, weight loss, hypotension, nausea, vomiting, diarrhoea and cutaneous and mucosal pigmentation. Pigmentation due to melanin deposition is thought to be caused by an increase in MSH, a pituitary hormone of unknown function in man, which accompanies the increased secretion of ACTH. Patients may comment on persistent tanning following exposure to the sun, but increased pigmentation develops on unexposed as well as exposed areas of the skin. Darkening also occurs in the areolae of the nipples.

Oral manifestations

The melanin pigmentation ranges from brown to blue-black on any area of the oral mucosa. Obviously it must be differentiated from physiological pigmentation seen in dark-skinned races or Caucasians with a dark complexion; this is based upon the appearance of new areas of pigmentation developing in contrast to its lifelong existence.

Immunological diagnosis

The immunological feature in the diagnosis of hypoadrenocorticalism is the presence of a circulating immunoglobulin reactive to adrenal cortical microsomes. As there may be coexisting endocrine disorders, it may therefore be appropriate to screen for antibodies to thyroid, parietal cells and gonads.

Laboratory tests

The diagnosis is confirmed by the presence of hypotension, hyponatraemia and hyperkalaemia. The serum level of cortisol is depressed, and this is ideally measured in the early morning as well as in the evening to examine for a circadian rhythm. Low urinary levels of 17-ketosteroids and 17-hydroxysteroids are also found. A useful test of adrenal function is to measure the serum cortisol levels before and 30 minutes after the intramuscular injection of 0.25 mg Synacthen. Finally, serum ACTH concentration can be measured directly.

WEGENER'S GRANULOMATOSIS

General considerations

Wegener's granulomatosis is an uncommon, granulomatous disease characterized by widespread necrotizing vasculitis. In the systemic form the tissues most commonly affected are the upper and lower respiratory tract and the kidneys. The disease occurs twice as commonly in males as females, and although it has been recorded from the first to the eighth decade it most commonly presents in middle age.

A more localized form of this condition with identical histology is the midline granuloma. In this disorder the inflammation and subsequent necrosis is limited to the tissues of the upper respiratory tract and face.

Immunological aspects of pathogenesis

The aetiology of Wegener's granulomatosis remains an enigma, although there is some evidence which may implicate immune complexes. Circulating immune complexes have been reported in a number of patients and in those with renal involvement, complexes have been observed in the basement membrane area of the glomeruli. However, immune complexes have not been detected in the arterial walls as they have in the vasculitis of polyarteritis nodosa. Serum complement levels tend to be lowered in immune-complex disease and in systemic lupus erythematosus but this is not the case in Wegener's granulomatosis: one study noted a raised level of C3 in half of their patients.

Serum concentrations of both IgA and IgM are elevated in some patients and circulating smooth muscle antibodies may be present. Furthermore, it has been suggested that anticytoplasmic antibodies may correlate with disease activity, but no other autoantibodies have been found to feature consistently in Wegener's granulomatosis.

Delayed hypersensitivity following intradermal injection of several antigens was reported as being depressed in one study, whereas this was not the conclusion in another. Likewise there has been the suggestion of an impaired response to antigens in the lymphocyte transformation test while that with PHA was variable. No abnormality could be detected using the macrophage migration inhibition test in a group of patients. Certain of these limited immunological findings would seem to merit further confirmation.

Systemic manifestations

Wegener's granulomatosis presents in previously healthy adults as persistent headache, sinusitis, rhinorrhoea and an otitis media which is often associated with hearing loss. Involvement of the lower respiratory tract leads to coughing, chest pain and haemoptysis. Albeit fever, arthralgia, malaise and anorexia are present, the severity of the active disease process is generally greater than the symptoms might indicate. Although the kidneys are almost always involved with a generalized glomerulonephritis, only about 10% of patients present in renal failure. With these patients the characteristic changes of proteinuria, haematuria and red cell casts are found.

Skin and eye involvement are reported in about 50% of cases with the generalized angiitis causing skin nodules and ulcers of the anterior ciliary body as well as granulomatous lesions in the cornea. Less frequently other organ systems are involved with coronary arteritis or cranial and peripheral nerve involvement being especially frequent. The tissue destruction of the facial skeleton can cause nasal septal perforation and saddle nose deformity. A widespread persistent sinusitis infected with *Staphylococcus aureus* or *Pseudomonas aeruginosa* is commonly present. Pulmonary changes recorded are transient but may show solitary or multiple nodules and cavitation. Lung biopsy in these patients often confirms the diagnosis.

Oral manifestations

Oral ulceration occurs at some stage of this disease in about 50% of cases and this presents as persistent ulcers especially in the palate and in the pharynx. Specific oral lesions in Wegener's granulomatosis are rare but a distinctive type of gingivitis can be the presenting symptoms; this has been described as 'strawberry gums' from their resemblance to an over-ripe strawberry.

The lesions arise in the interdental papillae as florid, proliferative magenta-red enlargements. The presence of multiple petechiae is found, the tissue bleeds very readily and the appearance has been likened to multiple pyogenic granulomata. Radiographs will show erosion and advanced bone loss in the area, and spontaneous exfoliation of the affected teeth has been reported. Delayed healing of the extraction sockets is almost inevitable.

Immunological aspects of diagnosis

In Wegener's granulomatosis the ESR and C-reactive protein are invariably raised during active phases of the disease and serve as useful markers of therapeutic efficacy. The role of anticytoplasmic antibodies in the diagnosis remains to be established.

Laboratory investigations

There is no specific laboratory investigation for this condition, and diagnosis is confirmed by biopsy of an affected area. The histology of the lesion is specific with vasculitis and granulomatous inflammation present. This distinguishes the disease from polyarteritis nodosa where only a vasculitis is present, and from the granulomatous diseases where the vasculitis is absent. Routine haematological screening will usually find a normochromic normocytic anaemia with leukocytosis, especially if there is a superimposed bacterial infection.

Midline granuloma

A localized form of non-healing granuloma has been recorded with localized inflammation, destruction and mutilation of the tissues of the upper respiratory tract and face.

The patient frequently presents with a persistent nasal obstruction associated with a watery discharge and recurrent sinusitis. In time this proceeds to necrosis of the mucosa and bone of the nasal skeleton, palate and pharynx. Although there is extensive tissue destruction, pain is not severe. Extension of the lesion to the retropharyngeal tissues and base of skull signal the lethal termination of the disease.

Although oral lesions are rare, extension of the necrosis to tissues of the maxillary sinus may cause the patient to present with toothache. Extraction of the loosened teeth is inevitably followed by delayed healing. Extensive ulceration of the hard palate is associated with perforation of the bone.

POLYARTERITIS NODOSA

General considerations

Polyarteritis (periarteritis) nodosa is a polymorphic disorder involving, segmentally, arterioles, small and medium arteries throughout the body in a necrotizing inflammatory process. The initial lesion consists of a focus of fibrinoid necrosis accompanied by an acute inflammatory infiltrate. Thrombosis or haemorrhage may occur at this stage, which subsequently is replaced by granulation and scar tissue.

Immunological aspects of pathogenesis

There is evidence to indicate that the pathogenesis of this disorder involves a Type III hypersensitivity reaction with deposition of immune complexes in the vessel walls. Immunoglobulins and complement have been demonstrated in the acute lesions, and in experimental animals an immune complex disease has been induced with vascular lesions resembling those of polyarteritis.

A specific antigen has not been identified in polyarteritis nodosa although the disorder may sometimes be a feature of systemic lupus erythematosus where complexes with DNA are well recognized. Up to 50% of patients have been found to be chronic carriers of hepatitis-B virus and have been shown to have circulating HBs antigen–antibody complexes. In addition this antigen has been demonstrated in the acute vascular lesions of some such cases. The occurrence of polyarteritis nodosa following ingestion of certain drugs raises the possibility that these act as haptens to initiate immune complex formation.

Systemic manifestations

The patients usually present with fever, weakness, anorexia and arthralgias. Aneurysms occur with rupture of small nodules in the vessel walls and disturbance of blood supply to the tissues. Most patients complain of abdominal symptoms, pain, nausea, vomiting, diarrhoea and bleeding. This is due to involvement of the mesenteric vessels. With involvement of the renal vessels glomerulosclerosis and hypertension with renal failure may occur.

Skin involvement results in the development of rashes, purpura and ulcers while rarely livedo racemos appears.

Oral manifestations

There are similar mucosal changes to those described on the skin, with single or multiple nodules along the vessels especially in the tongue. Other oral changes noted are erythema, papules, ulceration and haemorrhages.

Immunological aspects of diagnosis

There is no specific immunological diagnostic procedure for polyarteritis nodosa. However, the ESR is usually grossly elevated, a polymorpho-leukocytosis is common and eosinophilia is a further feature.

The serum immunoglobulin levels tend to be raised, especially in the acute phase, and complement levels may be normal or elevated.

Laboratory investigations

There is no specific laboratory test for this condition but histology of clinically involved tissue will confirm the presence of inflammation of the vessel walls with cellular infiltration. Due to the segmental nature of the condition examination of multiple sections may be necessary. Angiography of the affected vessels will demonstrate the presence of nodules and aneurysms, especially at the branching points of the vessels.

In view of the significant association between carrier status for hepatitis B and the development of polyarteritis nodosa patients should be screened for the presence of the antigen and appropriate precautions initiated to prevent transmission if positive.

MYASTHENIA GRAVIS

General considerations

Myasthenia gravis is a condition wherein defective neuromuscular transmission leads to excessive fatiguability. There are several forms of the disorder: the most frequent type is of juvenile/adult onset which has a peak incidence in early adulthood. At that point females are more commonly affected with this autoimmune disease, although after the age of 50 years males show a preponderance. Neonatal myasthenia gravis occurs in babies born to affected mothers, but after a short period there is complete recovery. This presentation has been attributed to the transplacental passage of anti-acetylcholine receptor antibody from maternal plasma. A third form of the disorder, termed congenital myasthenia gravis, manifests between infancy and adolescence but unlike the adult onset form it has been attributed to an inherent defect of the acetylcholine receptor rather than an autoimmune mechanism.

There is no strong hereditary pattern to myasthenia gravis although it occasionally develops either in siblings or in parent and child.

Immunological features

It has been proposed for many years that myasthenia gravis is related to a circulating factor and the presence of neonatal myasthenia gravis in the babies of affected mothers supported this concept. The basic defect in this condition is autoimmune, manifesting at the acetylcholine receptor of the neuromuscular junction. Autoantibodies have been demonstrated to striated muscle, specifically nicotinic acetylcholine receptors, as well as to thymic myoepithelium. Most of these patients have thymic pathology; about 80% show hyperplasia with the appearance of active germinal centres within the medulla, and 20% develop a thymoma.

It does not appear that the immunological abnormalities are secondary to the development of myasthenia. There is no evidence to suggest that the damage to the thymus results from autosensitization to breakdown products of muscle tissues. Similarly there does not appear to be any support for the suggestion that a neuromuscular junction blocking agent is involved. Although it has been suggested that a viral thymitis is the initial step in development of this condition this is not always the case. In young adult onset myasthenia gravis, the presence of HLA-A2, B8 and DR3 are reported in association with thymic hyperplasia, while in those older individuals with thymoma HLA-A2 and HLA-A3 are found more frequently.

A muscle-binding, complement-fixing immunoglobulin has been demonstrated in the serum of patients with myasthenia gravis. The gamma-globulins isolated from these patients appear to be heterogeneous, reacting with several contractile elements of skeletal muscle and also thymic tissue where, by immunofluorescence, this activity was localized to the epithelioid cells in fetal tissue. These cells contain myofilamentous elements and sarcoplasmic features identical with skeletal muscle. This antimuscular factor has been found in 95% of myasthenic patients with a thymoma but in only 30% of remaining patients.

The reaction of affected serum with skeletal muscle has been demonstrated also by agar double-diffusion, haemagglutination and complement fixation. This may reflect more than one type of reactivity and suggests that the anti-muscle factor reacts with the microsomal fraction of skeletal muscle rich in ribonucleoprotein, probably the sarcoplasmic reticulum. Serum from normal subjects can also bind to these sites but in low titres only, with reaction from any of the three major immunoglobulins and no fixation of complement. In contrast, myasthenic patients possess anti-muscle factor which will fix complement and is restricted to the IgG component only. This activity resides in the Fab part of the molecule but not the Fc portion. The reverse obtains in normal subjects and suggests that anti-muscle factor is a significant antibody.

By the use of an immunohistochemical technique it has been shown that serum from myasthenic patients blocks the binding of α-bungarotoxin to extra-junctional receptors: this neurotoxin has a particular affinity for acetylcholine receptors and elution of the serum blocking factor indicates that it is IgG.

In addition approximately 20% of myasthenic patients have anti-nuclear factor occurring in IgA, IgG or IgM and antibodies to double-stranded DNA occur with increased frequency, albeit in the absence of clinical evidence of systemic lupus erythematosus (SLE). However, in some patients myasthenia gravis and SLE do coexist. Overall 20% of myasthenic patients have autoimmune thyroid disease, but this is more common in those with the ocular form of myasthenia gravis.

There is a recorded variability in the complement activity of myasthenic patients. In the majority of the subjects a subnormal level of complement is found during active periods of disease and a low complement activity is also associated with the presence of anti-muscle factor.

The anti-acetylcholine receptor antibodies found in a large proportion of myasthenic patients have the ability to react in vivo at the neuromuscular junction with either nerve or muscle, producing both the defective transmission and morphological abnormalities. Although this hypothesis is gathering increased support from patient studies and animal experiments, the precise event which triggers off the autoimmune response is still unclear.

It may be speculated that environmental and infective agents can either cross-react with the acetylcholine receptor or modify it to become antigenic; this could be initiated at the peripheral neuromuscular junction or centrally within the thymus. In some patients there has been an association between D-penicillamine therapy and the onset of myasthenia gravis, but the mechanism remains unclear.

Although a condition resembling myasthenia gravis in clinical, physiological and pharmacological features has been described in dogs no immunological tests were documented. Injection of bovine thymus or skeletal muscle into guinea pigs has been claimed by one group of workers to cause a form of thymitis associated with alterations in electrophysiological parameters similar to those found in myasthenia gravis. These findings have not been confirmed, and accordingly this proposed model has lost favour.

By injecting acetylcholine receptor derived from the electric eel, *Electrophorus electricus*, into rabbits paralysis developed which frequently led to death. However, repeated stimulation of the peripheral nerves of these animals produced fatigue. The administration of cholinesterase inhibitors resulted in an improvement in the clinical weakness and measured fatiguability. A similar model using rats and guinea pigs has been described; these animals are injected with electric eel acetylcholine receptor as the antigen and have been shown to develop antibodies to this receptor protein. In the rat evidence of antibodies against their own muscle was found along with antibodies to the injected anguillal material. This antibody, presumably to the target tissue, is present in very low titre.

While no definite abnormality of cell-mediated immunity has been established in myasthenia gravis, thymic lymphocytes from patients have been reported to be cytotoxic to fetal muscle. Inhibition of leukocyte migration caused by unidentified muscle antigens has also been reported, and some patients may show a defect in the suppressor lymphocyte population.

Systemic manifestations

The onset of the disease is insidious, with progressive weakness being noted. Frequently the ocular muscles are first affected and the patients report drooping of the eyelids and diplopia. Involvement of the respiratory muscles may eventually necessitate the use of a mechanical ventilator with a consequential susceptibility to repeated chest infections.

The course of the disease is usually prolonged, with irregular progress and even long periods where the severity is stable. In the event of a fatal outcome this usually occurs in the first year of the disease although remission can be expected in about half of the patients with the remainder following a benign course.

The diagnosis of myasthenia gravis may be confirmed by requesting the patient to carry out repeated movement of the affected muscles, e.g. looking at the ceiling when the oculomotor nerves are involved. A similar effect can be elicited by repeated electrical stimulation of the nerve to the affected area.

Oral manifestations

Involvement of the pharyngeal muscles leads to choking and regurgitation of fluids. Abnormal speech with a feeble, mushy voice and nasal tone results; prolonged talking increases muscle weakness and speech then becomes unintelligible. In addition to difficulty with mastication, patients present with an immobile smooth facies. On smiling the lips elevate but do not retract, giving a resemblance to a sneer. The tongue may be weak and furrowed with muscle wasting giving an appearance of a 'trident' tongue on protrusion. Weakness of the masseter muscles may prevent closure of the jaw, and these patients habitually use a hand to support the mandible.

Immunological aspects of diagnosis

Demonstration of circulating anti-muscle and acetylcholine receptor antibody will support a diagnosis of myasthenia gravis.

Laboratory investigations

Biopsy of an affected muscle shows the presence of small round cells, probably lymphocytes, in the muscle fibres. In time areas of muscle degeneration and atrophy will develop with fat replacement of tissue. The motor end-plates are thin and unbranched, with a reduced surface area of filaments, increase in the width of synaptic clefts and reduction of the postsynaptic folds.

Nerve fibre biopsy vitally stained with methylene blue reveals dysplastic abnormalities with marked elongation of the terminal nerve endings and denervating processes. A dystrophic change is found with modification of the subterminal nerve fibres and disorganization of the terminal innervation pattern close to the lymphocyte accumulation at the necrotic fibres. Ultrastructural studies have demonstrated that the density of synaptic vesicles in the nerve endings and width of the synaptic cleft are normal. There is a quantitative reduction in the subneural membrane area with reduction in the secondary folding of the sacrolemmal membrane which is shallow and widened.

Diagnosis of the condition can be confirmed by slow intravenous injection of 10 mg of edrophonium chloride, which will cause a marked improvement in muscle power in the patient within 1 minute. For the test, respiratory resuscitation facilities should be immediately available.

FURTHER READING

Ferguson, M. M. and MacFadyen, E. E. (1986). Oro-facial granulomatosis – a ten year review. *Ann. Acad. Med. (Singapore)*, **15** (In press)

Gell, P. G. H., Coombs, R. R. A. and Lachmann, P. J. (1975). *Clinical Aspects of Immunology*. 3rd edn. (Oxford: Blackwell Scientific Publications)

Isrealson, H., Binnie, W. H. and Hurt, W. C. (1981). The hyperplastic gingivitis of Wegener's granulomatosis. *J. Periodont.*, **52**, 81–7

Scadding, J. G. and Mitchell, D. N. (1985). *Sarcoidosis*. (London: Chapman and Hall)

9
Haematological Diseases with Oral Manifestations

P.-J. LAMEY

PARAPROTEINAEMIAS

Introduction

The paraproteinaemias or monoclonal gammopathies all have in common the monoclonal production of immunoglobulins. Since the over-production is monoclonal from a single tumour stem cell, the immunoglobulins produced all have the same light chains, either kappa or lambda. The commonest paraproteinaemias produce IgG, or IgA or light chain (Bence-Jones) and come under the overall name of myelomatosis (multiple myeloma). The term macroglobulinaemia is used when IgM is produced. IgM paraprotein may be associated with malignant disease (non-Hodgkin's lymphoma, Waldenström's macroglobulinaemia and chronic lymphocytic leukaemia) or benign disorders (cold haemagglutinin disease, rheumatoid arthritis and some lymphoid disorders). In some elderly patients a benign monoclonal gammopathy may be found, and is not necessarily of any significance.

Myelomatosis (multiple myeloma)

General considerations

Myelomatosis is the result of a neoplastic proliferation of plasma cells. The plasma cells replace bone marrow interfering with normal haemopoiesis and produce lytic lesions and sometimes pathological fractures. The disease usually affects the 50–70-year-olds and is commoner in males. Staging of the disease can be undertaken in relation to the myeloma cell burden but complete remission is rarely achieved. Response to treatment can be gauged by clinical response or reduction in paraprotein. Irradiation, chemotherapy

187

and haemodialysis in cases of renal failure are still the treatment of choice. Irradiation aims to reduce the pain of local or extradural deposits. Drug therapy with alkylating agents such as cyclophosphamide or melphalon can be enhanced by corticosteroids. Other therapy may include plasmaphoresis for hyperviscosity. Untreated the median survival is about 12 months, which may be increased only to 24 months with treatment.

Immunological features

In around 50% of cases of myelomatosis it is monoclonal IgG which is produced, constituting the paraprotein (monoclonal gammopathy). The production of the paraprotein reduces normal immunoglobulin production and light chain (Bence-Jones) proteinuria impairs renal function. Interference with clotting factors is common and 15% of cases of IgG myeloma have haemorrhagic manifestations. In patients with IgA myeloma the incidence of haemorrhagic manifestations is 40%. Accompanying the paraproteinaemia is an increased plasma viscosity. Amyloidosis is also an associated feature occurring in 10% of cases.

Systemic manifestations

The clinical features of multiple myeloma result from proliferation of bone marrow plasma cells leading to lytic lesions and paraproteinaemia. Asynchronous production of light chains over heavy chains may result in the appearance of light chains in the urine (Bence-Jones protein). Osteolytic lesions of skull may be asymptomatic, whereas deposits in long bones or spine can produce pathological fractures and vertebral collapse. The hypercalcaemia of bone destruction is an important cause of renal failure. The accompanying hyperviscosity syndrome from high levels of paraprotein may lead to weakness, lethargy and a haemorrhagic tendency.

Oral manifestations

The oral manifestations of myelomatosis may be the result of generalized disease or due to localized plasma cell tumours (plasmacytomas). In myelomatosis a variety of oral changes have been reported. In some cases severe post-extraction bleeding has followed tooth extraction in patients with IgA (kappa light chain) myeloma. This finding is in keeping with the overall increase in bleeding disorders in patients with IgA gammopathy compared with patients with IgG gammopathy. Salivary gland involvement in multiple myeloma has also been described. Benign lymphoepithelial lesion complicating Sjögren's syndrome in a patient with IgG paraproteinaemia is recorded. Localized parotid lesions of plasmacytoma are known and cases of monoclonal B cell neoplasms of parotid gland in Sjögren's syndrome have also been reported, as described in the section on non-Hodgkin's lymphoma.

Amyloidosis may complicate myelomatosis and have oral manifestations. Rare cases of IgD myelomatosis have been associated with macroglossia secondary to amyloidosis. As in other cases of myelomatosis, serum immunoelectrophoresis has confirmed the diagnosis and antisera to light chains has shown the preponderance of kappa light chain production over lambda light chain production.

In some cases oral involvement in IgA–IgM gammopathy has manifested as a solitary tongue mass. Such biclonal gammopathies constitute around 5% of paraproteinaemias and have a known association with lymphoproliferative disorders. It is of interest that even in biclonal gammopathies identical light chains are produced suggesting a 'genetic switch' producing one or other immunoglobulin. A relationship between lymphomatous change and chronic mucocutaneous candidiasis is recognized but the mechanisms involved are unclear. One study showed the presence of a specific serum inhibitor of the immune response to candidal antigen.

Diagnosis and laboratory tests

Diagnosis is based on blood investigation, serum immunoelectrophoresis, urinalysis and skeletal survey interpretation.

The blood picture is of a normochromic normocytic anaemia, with neutropenia and thrombocytopenia in the later stages. Plasma cells may be seen on the blood film and a leukoerythroblastic picture may develop. The ESR is very high except in Bence-Jones myelomatosis. Bone marrow investigations show marrow infiltration with plasma cells. Other reported features include a generalized increase in total protein due to a raised globulin fraction of which the paraprotein is monoclonal on immunoelectrophoresis. Urinalysis may confirm Bence-Jones protein on immunoelectrophoresis. Another common finding on urinalysis is proteinuria.

Waldenström's macroglobulinaemia

General considerations

This rare condition usually affects a similar age group to myelomatosis and is also commoner in males.

The clinical course is variable and the disease may run a benign course for many years. Chlorambucil may be very effective, especially when combined with prednisolone. Initially treatment is aimed at reducing plasma viscosity by plasmaphoresis.

Immunological features

Haemorrhagic manifestations of malignant paraproteinaemias occur frequently. In Waldenström's macroglobulinaemia 60% of patients are likely to experience bleeding complications. Several factors contribute to this haemorrhagic tendency. Thrombocytopenia may be present but more important is abnormal platelet function. The altered platelet function is due to a surface membrane coating of IgG which is in proportion to the serum IgA concentration. A reduction in certain coagulation factors, mostly factor VIII, is also a recognized feature of Waldenström's macroglobulinaemia. The reason for this is unclear, but it is probably due to immunoabsorption by peripheral blood and splenic lymphoid cells. Even if levels of coagulation factors are normal, haemostasis may be impaired by the presence of specific and non-specific inhibitors. The best characterized of these inhibitors interferes with fibrin–monomer polymerization. It is thought that the Fab sites on certain paraproteins bind to fibrin, interfering with normal polymerization. Laboratory tests such as thrombin time become normal when paraprotein levels are reduced, such as by plasmaphoresis.

Systemic manifestions

A wide variety of accompanying clinical features are reported, often related to haemorrhagic tendency and hyperviscosity. The accompanying hyperviscosity can produce renal failure, neurological symptoms and visual disturbance. Other systemic features include lethargy and muscle weakness. In addition, proliferation of lymphoid cells with plasmacytoid features occurs, and lymphadenopathy and splenomegaly (sometimes massive) are commonly found. Unlike multiple myeloma, bony lesions are a rare feature.

Oral manifestations

The principal oral manifestation of Waldenström's macroglobulinaemia are haemorrhage, infection and oral ulceration. Non-specific changes such as oral mucosal pallor have also been reported. The haemorrhagic tendency can lead to gingival bleeding, purpura and prolonged post-extraction haemorrhage. Dental treatment of such patients is best delayed until immediately after plasmaphoresis when the plasma viscosity and subsequent bleeding tendency are optimized.

Mucosal infections have been reported in the condition, but generally are less severe than in leukaemia. Long-term treatment with alkylating agents such as chlorambucil, particularly if combined with corticosteroids, predisposes to viral infections. Viral infections such as herpes simplex should be sought in cases of atypical oral ulceration. Candidal infection can be difficult to eradicate and may require prolonged therapy.

Oral ulceration is a particularly distressing aspect of Waldenström's macroglobulinaemia. The ulcers generally follow accidental trauma such as lip biting and can take weeks to heal. Accompanying oedema is also a feature, and the ulcers are deep. Local measures such as the use of covering agents have limited success and Gram-negative organisms contribute in some cases. Regular chlorhexidine usage has been advocated but a few patients are sensitive to this agent.

Diagnosis and laboratory tests

Typically there is a monoclonal overproduction of IgM. Diagnosis depends on demonstrating serum IgM paraproteins on immunoelectrophoresis. A minority of patients also have Bence-Jones proteinuria. The peripheral blood picture is similar to multiple myeloma with normochromic normocytic anaemia and marked rouleaux formation secondary to protein changes. Bone marrow studies show an excess of plasmacytoid lymphocytes.

Amyloidosis

General considerations

It is now generally believed that amyloid deposition involves proteolytic cleavage of an abnormal precursor protein, but why susceptible patients develop amyloidosis is unclear. Once formed amyloid deposits were traditionally thought to be relatively inert, but well-documented cases of disappearance of AA amyloidosis have been reported.

The prognosis in systemic amyloidosis is poor and management centres around treatment of the associated disease. Drug regimes involving melphalan, prednisolone and fluoxymesterone have reported clinical and histological improvement. In cases of renal failure, renal transplantation may be indicated.

Immunological features

Amyloidosis is currently classified into a systemic and localized form. This classification has replaced older clinical classifications and is based on biochemical knowledge of the composition of amyloid fibrils (Table 9.1). In paraproteinaemias the amyloid light chains (AL) are whole immunoglobulin light chains or fragments of it. The amyloid protein AA, and its serum counterpart SAA, are most commonly seen in conditions such as rheumatoid arthritis and Crohn's disease and may play a role in the pathogenesis of these conditions. Other amyloid fibril proteins have been found in familial studies (AF). In localized amyloidosis secondary to medullary carcinoma of the thyroid (AE_t) the amino acid sequence shows homology with calcitonin. Fibrinogen, complement and lipoprotein are also found in amyloid deposits.

Systemic manifestations

Since the extracellular deposition of amyloid protein can occur in any tissue there are many reported systemic manifestations. Deposition in vital organs is considered irreversible and therefore systemic amyloidosis is usually fatal. Clearly patients may have symptoms from the conditions accompanying amyloidosis.

Table 9.1 Classification of amyloidosis based on amyloid fibril protein composition (after Hind and Pepys, 1984)

	Amyloid fibril	Serum protein
1. Systemic amyloidosis		
A. Immunocyte dyscrasia	AL	Ig light chain
Monoclonal gammopathy		
Multiple myeloma		
Waldenström's macroglobulinaemia		
B. Reactive systemic amyloidosis	AA	SAA
C. Heredofamilial systemic amyloidosis		
Neuropathic forms		
Non-neuropathic forms	AF	Prealbumin
Familial Mediterranean fever	AA	SAA
2. Localized amyloidosis		
Plasmacytomas	AL	Ig light chain
Endocrine (medullary carcinoma,		
thyroid, insulinoma)	AE_t	Calcitonin

Renal involvement may take the form of nephrotic syndrome or renal failure. Gastrointestinal involvement can lead to malabsorption and weight loss. Hepatomegaly is common, as is pulmonary involvement, but this is usually asymptomatic. Skin lesions are seen as waxy lesions around the perineum, axilla or eyelids which may bleed on pressure.

Oral manifestations

The orofacial region may show features of skin involvement in amyloidosis. Cranial nerve lesions have also been described. Intra-orally xerostomia is said to be a feature following salivary gland involvement and one case of localized amyloidosis presented as apparent Sjögren's syndrome. Gingival involvement with hypertrophy and haemorrhagic bullae may be present, which rupture producing ulcers. Tongue involvement is probably the commonest intra-oral feature with macroglossia and reduced tongue mobility often being described. Localized amyloid deposits can affect any part of the oral cavity.

Diagnosis and laboratory tests

Biopsy of an affected site, e.g. tongue or salivary gland, stained with Conga Red shows the characteristic apple-green birefringence when viewed in polarized light. Other stains such as thioflavine T have been used, but are not specific. At the ultrastructural level the deposits consist of paired filaments, and binding to elastin has been demonstrated. Of interest in relation to the pattern of amyloid deposition is the finding that the nonfibrillar glycoprotein known as amyloid P is a normal feature of glomerular basement membranes and elastic microfibrils in blood vessel walls.

Heavy chain disease

General considerations

This disease is extremely rare in the Western world and is more often seen in patients of Middle Eastern descent. Three variants are recognized namely γ chain disease, α chain disease and μ chain disease. The α chain disease variant is more common. Heavy chain disease is basically a variant of myelomatosis.

Immunological features

The disease itself is the result of the production of abnormal heavy chains of immunoglobulins in some cases related to chronic lymphatic leukaemia (μ chain disease) or to a lymphoma-type illness (α chain and γ chain disease). Eventually the disease is fatal in most cases and is almost always associated with malignant B-cell neoplasia which is then treated on its merits.

Systemic manifestations

In γ chain disease recurrent infections occur and clinically patients have a painful lymphadenopathy. The condition often presents as a malignant soft-tissue plasmocytoma. Hepatosplenomegaly is another feature of γ chain disease and this does not occur in α chain disease. In the latter condition patients present with severe malabsorption syndrome and barium follow-through studies show a stove-pipe-like involvement of the small intestine. Intestinal lymphomas have also been reported. In addition, these patients have a high serum IgA with almost absent IgG and IgM. Spontaneous remission has been noted in some patients. The μ chain disease may be another finding in patients with otherwise typical chronic lymphatic leukaemia.

Oral manifestations

There are no specific oral manifestations of heavy chain disease but a peculiar form of palatal oedema has been noted in cases of γ chain disease. The α chain disease protein has been detected in saliva. In μ chain disease the oral changes would be expected to be those of chronic lymphatic leukaemia. Since the patients are unable to produce antibodies normally, they are prone to infection.

Diagnosis and laboratory tests

Diagnosis depends on the demonstration of an abnormal protein in serum and urine. The protein produced consists of the heavy chains of the IgG molecule which are secreted unconjugated into the circulation. Bone marrow investigations may demonstrate atypical plasma cells.

Cryoglobulinaemia

General considerations

This condition occurs in association with various underlying diseases and treatment is aimed at the underlying disease. Several types of cryoglobulins are recognized but all have the property of precipitation or gel formation at temperatures below 37 °C. The globulins may or may not be monoclonal.

The management of patients with cryoglobulinaemia is currently unsatisfactory but in severe cases splenectomy has been effective, particularly if preceded by plasmaphoresis.

Immunological features

Type I, in which isolated monoclonal paraproteins or light chains are found, is associated with myelomatosis and macroglobulinaemia. In Type II a mixture of cryoglobulins and immunoglobulins is found which may be monoclonal, and this type is nearly always associated with non-Hodgkin's lymphoma. Type III disease has a mixture of several classes of polyclonal immunoglobulins and non-immunoglobulin molecules including complement. The disease is associated with systemic lupus erythematosus (SLE) but may also be associated with certain infections.

Cryoproteins in patients with SLE are known to be rich in antibodies to single-stranded DNA (ss-DNA) and double-stranded DNA (ds-DNA). The detection of cryoproteins in patients with viral hepatitis and infectious mononucleosis has led to the suggestion that serum cryoprecipitation is related to the presence of immune complexes. An association between cryoproteins and hypocomplementaemia is recorded, possibly because cryoprecipitates activate complement by the classical and alternative pathway at least *in vitro*.

Systemic manifestations

The clinical features of cryoglobulinaemia are due to circulating abnormalities induced by cold or due to the hyperviscosity syndrome. In severe cases Raynaud's syndrome or even gangrene may be clinical features. The hyperviscosity syndrome is again associated with a haemorrhagic tendency since high serum paraprotein levels result in platelet coating with resultant abnormalities in platelet function. Such patients have low platelet adhesion, impaired clot retraction and a long bleeding time. General management involves keeping the patient warm and avoiding unnecessary cold exposure. Cytotoxic drug therapy improves about one-third of patients. Patients who have the disease for 10 years or more may develop lymphoma.

Oral manifestations

Since cryoglobulinaemia has several recognized types, the manifestations of the associated disease may be present. Type I oral manifestations in myelomatosis and macroglobulinaemia are discussed elsewhere. The Type II form of the disease has the orofacial manifestations of non-Hodgkin's lymphoma. These include oral change due to anaemia and thrombocytopenia secondary to bone involvement. Secondary immune deficiency predisposes to infection with viruses and opportunistic organisms. Rarely tumour deposits themselves may present in the oral cavity as submucosal swellings or rapidly growing neoplasms. The association of Type III lesion with connective tissue disease including systemic lupus erythematosus (SLE) means that the oral features are those of the underlying disease. In SLE the oral features are of white lesions and oral ulceration. Antinuclear factor (ANF) has long been recognized as a major immunological abnormality in SLE, and as such is a routine investigation.

Diagnosis and laboratory tests

Study of the cryoprecipitates of patients with rheumatoid arthritis and Sjögren's syndrome has characterized the cryoproteins as containing IgG, IgM, IgA and the complement proteins C1q, C4, C3 and Factor B (hence haemolysis). It has been proposed that the immune complex nature of these cryoglobulins may be responsible for clinical features of vasculitis. Other reports of patients with vasculitis, Sjögren's syndrome and IgA–IgG cryoglobulinaemia terminating in immunoblastic sarcoma have appeared in the literature.

Rarely patients with IgG cryoglobulinaemia are described in which the patient's only oral symptoms have been of recurrent aphthous ulceration. In such cases of 'essential cryoglobulinaemia' the oral ulcerations have been assumed to be a manifestation of cold sensitivity. Similar cryoglobulins have been described in patients with Behçet's syndrome.

LEUKAEMIA

General considerations

The aetiology of leukaemia in man is currently unknown, but various factors have been proposed. Genetic studies have shown a slight familial tendency and a high concordance in monozygotic twins. In patients with known chromosomal abnormalities such as Down's syndrome (trisomy of chromosome 21), the incidence of leukaemia is about 30 times that expected. Irradiation damage following excessive exposure or atomic bomb blasts is associated with an increased incidence. Radiotherapy, especially combined with chemotherapy, has led to leukaemia in some patients with malignant disease and with ankylosing spondylitis. In cats leukaemia virus is a well-documented cause of the disease but evidence in man for a viral aetiology is also accumulating.

Leukaemias arise from a malignant clone of myeloid or lymphoid stem cells. They are divided into acute and chronic types and arise during the process of differentiation of stem cells. In acute leukaemias the clone of cells is primitive (blast cell) involving the myeloid series (acute myeloblastic leukaemia or AML) or the lymphoid series (acute lymphoblastic or ALL). AML can be divided into seven types using morphological criteria (Table 9.2). ALL is also divided into several categories on the basis of cytochemical techniques and certain immunological cell membrane characteristics.

Table 9.2 Morphological classification of oral myeloblastic leukaemia (after Chessels and Pawles, 1983)

Subcategory	Cell characteristics
M0	Undifferentiated (AUL)
M1	Undifferentiated with few cells differentiated (AUL)
M2	Acute myeloblastic leukaemia (AUL)
M3	Promyelocytic leukaemia (A Prol L)
M4	Acute myelomonoblastic leukaemia (AMML)
M5	Acute monoblastic leukaemia (AMoL)
M6	Erythroleukaemia (EL)

For acute myeloid leukaemia (AML) combination chemotherapy with daunorubicin, cytosine arabinoside and 6-thioguanine has been widely employed but some centres favour a four-drug regime in combination; an anthracycline (daunorubicin or adriamycin) cytosine arabinoside, vincristine and prednisolone. The results of these regimes have meant complete remission rates for AML of 75%, although older patients tend to have a poorer prognosis. Other figures suggest that around 45% of patients will remain in remission for 3 or more years and 20% of patients continue in complete remission for 3–10 years.

In acute lymphoblastic leukaemia (ALL) the prognosis is less favourable than for patients with AML. Five years survival studies of 60% have been quoted but other groups report the duration of first remission to be 10–25 months even with prophylactic cerebrospinal chemotherapy in addition to conventional chemotherapy. Clearly, the understanding of the HLA system has been of immense significance but various techniques such as depletion of alloreactive T cells from the graft *in vitro* are being studied, since in almost 50% of patients an HLA identical sibling donor is not available.

Prognosis within childhood ALL depends to some extent on the type of ALL. In B-cell ALL the 5-year survival is zero compared with 70% of patients with C-(common)-ALL. Many trials are currently evaluating the wider use of bone marrow transplantation (BMT) and in particular hope to reduce the incidence of graft-versus-host disease (GVHD) with allogenic transplantation.

Radiotherapy seeks to aid eradication of leukaemic tissue just as bone marrow transplantation (BMT) aims to completely ablate normal and leukaemic marrow prior to infusing compatible bone marrow. Bone marrow transplantation is used in AML, ALL and acute non-lymphoblastic leukaemia (ANL), but is also of value in a range of otherwise fatal congenital and acquired haemopoieitic and lymphoid diseases. There is current debate about the relative effectiveness of BMT over prolonged chemotherapy in acute leukaemia. Immunosuppression generally is also said to be associated with an increased incidence of leukaemia.

Of chronic myeloid leukaemia (CML), chronic granulocytic (CGL) is the commonest, although it only accounts for about 15% of all cases of leukaemia. It is thought to arise by somatic mutation of a pluripotential haemopoietic stem cell.

Chronic lymphatic leukaemia (CLL) constitutes about 25% of all leukaemias and is twice as common in men than women. It has no known aetiology and is the one major type of leukaemia not associated with ionizing radiation.

Prognosis in CGL and CLL is variable with a range of months to more than 10 years. Busulphan is the treatment of choice in CGL and whole-body irradiation with BMT has yielded disappointing results. In CLL, chlorambucil is widely used and corticosteroids undoubtedly reduce the leukaemic cell mass but at the risk of infections. Death in CLL is usually due to infection as a result of bone marrow failure and combined cell-mediated and humoral immunodeficiency.

Immunological features

In acute myeloid leukaemia blast cells react positively for an anti-Ia-like antigen. Detailed studies of platelet function in acute leukaemia and myelodysplastic (preleukaemia) syndromes have shown morphological abnormal granules, defective thromboxane A_2 synthesis and deficient binding sides for thrombin. A factor V deficiency has been described in patients with untreated chronic myeloid leukaemia and correction of this defect may allow control of intractable bleeding. The immunological features of ALL depend on the type of ALL, and there are differences between the childhood and adult (>15 years) forms of the disease. Thus in common-ALL reaction with anti-ALL antiserum is positive whilst it is negative in null-ALL. In both these forms cells are negative for B and T cell markers which would be positive in T-ALL.

Morphologically the lymphocytes in CLL are identical to normal small lymphocytes but are obviously present in greater numbers. In nearly all cases the lymphocytes are B-cell in nature having surface bound IgM and IgD and membrane receptors for the Fc fragment of IgG and C3.

Systemic manifestations

The symptoms of acute leukaemia arise acutely or subacutely. Nearly all symptoms arise as a result of bone marrow replacement. Patients have visual disturbance from retinal haemorrhages, exhibit purpura, or are pyrexial from infection or even septicaemic. Other complaints include bone pain, joint pain due to hyperuricaemia, headaches from meningeal deposits, or have non-specific complaints such as weight loss, anorexia or weakness. Rare cases of recurrent parotid enlargement in children have been reported as the initial presenting feature of acute myeloid leukaemia. On examination, lymphadenopathy is common, as is splenomegaly and tonsillar enlargement, especially in ALL patients who may be found in addition to have a mediastinal mass.

In chronic myeloid leukaemia the onset is insidious with lethargy, weakness, anorexia and bone pain. Abnormal bleeding due to abnormal platelet function can occur, as can gout (rarely) and abdominal discomfort due to splenomegaly or splenic infarct. As many as 10% of cases of chronic leukaemia are diagnosed by routine blood tests done for other reasons. In CLL, physical examination may be entirely negative.

Oral manifestations

Oral manifestations of leukaemia are amongst the commonest features of acute leukaemia and are also a feature of chronic leukaemia. The principal oral lesions encountered in acute leukaemia are mucosal infections, oral ulceration and haemorrhagic phenomena. The gingival tissues may be infiltrated with leukaemic cells and be obviously enlarged, and this phenomenon may lead to local circulatory stasis and thrombosis. Clearly such changes would further compromise tissue resistance.

Gingival enlargement in leukaemia arises from infiltration of the tissues with leukaemic cells. It is said particularly to occur in acute monocytic leukaemia but also occurs in other forms of acute leukaemia and in chronic leukaemia. Histological studies on gingival biopsy specimens have, however, suggested that leukaemic infiltration of gingival tissues is uncommon, occurring only in around 4% of patients. Gingival infiltration, although more commonly found in dentate patients, has also been reported in edentulous patients. Patients with gingival enlargement usually also complain of gingival pain. A feature of patients with leukaemia is the relative lack of inflammatory response even in cases with poor oral hygiene. Other gingival changes have been reported in leukaemia treated with chemotherapy, and take the form of a generalized white appearance, perhaps due to altered cell turnover.

In the pre-antibiotic era extensive tissue necrosis and osteomyelomitis were common after dental extractions. With the widespread use of chemotherapeutic agents in the treatment of leukaemia an additional factor, namely drug-induced mucosal toxicity, has also to be considered. Rather surprisingly, scant attention has been paid to the relationship between oral mucosal lesions and circulatory leukocyte function or the thrombocytopenia which often accompanies leukaemia, even though remission of leukaemia is accompanied by resolution of the oral lesions. One author has recently described a specific form of oral ulceration, 'neutropenic ulceration', in patients with leukaemia.

The importance of oral infections in leukaemic patients cannot be underestimated and many centres liaise with Oral Medicine Units in the management of such patients. The oral cavity may be a source of serious, even fatal, infections in such patients but conclusive proof is lacking. Fungal infection due to *Candida* species or more rarely *Aspergillus flavus* and *Cryptococcus neoformans* are common, both in BMT patients and in leukaemics receiving chemotherapy. Established oropharyngeal fungal infections should be eliminated as a relationship between disseminated fungal infections, including those of the lower gastrointestinal tract, has been postulated.

Viral infections, particularly those of the herpes virus group (herpes simplex, herpes zoster, cytomegalovirus and Epstein–Barr virus), occur in patients with acute and chronic leukaemia. Two extensive series of leukaemic patients reported an incidence of approximately 60 per 1000 patients. Diagnostic difficulty can arise, however, as the presentation can be atypical with superimposed infection with *Candida* species and Gram-negative bacteria. Careful methods of virus detection therefore need to be employed, and virus infection should be suspected in patients with oral ulceration which shows little tendency to heal. Some patients suffer severe herpes simplex infections with each bout of chemotherapy, and may require prophylactic antiviral therapy.

Haemorrhagic disorders affecting the oral cavity are common in leukaemic patients. Infection also contributes towards abnormal bleeding, as with a given platelet count bleeding is more likely if the patient has a serious infection. A figure of 60% has been quoted, and oral bleeding and bruising is a reasonable indicator of thrombocytopenia. Other factors may also be operating to enhance the likelihood of oral bleeding; for example platelet dysfunction in disseminated intravascular coagulation.

In BMT patients, GVHD may have other oral complications. Reduced salivary gland function with xerostomia and rampant dental caries has been reported, as have oral lichenoid reactions.

Diagnostic and laboratory tests

Blood and bone marrow investigations are clearly central to the diagnosis of leukaemia. Thus in C-(common)-ALL, which is the commonest type in children, the leukaemic blast cells resemble neither T nor B lymphocytes, but react with antisera against non-T and non-B-ALL. In contrast, in T-cell

ALL blasts react like mature T cells with sheep erythrocytes to form E rosettes. In both these forms of ALL the blast cells have high levels of the enzyme terminal deoxynucleotidyl transferase (TdT). In the rare B-cell ALL, which is refractory to chemotherapy, the blast cells show monoclonal surface immunoglobulins. In acute myeloid leukaemia so-called Auer rods in the cells are unique to AML. Cells in AML exhibit no response to common-ALL antiserum and carry no surface immunoglobulin or E receptors, therefore no rosette formation with sheep red cells.

In chronic myeloid leukaemia, karyotypic analysis often shows the Philadelphia chromosome (Ph') in which chromosome 22 has lost part of the long arm and it is usually translocated to chromosome 9. The Ph' chromosome characterizes leukaemic precursor cells of granulocytes, erythrocytes, megakaryocytes and monocytes. The differential count shows greatly increased absorbed numbers of neutrophils, metamyelocytes, myelocytes, promyelocytes and blast cells. Other blood investigations show high serum vitamin B_{12} levels as a result of increased production of transcobalamin 1 by the expanded granulocyte mass. Other variants of CML are recognized such as atypical (Philadelphia chromosome negative) CGL, chronic neutrophilic leukaemia and eosinophilic leukaemia, but all are rare.

LYMPHOMA

It is convenient to consider leukaemias and lymphomas together since both can be thought of in terms of the development of the lymphocyte from a primitive lymphoid precursor in the bone marrow to the mature T and B cell. Leukaemias are tumours which occur during the differentiation process; that is the process of moving through immature stages before reaching the mature phenotype. Lymphomas are tumours which arise during the transformation process; that is the functional development of the cell once it has achieved the mature phenotype. Overlap between leukaemia and lymphoma occurs in a malignant leukaemia–lymphoma of mature T cells. This condition has an acute onset in adults and is associated with a retrovirus (HTLV).

Hodgkin's disease

General considerations

Lymphomas are currently the seventh commonest malignancy in Britain. The diagnosis of Hodgkin's disease requires lymph node biopsy which allows histological classification (Table 9.3) and demonstration of Reed–Sternberg cells. Staging of the disease is then undertaken, usually involving a laparotomy (pathological staging) and a skeletal survey with chest radiographs. A complete clinical examination with careful attention to Waldeyer's ring is also undertaken. Disease extent is designated Stage I if a single lymph node region is involved, Stage II involves two or more lymph node regions on the same side of the diaphragm, Stage III involves both sides of the diaphragm and Stage IV indicates disseminated involvement. Staging decides treatment, as Stage I disease usually involves radiotherapy only and all other stages involve irradiation with combination therapy. The cure rate in Stage I disease approaches 100% and even in Stage IV disease is of the order of 20–40%.

Table 9.3   Histological classification of Hodgkin's disease (after Lukes and Collins, 1975)

Classification	Prognosis	Incidence in Europeans (%)
Lymphocytic predominance	Good	10
Nodular sclerosis	Good	60
Mixed cellularity	Good	25
Lymphocytic depletion	Poor	5

Immunological features

The histogenesis of Hodgkin's disease is still not fully understood. Previously Reed–Sternberg cells were considered similar to transformed lymphocytes which, since they contained cytoplasmic immunoglobulin, favoured a B-lymphocyte origin. Later studies, however, showed the immunoglobulin to include both light chains and to probably result from cell uptake along with other serum proteins. Immunohistochemical studies of fibronectin and α_1-antitrypsin are more suggestive of the Reed–Sternberg cells being derived from monocytes. Accompanying Hodgkin's disease are disturbances of T lymphocyte function which are restored by successful treatment.

Systemic manifestations

The commonest presentation of Hodgkin's disease is of painless enlarging cervical, axillary or inguinofemoral lymphadenopathy. The age groups most affected are early adult life and a second peak after the age of 50. Less commonly lymphatic enlargement causes pain or venous or tracheal compression. Other features on presentation are weight loss, fever, night sweats and fatigue. Alcohol ingestion may make the lymphadenopathy painful, possibly due to hyperaemia of the affected nodes.

It is common for patients to suffer from a variety of infections, such as herpes zoster associated with the disease itself or to its treatment.

Oral manifestations

The oral mucosa is rarely directly involved in Hodgkin's disease, although, of course, cervical lymphadenopathy is common. Rare cases of Hodgkin's disease presenting with an oral ulcer or swelling are reported, and intra-bony involvement is also recorded. Oral infections can, however, arise in patients with Hodgkin's disease secondary to a reduced immune response or to the effects of radiotherapy or chemotherapy. In particular, T cell deficiency seems likely on clinical grounds because of the susceptibility of these patients to tubercle infections and herpes zoster infections.

A recent prospective study of patients with Hodgkin's disease reported 16% of patients to have histological involvement of Waldeyer's lymphoid tissue. Some centres now advocate such a biopsy to be routinely included in the staging procedure.

Diagnosis and laboratory tests

The diagnosis of lymphoma is made by means of lymph node biopsy, by bone marrow biopsy or less commonly by biopsy of an extranodal tumour. Typically Reed–Sternberg cells are present on lymph node biopsy. The other histological features allow categorization into the four histological types of lymphocyte predominant, nodular sclerotic, mixed cellularity and lymphocyte depleted. Other laboratory tests are often normal but a moderate normochromic normocytic anaemia may be present, as may autoimmune haemolytic anaemia. Analysis of the white cell series commonly shows neutrophilia, lymphopenia and occasionally eosinophilia. Marrow infiltration would be suspected if a blood film showed a leukoerythroblastic picture. An elevated ESR usually indicates disease activity. Hyperuricaemia reflects cell proliferation and catabolism. Other investigations are required for staging, such as a chest radiograph, skeletal survey or abdominal lymphangiogram.

Non-Hodgkin's lymphoma

General considerations

The currently used classification for non-Hodgkin's lymphomas is shown in Table 9.4. The majority of non-Hodgkin's lymphomas are B cell in type but others, such as Sezary syndrome and mycosis fungoides, are T cell. Although the term histiocytic is retained it is now recognized that most cells thus designated are not true histiocytes but are of lymphoid origin. In general, those tumours which are either lymphocytic diffuse or lymphocytic nodular carry the best prognosis.

Immunological features

The cutaneous T cell lymphomas will not be discussed in detail since, for example, only 1% of all lymphoma deaths are due to mycosis fungoides. Oral involvement in mycosis fungoides has been reported but only occurs in

202

Table 9.4 Histological classification of non-Hodgkin's lymphoma

Old terminology	New simplified terminology
Lymphosarcoma	Lymphocytic lymphoma (diffuse)
Follicular lymphoma	Lymphocytic/lymphohistiocytic lymphoma (nodular)
Reticulum cell sarcoma	Histiocytic lymphoma
Chronic lymphocytic leukaemia	Chronic lymphocytic leukaemia
Waldenström's macroglobulinaemia	Macroglobulinaemia
Mycosis fungoides	Mycosis fungoides
Sezary syndrome	Sezary syndrome
Burkitt's lymphoma	Burkitt's lymphoma

advanced disease in previously diagnosed patients. Immunological studies of such T cell tumours has provided two contrasting theories on aetiology. One theory suggests that such neoplasms are from the outset malignant, and that the thymus may play a role. The implication of this theory is that the skin is an important physiological site for T cells and may be responsible for post-thymic differentiation of T cells. Another theory proposes that the T cells are persistently activated by antigen after immunological presentation by Langerhans cells. Chronic and continual immunological stimulation of T cells then produces a malignant clone of T cells which eventually predominate the histological picture.

Burkitt's lymphoma, although a B cell neoplasm, will also not be discussed in detail. The orofacial manifestations of the condition are well documented. A relationship to Epstein–Barr (EB) virus is well described. One suggestion is that EB virus enters B lymphocytes (T cells do not have the necessary receptors to allow entry of the virus) and on reaching the nucleus the B cells demonstrate surface EB virus antigens. Since affected patients are also malnourished and have other chronic conditions such as malaria, the EB virus takes over a population of B lymphocytes and uncontrolled growth of B cell clone gives rise to a tumour population presenting clinically as a B cell lymphoma.

Systemic manifestations

As in other lymphomas patients with non-Hodgkin's lymphoma may present with lymph node enlargement including Waldeyer's ring. The lymphocytic nodular form of the disease usually occurs in middle-aged adults. Unlike in Hodgkin's disease, it is uncommon for one lymph node group to be involved, and widespread lymph node enlargement including retro-peritoneal or mesenteric nodes is more usual. The lymphadenopathy is painless and may have been present for years before medical attention is sought. Enlargement of the spleen is common but usually asymptomatic. Bone marrow is involved in 70% of cases on trephine iliac crest biopsy. Other symptoms of fever, night sweats and weight loss may appear.

Oral manifestations

There are no specific oral manifestations of non-Hodgkin's lymphoma. Rare cases have been reported of patients presenting with pericoronitis and tooth displacement, and even with toothache alone. As in leukaemia, anaesthesia or parathesiae of the lip may be presenting features and always warrant further investigation. In fact, any oral complaint or multiple complaints which do not appear typical should raise the suspicion of underlying systemic disease.

Another group of patients in whom non-Hodgkin's lymphoma is important are patients with Sjögren's syndrome. Many reports in the literature have shown a relationship between the development of malignant lymphoma and Sjögren's syndrome. In these patients lymphomas appear to arise in the parotid salivary glands, particularly in patients with previous parotid gland enlargement treated with radiotherapy. Generally, immunohistochemical studies have shown the lymphomas to be B cell lymphomas. Many of these patients later develop extrasalivary malignant lymphoma of the same histology. Other lymphomas, some monoclonal, have also been reported, as have pseudolymphomas in this group. Occasionally, Sjögren's syndrome and paraproteinaemia are present in the same patient. Since the parotid gland developmentally includes intrasalivary lymph nodes it is not surprising that the malignant lymphomas, including Burkitt's lymphoma, have arisen at this site. In such cases, however, there is no evidence of the salivary histological change usually seen in Sjögren's syndrome.

Diagnosis and laboratory tests

Biopsy of the affected lymphoid tissue is essential to allow classification of the type of non-Hodgkin's lymphoma. Staging of the disease is of less value than in Hodgkin's disease, as it is usually disseminated. Other laboratory investigations are as for Hodgkin's disease. Anaemia may be an accompanying feature and a raised ESR crudely reflects disease activity. A blood film may show atypical lymphocytes and perhaps circulating malignant lymphoid cells.

IDIOPATHIC THROMBOCYTOPENIC PURPURA

General considerations

Idiopathic thrombocytopenic purpura (ITP) or, as some authors prefer, autoimmune thrombocytopenic purpura, occurs in acute, chronic and hereditary forms. Patients with the condition have a thrombocytopenia of varying severity and normal or increased megakaryocytes in the bone marrow. In other respects the cellular constituents of the blood are normal.

In acute ITP rapid recovery occurs in 80–85% of cases. Bed rest is often advocated and some patients require steroid therapy for overt haemorrhage or persistently low platelet counts (less than 10×10^9/l). Platelet transfusion has a place in the acute management of severe or life-threatening haemorrhage. Intravenous immunoglobulin is another treatment option.

For chronic ITP systemic steroids also have a role, but splenectomy is regarded as the treatment of choice (except in mild cases) because the spleen is an important site for anti-platelet autoantibody production. Splenectomy is contraindicated in acute ITP in children because of the likelihood of serious infections developing. The clinical course of chronic ITP is unpredictable and lasting remission is less common than in acute ITP.

In Wiskott–Aldrich syndrome prognosis is poor and bone marrow transplantation only cures a small number of cases. Survival has, however, been improved in splenectomized children given long-term prophylactic antibiotics. Splenectomy normalizes platelet count and survival but the prophylactic antibiotics are essential to decrease the risk of infection, particularly with *Haemophilus influenzae*.

Immunological features

The acute form of ITP occurs in children, usually aged 2–6 years, and affects males and females equally. The condition is of sudden onset and in preceding 1–2 weeks patients have often suffered from a viral infection. Some authors have demonstrated that following viral infection, e.g. mumps, the platelet membrane has soluble immune complexes attached to it consisting of viral particles and antiviral immunoglobulin. The immune complexes either directly damage platelets or cause them to be destroyed by the reticuloendothelial system. Over 80% of cases of acute ITP resolve in 2–3 weeks but a proportion of the remainder may progress to chronic ITP.

Chronic ITP principally affects adults, is commoner in females than males (3 : 1) and has an insidious onset over several years. This form is considered to be an autoimmune disorder in which autoantibodies, mainly of the IgG class, are formed to constituents of the platelet surface. It appears that platelet production in chronic ITP is not depressed but platelet survival is markedly shortened from the normal 6 10 days to only a few hours.

Hereditary thrombocytopenia comprises a group of syndromes which present early in life and are all exceedingly rare. The best characterized of this group of conditions is the Wiskott–Aldrich syndrome. In this disorder prognosis is poor and platelets show a decreased survival time as well as deficient production. The bone marrow shows normal megakaryocyte numbers.

Systemic manifestations

Acute ITP, since it commonly follows viral infection (in 85% of cases) is more common in Spring when viral infections are prevalent. A wide variety of viral illnesses has been reported, including mumps, infectious mononucleosis, rubella and chickenpox; vaccination against measles, tetanus and pertussis has also been implicated in acute ITP. Haematemesis, haematuria, melaena, epistaxis and petechiae on non-exposed body surfaces are all common presentations. The clinical features may initially suggest non-accidental injury. Intracranial haemorrhage is a rare presentation, and in these cases platelet levels are very low. Physical examination is frequently unremarkable with only minimal lymphadeno-pathy and splenomegaly. This is in contrast to children with thrombocyto-penia secondary to acute leukaemia or aplastic anaemia.

Chronic ITP may have clinical features similar to acute ITP but it is insidious in onset and a precipitating cause has not been identified (Table 9.5). In addition to the clinical features of acute ITP in childhood, menorrhagia is common. Physical examination is unremarkable and the patient feels generally well.

Table 9.5 Summary of acute and chronic ITP

Patients affected	Acute (children)	Chronic (adults)
Female to male ratio	1:1	3:1
Duration of condition	Weeks	Years
Onset	Sudden	Insidious
Clinical course	Recovery	Unpredictable
Immunology	Viral immune complexes	Anti-platelet antibody

Hereditary thrombocytopenias are all rare and tend to present in the neonatal period. The best characterized, Wiskott–Aldrich syndrome, is an X-linked recessive condition and therefore occurs in boys. Clinical features include bloody diarrhoea and purpura, although susceptibility to a variety of infections and eczema later develop. There is also a tendency to lymphoproliferative malignancy. Recently bone marrow transplantation has been successful in a small number of such cases.

Oral manifestations

The oral manifestations are due to thrombocytopenia and can resemble thrombocytopenia from other causes, e.g. leukaemia. In acute ITP areas of palatal or buccal submucosal purpura or petechiae have been reported at the time of presentation in these patients.

In patients with chronic ITP wearing complete dentures, petechiae and ecchymoses may occur beneath the denture-bearing area. Like acute ITP, excessive bleeding after trauma or surgery is an important presentation in chronic ITP.

Diagnosis and laboratory tests

In acute ITP a blood count shows quite severe thrombocytopenia, i.e. below $50 \times 10^9/l$. Characteristically bone marrow examination shows normal or increased numbers of megakaryocytes. These megakaryocytes tend to show increased immature forms together with a variety of morphological abnormalities of size and vacuolation. Clinical examination and blood film examination exclude other causes of thrombocytopenia such as aplastic anaemia, leukaemia and haemolytic uraemic syndrome. In the differential diagnosis, disseminated intravascular coagulation will show a prolonged prothrombin time, thromboplastin time and thrombin time, all of which are normal in ITP.

Chronic ITP has a picture similar to acute ITP but the magnitude is usually less severe $(50-100 \times 10^9/l)$. Other investigations are as for acute ITP, and as always a drug history is important since many drugs can produce thrombocytopenia (Table 9.6). It is appropriate to perform an antinuclear and DNA antibody screen for systemic lupus erythematosus (SLE) since the overlap between ITP and SLE is strong and ITP may antedate SLE. Thrombocytopenia is, however, uncommon in SLE, occurring in less than 5% of cases. Specialized tests have demonstrated platelet autoantibodies but are not in routine clinical use, and the diagnosis of ITP remains one of exclusion.

In the Wiskott–Aldrich syndrome purpura is usually present in the neonatal period or even at birth. Thrombocytopenia is present and the platelets themselves are smaller than normal. Bone marrow investigations show normal or reduced megakaryocyte numbers.

Table 9.6 Drugs causing thrombocytopenia by antibody-mediated and non-antibody-mediated mechanisms (after Miescher and Graf, 1980)

Drug class	Antibody-mediated	Non-antibody-mediated
Antimicrobials	Penicillin Sulphonamides Trimethoprin Rifampicin Cephalothin	Streptomycin Tetracyclines Methicillin Chloroquine
Antidiabetic		Tolbutamide Chlorpropamide
Diuretics	Chlorthiazide Frusemide	
Antithyroid		Propylthiouracil
Antidepressants	Phenothiazine	Chlorpromazine
Others	Acetazolamide Heparin	Methyldopa L-dopa

PERNICIOUS ANAEMIA

General considerations

Pernicious anaemia (PA) is a worldwide disease but appears to be more common in northern Europe. The incidence increases with age, reaching 2–3 per 100 in patients in their 70s. Females are more commonly affected than males. The vast majority of patients are diagnosed after the age of 40.

The prognosis in PA is good. A small proportion of patients, however (5–8%) develop gastric carcinoma. Replacement vitamin B_{12} therapy is given by injection for life. With B_{12} treatment the patient feels better very quickly (1–2 days) and bone marrow returns to normal in the same period. The macrocytosis may take weeks (up to 10 weeks) to disappear. Oral symptoms also rapidly improve but neurological changes may be slow to resolve and may even be permanent.

Immunological features

Approximately one-third of patients' relatives have a history of PA or other autoimmune disease, such as thyroid disease. There is a known association with HLA-B7. The autoimmune nature of PA is shown by the finding that 80–90% of patients have parietal cell antibodies and over 50% have antibodies to intrinsic factor. Vitamin B_{12} needs to bind to the glycoprotein called intrinsic factor (IF) produced by parietal cells for later ileal absorption. Hydrochloric acid is also produced by parietal cells, and loss of hydrochloric acid parallels loss of IF secretion. The symptoms of the disease are the result of a megaloblastic anaemia, secondary to atrophic gastritis and low intrinsic factor levels.

Systemic manifestations

Patients usually complain of lethargy, tiredness, breathlessness or tongue discomfort. Other complaints may be of symmetrical peripheral neuropathy and on testing loss of vibration sense is present. Rarely, subacute combined degeneration of the cord may complicate PA.

Oral manifestations

Approaching 25% of patients with pernicious anaemia have tongue discomfort of fluctuating severity, particularly on eating hot or spicy foods. Clinically there is a marked atrophic glossitis. In early stages only tongue discomfort may be present, but latterly progressive atrophy of filiform, fungiform and circumvallate papillae occurs. The other oral feature of pernicious anaemia is recurrent oral ulceration.

Diagnosis and laboratory tests

Blood examination in a patient with pernicious anaemia (PA) will show a macrocytic anaemia with raised mean corpuscular volume and mean corpuscular haemoglobin. The reticulocyte count may be normal as reticulocytes enter the circulation late in PA. A low serum B_{12} level is present but folic acid levels are normal. The marrow red cells show delayed condensation and extrusion of the nucleus (megaloblastic change) and circulating red cells are usually large (macrocytosis). Other causes of a megaloblastic blood picture are shown in Table 9.7. Diagnosis of a megaloblastic blood picture PA is established by showing that there is impaired vitamin B_{12} absorption and that it improves with the addition of extraneous intrinsic factor. The Schilling test of B_{12} absorption involves giving the patient 1.0 μg B_{12} of isotopically labelled cobalt 57 (usually) orally. The patient is given 1000 μg of 'cold' B_{12} by injection, which encourages urinary excretion of the isotope. A 24 hour urine collection is undertaken and normal individuals excrete more than 10% of the oral dose. When there is shortage of intrinsic factor, as in PA, the absorption is improved by repeating the test with a source of intrinsic factor.

Table 9.7 Causes of a megaloblastic blood picture

Vitamin B_{12} deficiency
Folic acid deficiency
Orotic aciduria
Lesch-Nyhan syndrome

AUTOIMMUNE NEUTROPENIA

General considerations

There is some overlap between neutropenia as a result of drug ingestion and autoimmune neutropenia. The mechanism whereby drugs induce neutropenia is still largely speculative and an immune-mediated phenomenon may well apply in some cases. Other causes of neutropenia have also to be considered, such as defective granulopoiesis (as a result of B_{12} or folate deficiency or malignant proliferation), removal of neutrophils from the circulation (as in hypersplenism) or certain infections (such as typhoid, typhus or malaria).

Immunological features

Neutropenia may develop in conditions known to have an autoimmune basis. The most common of these are systemic lupus erythematosus and rheumatoid arthritis. In rheumatoid arthritis some patients develop splenomegaly and neutropenia (Felty's syndrome). The reason for this is not clear, although an antineutrophil antibody has been assumed but positive proof is lacking. Studies of neutrophil kinetics have given highly variable results. Splenectomy in Felty's syndrome produces variable results. Other splenic disorders, such as congestive splenomegaly secondary to liver cirrhosis, also produce a neutropenia for uncertain reasons, as the spleen is not normally an important site of neutrophil destruction. In this condition also blood neutrophil turnover rate is markedly increased.

One other type of autoimmune neutropenia, of which there are at least three forms, is dominant-inherited neutropenia. This condition is usually benign. Neonatal neutropenia is occasionally due to transplacental transfer of antibody directed against fetal neutrophils from the mother. In these cases the mother has always been exposed to fetal neutrophils antigenically different from her own by prior pregnancy or transfusion.

Systemic manifestations

Autoimmune neutropenia is generally of gradual onset. The systemic manifestations are often of infections, principally of the lungs and oropharynx. Septicaemia can complicate some cases, and the paucity of neutrophils may result in infections such as pyelonephritis being diagnosed late since urinary neutrophils may be absent. In patients who have the condition of cyclic neutropenia, fever, malaise, pyrexia and joint pains may be prominent systemic features.

Oral manifestations

The two principal oral manifestations of neutropenia are infection and non-specific oral ulceration. In the rare condition of cyclic neutropenia, periodontal destruction is out of proportion to the degree of oral hygiene. The aetiology is unknown but presumably minimal infection is allowed to produce significant periodontal destruction against a background of neutropenia. Similar mechanisms are presumed to permit candidal proliferation and infection. The oral ulceration of cyclic neutropenia occurs during the period of neutropenia and usually heals in 10–14 days, sometimes with scarring. A similar mechanism may account for the oral ulceration which occurs in patients receiving chemotherapy with a resultant neutropenia.

Diagnosis and laboratory tests

The diagnosis of neutropenia is clearly made by analysis of a differential white blood cell count. As mentioned, a level of neutrophils below $2.5 \times 10^9/l$ is termed neutropenia. The diagnosis of autoimmune neutropenia is more difficult, and general aspects of the patient's condition need to be considered as well as other factors such as whether the neutropenia is part of a pancytopenia or is part of a syndrome of aplastic anaemia. A physiological neutropenia can occur in individuals in isolated communities, e.g. Polar base.

Pathological neutropenia can result from bone marrow damage by irradiation or tumours, or severe infections, or drugs, including alcohol. Appropriate bone marrow and microbiological studies should eliminate these causes as well as detailed clinical history. Other blood parameters, such as vitamin B_{12} and folic acid, may need to be performed to eliminate deficiencies as a cause. Studies aimed at demonstrating Felty's syndrome, where one-third of cases have subnormal neutrophil production, will require analysis of rheumatoid factor and antinuclear factor with DNA binding capacity.

Family studies to confirm either familial cyclic neutropenia or benign familial neutropenia may be relevant, as both have an autosomal dominant inheritance. Rarely other conditions may coexist, such as the autosomal recessive condition of infantile genetic agranulocytosis or the Chediak–Higashi anomaly in which neutropenia is associated with an increased granulocyte turnover.

In some cases of true autoimmune neutropenia it has been possible to demonstrate antibodies promoting a decrease in neutrophils. The complexity of diagnosing autoimmune neutropenia means that largely it is a diagnosis by exclusion of other causes of neutropenia.

DRUG-INDUCED NEUTROPENIA

General considerations

A large number of drugs can produce defects in red blood cells, the white cell series or platelets. Generally such reactions are uncommon; however, they require prompt recognition and often withdrawal of the drug will resolve the condition. In aplastic anaemia, however, the condition may become more severe on withdrawal of the drug. The more common side-effects of drug therapy are agranulocytosis and thrombocytopenia. Deficiency anaemias such as folic acid may follow phenytoin or sulphasalazine therapy, and haemolytic anaemias can result from methyldopa therapy. Less poorly understood are alterations in neutrophil function by high-dose corticosteroids and defective platelet function induced by ibuprofen, aspirin and other non-steroidal anti-inflammatory drugs.

Immunological features

The mechanism whereby drug ingestion leads to a reduction in neutrophil count is still not clear. It may be that the condition results from immune complex formation, as has been suggested in drug-induced systemic lupus erythematosus. Patients with the latter usually have circulating antinuclear factor which can be of IgG, IgA or IgM. Antibodies to double-stranded DNA are not a feature in iatrogenic disease and this factor can help differentiate drug-induced disease from the idiopathic variety.

Theories of how drugs induce neutropenia include a direct effect of the drug or the drug acting as a hapten, or physical effects such as ultraviolet light altering skin protein antigenicity when exposed to the drug.

Systemic manifestations

The systemic manifestations of neutropenia are often non-specific and include malaise, joint aches and fever. Infections of the skin are commonly present, and the reduction in neutrophil levels facilitates invasion by bacteria and fungi. Skin rashes may also be a feature.

Oral manifestations

The main oral features of drug-induced neutropenia are non-specific oral ulceration and a predisposition to oral infections and periodontal disease. Clearly early recognition of the cause is imperative, and discontinuation of drug therapy mandatory. The oral ulceration usually affects the buccal mucosa and is persistent.

Diagnosis and laboratory tests

By definition a patient has agranulocytosis if the blood neutrophil count is less than 0.5×10^9/l. Lesser degrees of a reduction in neutrophil count (less than 2.5×10^9/l are termed neutropenia. Clinical suspicion of the condition and a differential white blood cell count are therefore required for diagnosis. Analysis of other blood constituents will differentiate the neutropenia from an aplastic anaemia-type picture.

Bone marrow investigations are also helpful in achieving a diagnosis. In drug-induced agranulocytosis marrow aspirates show an increased number of promyelocytes and myelocytes.

Table 9.8 Some of the more commonly prescribed drugs which can cause drug-induced neutropenia and agranulocytosis

Amidopyrine	Phenothiazines
Amodiaquine	Phenylbutazone
Barbiturates	Prochlorperazine
Carbimazole	Quinine
Chloramphenicol	Sulphonamide
Gold and its salts	Thiourea
Isoniazid	Thiouracils
Meprobamate	Tolbutamide
Phenacitin	

Since only fatal cases of drug-induced neutropenia are reported, the true incidence of drug-induced neutropenia is probably higher than currently assumed. Some of the more common drugs implicated are listed in Table 9.8. Agranulocytosis is often fatal; therefore discretion must be exercised in prescribing high-risk drugs, and regular blood counts should be performed on all patients receiving such drugs on a long-term basis.

INFECTIOUS MONONUCLEOSIS

General considerations

Infectious mononucleosis is an endemic disease caused by the DNA virus termed the Epstein–Barr virus (EBV). The disease has its highest incidence in the late teens and early 20s period. Prospective studies, using sero-conversion studies, have suggested that infectious mononucleosis is one of the commonest infectious diseases. The condition affects males and females equally and is spread by intimate oral contact. In some cases the disease is spread by chronic carriers of the infection who lack EBV antibody. The incubation period of the condition is 4–7 weeks.

Immunological features

When a virus enters a cell, generally speaking it can replicate completely (permissive infection) or incompletely. When a virus replicates completely it codes for nuclear proteins then capsid proteins, in that order. In EBV infections it is not understood why antibodies to viral capsid antigen (VCA) always precede antibodies to the early antigen (EA) complex. As previously mentioned the EBV can enter B lymphocytes but not T lymphocytes (which do not have the necessary receptors to allow entry of the virus). Like many herpes viruses latency is a feature, and reactivation can occur for example in immunosuppressed patients.

Systemic manifestations

There is a spectrum of host response to EBV infection ranging from inapparent infection to fatal infection. Clinically most patients experience mild infection with pharyngitis, cervical lymphadenopathy and less commonly splenomegaly and hepatomegaly. Serological evidence of abnormal liver function is a regular feature, although jaundice is uncommon. Rarely encephalitis, Guillain-Barré syndrome, thrombocytopenic purpura, myocarditis and nephritis may be present.

213

Oral manifestations

Like many viral infections non-specific oral ulceration can be present in infectious mononucleosis. The general reduction in host reponse may predispose on occasion to oral infections. Petechiae on the hard palate are said to be a fairly common accompaniment. EBV can also produce acute salivary gland enlargement which may mimic infectious parotitis (mumps). A relationship between nasopharyngeal carcinoma and EBV infection has been proposed, as has a relationship to Burkitt's lymphoma (see above). Epidemiological studies have also supported a link between virus infection and Hodgkin's disease.

Diagnosis and laboratory tests

In common with other herpes viruses, EBV can be isolated in tissue culture, although because its isolation is technically difficult, it is usually a research tool only. Serological antibody studies of EBV infection are generally not of value as an indication of acute infection. The reason for this is partly because many patients already have such antibodies at presentation and rises in antibody titre occur in only 15–20% of cases. For these reasons other diagnostic tests are usually employed.

The main laboratory technique for diagnosis is the IgM heterophil antibody technique usually employing sheep or horse agglutination tests after adsorption. In essence EBV attaches to B lymphocytes which are antigenically altered, resulting in lymphocyte proliferation of 'atypical mononuclear cells' (T lymphocytes). The cytotoxicity of the T lymphocytes for B lymphocytes infected with EBV releases antigen which stimulates IgM antibodies against EBV. This antibody agglutinates sheep or horse red cells (Paul-Bunnell test). Other blood investigations usually show a leukocytosis and a shift to the left of neutrophils. This blood picture fits with other features of the condition such as transient depression of delayed hypersensitivity and depressed T-cell stimulation. In addition, atypical lymphocytes are a feature and a thrombocytopenia indistinguishable from ITP may be present. Some patients develop a haemolytic anaemia.

FURTHER READING

Chessels, J. D. and Pawles, R. (1980). Acute leukaemia. *Medicine*, **29**, 1477–82

Hind, C. R. K. and Pepys, M. B. (1984). Amyloidosis: classification and pathogenesis (1). *Hospital Update*, **10**, 593–8

Hobb, J. R. (1974). Paraproteins. In Hardisty, R. M. and Weatherall, D. J. (eds) *Blood and its Disorders*. pp. 1343–73. (Oxford: Blackwell Scientific Publications)

Lukes, R. J. and Collins, R. A. (1975). New approaches to the classification of lymphoma. *Br. J. Cancer*, **31**, (suppl. II) 1–28

Miescher, P. A. and Graf, J. (1980). Drug induced thrombocytopenia. *Clinics in Haematology*, **9**, 505. (London: Saunders)

Mikåelian, D. O. *et al.* (1981). Primary T-cell lymphoma of oral cavity. *Otolaryngol.–Head–Neck–Surg.*, **89**, 742–5

Robins-Browne, R. M., Green, R., Katz, J. and Becker, D. (1977). Thymoma, pure red cell aplasia, pernicious anaemia and candidiasis: a defect in immunohomeostasis. *Br. J. Haematol.*, **36**, 5–13

10
Oral Neoplasia

W. D. ROBERTSON and J. C. SOUTHAM

GENERAL CONSIDERATIONS

Oral cancer comprises approximately 2% of the total malignant tumours in Western Europe and North America, with an incidence of about four new cases per 100 000 population per annum. The incidence varies throughout the world, however, and cómprises approximately 40% of the total malignant tumours in India. Up to 90% of human cancer is thought to be determined environmentally, and the wide variation in incidence of oral carcinoma in different countries is related to environmental factors. Squamous cell carcinoma accounts for over 90% of oral cancer and this chapter is primarily related to primary squamous cell carcinoma of the oral mucosa. Oral carcinoma occurs more commonly in men than in women, although in recent years this difference has been much less marked in England and Wales. It may occur on any part of the oral mucosa, but in Western Europe the lip and tongue are the two commonest sites with the cheek the most common site in India. Over 90% of cases occur in patients over 40 years of age.

The prognosis of oral carcinoma depends on a number of factors, by far the most important being early diagnosis. The site of the tumour is also a factor; the further back in the mouth the tumour is then the worse is the prognosis. This is mainly because tumours in the posterior part of the mouth are diagnosed later and are more difficult to treat than tumours in the anterior part. The prognosis in females is generally better than in males, probably because of earlier diagnosis and treatment, and age affects prognosis because the elderly are less able than the young to withstand extensive surgery and radiotherapy. The degree of histological differentiation of the carcinoma does not significantly affect the prognosis. Statistics for the prognosis for patients with oral carcinoma vary between different centres. In general a 5-year cure rate of about 80% is reported for carcinoma of the lip, with about a 30% 5-year cure rate for carcinoma of the tongue.

A premalignant lesion is a lesion which precedes or coexists with a tumour more frequently than would be expected by chance alone. While the majority of oral carcinomas clinically appears to arise *de novo*, recognized premalignant lesions are leukoplakia, erythroplakia, chronic hyperplastic candidosis, lichen planus, and oral epithelial atrophy occurring in syphilis, oral submucous fibrosis, sideropenic dysphagia and possibly some vitamin deficiencies. Leukoplakia is defined for epidemiological purposes as a white patch on the oral mucosa which cannot be removed by scraping and cannot be attributed to any other diagnosable disease. It has an unpredictable tendency to undergo malignant transformation but in Western Europe a figure of 4% malignant transformation over a prolonged period is likely to be a reasonable estimate. High-risk sites of oral leukoplakia have been identified; these are the ventral tongue, floor of mouth and lingual aspect of the lower alveolar mucosa. Such lesions are often designated sublingual keratoses. It is generally regarded that a leukoplakia showing histological features of epithelial dysplasia is more likely to undergo malignant transformation than a leukoplakia not showing such features, and that malignant transformation is increasingly likely to occur as the degree of dysplasia increases. However, malignant transformation of sublingual keratoses does not appear to be related to the degree of dysplasia present.

Related to leukoplakia is erythroplakia, which may be defined as a bright red velvety plaque on the oral mucosa which cannot be categorized clinically or pathologically as being due to any other condition. Areas of erythroplakia may be intermingled with patches of leukoplakia and such lesions are often described as speckled leukoplakias. The lesions of chronic hyperplastic candidosis may present as a speckled leukoplakia. Erythroplakia, especially when associated with candida infection, is particularly prone to undergo malignant transformation.

Malignant transformation is thought to occur in up to 1% of cases of oral lichen planus, the erosive forms being particularly liable to undergo malignant transformation.

The relationship between neoplasia and the immune system has been extensively investigated in recent years, but the subject remains confused and controversial. Much of the data on which current ideas are based is derived from studies of experimentally induced or transplanted tumours, and the behaviour of spontaneous tumours appears to differ in a number of respects. The concept of immunological surveillance in neoplasia is based on the belief that malignant cells arise as a result of somatic mutation and that tumour antigens on the malignant cell are recognized as 'non-self' by the immune system, this recognition being followed by destruction of the cell. Overt tumours arise because they are non-antigenic or because in some way the tumour cells avoid the surveillance, either by overcoming the immune mechanisms or because the appropriate immune mechanisms are deficient.

It is now realized that the deficiency or absence of one of the various types of immune or natural resistance does not necessarily lead to enhanced tumour growth and the resistance mechanisms have not been shown to be capable of killing all types of tumour cells. The concept of immunological surveillance in neoplasia has therefore been questioned, despite the fact that malignant transformation of cells has been shown to be associated with a change in cell surface antigens.

When compared with normal cells in tissue culture, malignant cells show a lack of stable adhesion formation, contact inhibition of movement, and contact inhibition of mitosis. A malignant cell present in otherwise normal tissue is not therefore subject to the restraints which operate to inhibit non-malignant cells. Both chemical and biophysical changes at the cell surface are likely to be present in malignant cells, such changes being ill understood at present. The chemical changes will be recognized by a change in antigenic structure but the biophysical changes provide a powerful barrier against cell to cell contact. It is interesting that lymphocytes possess a cellular process with low electrostatic forces which allows them to contact a target cell, and it could be that the immunosensitivity of a tumour depends as much on its biophysical structure determining its electrostatic force as it does on its antigenic structure.

The objective of this chapter is to provide a review of current knowledge and opinion on the relationship between neoplasia and the immune system in general, with a subsequent short account of work particularly related to oral carcinoma.

IMMUNOLOGICAL SURVEILLANCE OF TUMOURS

The concept of immunological surveillance of tumours is based on the premise that malignant change in a cell involves a somatic mutation which is associated with major structural alterations in the cell surface which the immune system detects as a change in antigenic structure. The immune response which follows leads to destruction of the malignant cell. If the concept is correct, it means that individuals with congenital or acquired defects in immunological responsiveness should show a greatly increased incidence of malignant tumours. While patients with a congenital immunodeficiency or receiving immunosuppressive therapy show an increased incidence of lymphoreticular tumours (lymphomas and leukaemias), they do not show a general increased incidence of other types of tumour. Such patients may have an increased susceptibility to oncogenic viruses, and this could account for the increased incidence of certain types of tumour reported in some studies. Other patients with defective immunological responses, for example patients with chronic renal failure or leprosy, do not show an increased incidence of tumours.

Immunosuppressed animals do not show an increased susceptibility to chemically induced tumours, although both the incidence and rate of growth of virally induced tumours in such animals are increased. Nude (athymic) mice which show no detectable delayed hypersensitivity reactions and fail to reject allografts or xenografts (i.e. show no cell-mediated immune responses) should show an increase in the incidence of spontaneous tumours and an enhanced susceptibility to chemical carcinogenesis if the immunological surveillance theory is correct. That such mice do not do so is strong evidence that the concept of immunological surveillance of tumours needs to be reappraised.

The original concept of the immunological surveillance of tumours was based on the supposition that tumour cells arise frequently. For example, the frequency of a spontaneous mutation arising for a diversity of human properties is approximately 1 in 5×10^4 cells, and it is unlikely that this figure is greatly divergent in carcinogenesis. About 10^{10} new cells arise daily in the human adult body which means that 2×10^6 new tumour cells would arise daily if only one mutation were needed. As described later, there are a number of different effector mechanisms for the immunological control of tumours and if it is assumed that each of these mechanisms kills 50% of all newly arising tumour cells (thought to be a reasonable estimate with present knowledge), then 1 out of about 2^{10} (1024) tumour cells would escape the antitumour mechanisms. This would mean that tumours should develop frequently during a lifetime even with effective immunosurveillance mechanisms against tumours. Tumours do not in fact occur frequently during a lifetime, and it must be presumed from this that the majority of malignant mutations do not progress to overt tumours for a variety of reasons. For example, damage to DNA can be repaired before a fixed mutation is produced, as shown by the high incidence of squamous cell carcinoma of the skin in patients with xeroderma pigmentosa who have a congenital inability to excise thymine dimers formed in DNA after ultraviolet irradiation.

A more realistic way at present of looking at the immunological surveillance of tumours is to say that tumour cells originate rarely, that when they do originate the tumour antigens may or may not be immunogenic, but if they are immunogenic they will induce an immune reaction which may lead to destruction of the tumour cells.

TUMOUR ANTIGENS

The antigenicity of tumours was first demonstrated in genetically uniform strains of inbred mice whose isoantigenic homogeneity permits the identification of new antigens in tumour cells by methods involving transplantation. It is also now possible to demonstrate immune responses to primary tumours both in experimental animals and in man, using both *in vivo* and *in vitro* techniques. There is no clear evidence yet that human tumours possess tumour-specific antigens, i.e. antigens which are present and expressed only when malignant transformation has occurred in a cell and which are never found in the normal cell. What are described are tumour-associated antigens, which are antigens expressed in minute quantities in normal cells but in much greater quantity when malignant transformation has taken place. Tumour-associated antigens may be related to factors such as the rate of cell division or the degree of cellular differentiation.

Transplantation experiments have demonstrated that several distinct patterns of antigenicity are present in experimental tumour systems. Transplantation tumour antigens are those antigens detected by transplantation experiments and which have been shown to be individually specific for chemically induced tumours even when induced by the same chemical carcinogen to the extent that two tumours induced in the same animal by the same carcinogen have unique and distinct antigenic properties. This contrasts with virally induced tumours which have common transplantation antigens if induced by the same virus. Infection of adult animals with an oncogenic virus induces resistance to transplants of tumours induced by the same virus, suggesting that infection of normal cells by virus is followed by antigenic changes characteristic of malignant cells. Spontaneous tumours in experimental animals, i.e. those which arise without the deliberate use of any carcinogenic stimulus, are generally much less immunogenic than chemically or virally-induced tumours when transplanted.

In vitro techniques such as complement-mediated cytotoxicity, lymphocyte cytotoxicity and immunocytochemistry can now be used to demonstrate tumour antigenicity. For example, lymphocytes taken from tumour immune animals or tumour patients can inhibit the growth of, or lyse, tumour cells grown in culture. Tumours which, by transplantation techniques, appear to be non-antigenic can in fact be shown by *in vitro* studies to have distinctive membrane and cytoplasmic antigens. Specific antigens can be demonstrated similarly in virally-induced experimental tumours, and common antigens can be demonstrated in chemically-induced tumours.

Tumours in experimental animals may also have 'inappropriate' normal tissue antigens, inappropriate in that the antigens are normally found only in embryonic or differentiating cells. They are rather weak antigens and are probably not very important in tumour rejection.

Most studies of the antigenicity of human tumours have used *in vitro* techniques, *in vivo* techniques generally being ethically dubious or difficult to interpret. The *in vitro* techniques consist largely of the examination of the interactions of tumour cells with the various effector limbs of the immune response.

The humoral responses to human tumours do not show individual specific tumour antigens such as are seen with chemically-induced experimental tumours, but show a histogenic cross-reactivity in which all tumours derived from a particular tissue have a similar antigenic structure. For example, common tumour antigens have been identified in malignant melanomas, these cross-reacting antigens being present on all melanoma cells.

Inappropriate antigens may also be found in some human tumours. For example, an antigen has been identified in human colonic tumours which is also present in fetal endodermal gut. This has been called carcinoembryonic antigen (CEA) and it is a complex glycoprotein molecule synthesized by the tumour cells and also by normal colonic epithelium. It is carried on the surface membrane of these cells and shed into the surrounding medium (and therefore detectable in serum and serous fluids) in patients with colonic cancer. CEA is a potential marker substance in immunodiagnosis but there is no evidence that it is immunogenic in the host and so is not related to tumour immunity.

Monoclonal antibodies have now been raised to various tumours, and this

221

has helped greatly in detection and characterization of human tumour antigens. An interesting finding from the great majority of immunocyto-chemical studies using monoclonal antibodies raised against human epithelial tumours is that the antibodies bind to only some of the cells in a tumour, other cells of apparently identical morphology showing no antibody binding. Positive and negative staining cells may be quite evenly mixed together, or staining may be focal, or whole regions of a tumour may be largely positive while other apparently similar areas are negative. This heterogeneity of antigen expression shown by tumour cells is also shown by cell lines and clones of epithelial cells in culture, as well as by normal epithelia. The antigenic structures to which the antibodies bind are probably the carbohydrate part of a cell surface glycoprotein. It is not known whether the variations in antigen expression reflect variations in the differentiated state of the cells, or variations in the carbohydrate structures of otherwise identical cells. The protein part of the cell surface glycoprotein may not have the heterogeneity of the carbohydrate part and monoclonal antibodies to glycoproteins stripped of their carbohydrates are now being raised. It will be interesting to see whether or not they display the heterogeneity of staining seen with antibodies raised against the carbohydrate component. All the monoclonal antibodies produced so far cross-react to a differing extent with some normal tissue and no truly specific tumour antigens have been identified.

Studies of cell-mediated reactions to human tumours are less numerous than those of humoral reactions, but the results are similar in showing a histogenic cross-reactivity.

In summary, at least four different types of tumour antigen have been described. These are idiotypic antigens found in experimental tumours induced by chemical agents; cross-reacting virally controlled antigens; embryonic antigens associated with an earlier, fetal stage of the cell; and antigens which are the carbohydrate part of surface membrane glyco-proteins that may change during cell division.

MECHANISMS OF ANTITUMOUR IMMUNITY

There are a number of ways in which tumour cell growth can be controlled by the immune response and which have been confirmed by *in vitro* studies, but this does not necessarily mean that such mechanisms operate *in vivo*. Although cell-mediated immune mechanisms are generally considered to be of prime importance for the initiation and perpetuation of tissue-damaging immune responses, the absence of a thymus has not been associated with an increased susceptibility to all types of tumour, suggesting that T cell immunity has in fact only a limited role in tumour surveillance. It must be remembered that immune reactions to tumours involve both initial sensitization and interaction of immune cells with tumour cells or tumour-derived material. Rejection of a tumour is the end-result of a variety of effector mechanisms and is a complex process. It is now realized that discrimination between one cell type and another in preparations of mononuclear cells from peripheral blood or spleen may not be possible at present, as morphological criteria are far from adequate and the derivation of certain cells involved in tumour immunity is therefore not always clear. Natural resistance (resistance that is not induced by antigens on tumour cells) is also involved in tumour rejection and may be closely involved with immune resistance, and so some mechanisms of natural resistance are also described in this chapter.

Antibody-mediated mechanisms

Tumour cells may be lysed as a result of complement activation in the presence of complement fixing antitumour immunoglobulin. *In vitro* studies have shown that lymphoma and leukaemia cells are very sensitive to treatment with cytotoxic antisera whereas sarcoma cells are very resistant to such treatment, but the *in vivo* role of complement-dependent cytotoxic antibody is uncertain. Tumour cells may also be killed as a result of antibody-dependent cellular cytotoxicity (ADCC), the immunoglobulin responsible often being referred to as lymphocyte-dependent antibody (LDA) and is generally found to be of IgG class. The effector cells have surface Fc receptors for IgG which interact with the IgG bound to the target cells. The effector cells are not thought to be T cells and there may be a collaborative cytotoxicity involving K cells, monocytes, macrophages, neutrophils and eosinophils. ADCC is an efficient cytotoxic mechanism in terms of the amount of immunoglobulin required; relatively few immunoglobulin molecules being required for target cell lysis to occur. Alternatively antibody binding may inhibit cell division or the mobility of tumour cells. Large numbers of mast cells are seen in some animal tumours and a role for reaginic antibody in tumour immunity has been suggested, but supporting evidence is meagre.

It is thought that senescent erythrocytes may be removed by liver and spleen macrophages following opsonization with natural antibody to the erythrocytes due to the exposure of a surface antigen associated with increasing age of the cell. Similar defective cell surface antigens could be present on some tumour cells which could then be removed by macrophages following natural opsonization.

Cell-mediated mechanisms

Evidence indicates that T cell-mediated immunity plays a central role in protection against tumours induced by oncogenic viruses but not for spontaneous or chemically-induced tumours when cells associated with natural resistance are likely to be more important. T cells elaborate lymphokines which are non-immunoglobulin secretory products of activated lymphocytes with a wide range of potent physiological effects in inflammation and immunity. Factors resembling lymphokines are also produced by macrophages and fibroblast cell lines, these factors being called cytokines.

223

Lymphokines

These various chemical mediators of immunity are synthesized by T and B cells and released in response to immunologically specific stimulation, but the effects of lymphokines are non-specific. Lymphokines have many types of activity but ones which have been described and which may be relevant to antitumour activity are:

1. Inhibition of movement of macrophages and neutrophils (macrophage inhibition factor – MIF).
2. Differentiation of macrophages (macrophage activation factor – MAF).
3. Chemotactic activity which is attractive to macrophages.
4. Production of vascular dilatation and increased capillary permeability.
5. Blastogenic effect on lymphocytes with increased DNA synthesis and cell division.
6. Recruitment of other T cells into the immune response (interleukin-2 or IL-2).
7. Humoral cytotoxic factor (lymphotoxin or LT) capable of lysing target cells.
8. Interferon (IFN) (see page 226).

Cytotoxic T lymphocytes

These antibody-independent cytotoxic T cells (CTL) are equipped with specific receptors for the tumour cells, one effector cell being able to kill several target (tumour) cells. T cells only recognize foreign antigen when it is associated on the surface of a cell with a molecule encoded by the major histocompatibility complex (MHC) – this is called MHC restriction. Cytotoxic lymphocyte progenitors are small lymphocytes which enlarge after stimulation, but appear as small lymphocytes later in the immune process, with memory cells present as well as effector cells.

K (killer) cells

These effector cells in the immune response possess surface Fc receptors which interact with immunoglobulin bound to the target cells with subsequent lysis of the target cells (ADCC). K cells are readily detectable in the peripheral blood in man, and were originally thought to be lymphocytes. Their derivation is now less clear but they seem to be related to monocytes.

NK (natural killer) cells

These cells comprise a heterogeneous subpopulation of lymphoid cells that possess spontaneous cytolytic or cytotoxic activity against a variety of cellular targets. No apparent previous sensitization of the target cell is required for this activity, which is not MHC restricted. NK cells may be active against tumour cells, virus-infected cells and even some normal cells (e.g. haemopoietic bone marrow cells). Animal experiments suggest that they are particularly important in the control of metastasis by acting during the phase of haematogenous dissemination, presumably by their ability to rapidly eliminate the tumour cells from the circulation in capillary beds. NK cells have the morphology of large, granular lymphocytes and represent about 5% of the mononuclear cells in the peripheral blood or spleen, but they are not found in lymph and so cannot be truly described as lymphocytes. Interferon increases both the number and cytotoxicity of NK cells, as do agents such as BCG and a diphtheroid organism, *Corynebacterium parvum*. Susceptible tumour cells have one or more surface structures in common, recognizable by NK cells which then bind to the tumour cell via corresponding receptors. This close apposition leads to cell death but the mechanism is not understood. The surface structures recognized by NK cells are not conventional tumour antigens and may be shared by certain non-tumour cells. It is interesting that some chemical carcinogens, e.g. dimethylbenzanthracene, cause a profound depression of NK cell activity.

Both K and NK cells have been reported to possess identical organ distribution. This raises the question whether a K cell is an NK cell with an Fc binding site for cytophilic antibody.

LAK (lymphokine activated killer) cells

It has recently been shown that when lymphoid cells from normal individuals are incubated with the lymphokine interleukin-2, they acquire the ability to kill tumour cells in culture. The cells responsible are not conventional T cells or NK cells and have a remarkable ability to distinguish in culture between freshly isolated tumour cells, which they kill, and normal cells from the same donor, which are not killed. LAK cells in culture are active against carcinomas, sarcomas and lymphomas. *In vivo* experiments in animals suggest that administration of LAK cells and interleukin-2 in combination can result in significant tumour cell death.

Macrophages

Macrophages are involved in both the afferent and efferent limbs of the immune response. In the afferent limb, thymus-dependent antigen is phagocytosed and mostly degraded by macrophages, with a proportion of antigen surviving either intact or as antigenic fragments. This is then presented to antigen-specific helper T cells in association with an MHC molecule on the surface of the macrophage. At the same time the macrophages produce interleukin-1, which binds to receptors in T cells, and is mitogenic for thymocytes and apparently essential for the response of helper T cells to macrophage-associated antigen. The helper T cells respond by releasing a non-specific factor involved in the stimulation of B cells, and also produce a second factor (interleukin-2) which promotes the proliferation of T cells, including cytotoxic T cells.

Present in epidermis and oral epithelium are a small population of dendritic cells, the Langerhans cells, which have migrated from the bone marrow. Langerhans cells are responsible for the immunizing capacity of topically applied antigen, being able to present antigen to appropriate T cells in a similar manner to macrophages. The antigen is presented in such a way that T helper cells are preferentially activated. This function of Langerhans cells can be abolished by sufficient quantities of ultraviolet energy, following which topically applied antigen is non-antigenic. It has recently been suggested that another type of antigen-presenting dendritic cell is also present in epidermis, this cell interacting with suppressor T cells rather than with helper T cells and not being as sensitive to ultraviolet energy. This so-called Granstein cell may account for the general state of immunosuppression which is sometimes seen following injury to the skin.

Other macrophages, however, are involved in the effector limb and described as natural cytotoxic macrophages as they are directly cytostatic or cytotoxic for some tumour cell types. The surface structures on the tumour cells which are recognized are not the usual tumour antigens and are different from the structures recognized by NK cells. This antitumour activity of macrophages may be enhanced by macrophage inhibition factor, interferon and certain bacterial substances. The tumour cells are killed by an extracellular mechanism not involving phagocytosis, a soluble mediator probably being involved. The effects on tumour cells are non-specific in that cytotoxic macrophages are active against a variety of unrelated tumour cells *in vitro*.

Interferon

Interferons are a class of glycoproteins produced by certain cells in response to a variety of stimuli. There are three general types of human interferon, alpha being produced by leukocytes, beta by fibroblasts, and gamma by T lymphocytes in response to mitogens or exposure to antigen to which the cells are already sensitized. Gamma interferon therefore is a lymphokine and plays a role in the regulation of the immune system. Macrophages must be present for the production of gamma interferon by normal T cells, and a T to T cell interaction involving interleukin-2 may also be required. Interferon has numerous actions but in general produces a shift from antibody- to cell-mediated immune mechanisms. In relation to antitumour immunity, the important actions of interferon are enhancement of the phagocytic action of macrophages and non-specific tumour cell killing, augmentation of NK cell activity, and it is possibly a key factor in the induction of cytotoxic T cells. In tissue culture experiments, interferon inhibits cell proliferation, especially of tumour cells.

IMMUNOLOGICAL ESCAPE

Many tumour cells are antigenic in the host and immune mechanisms exist whereby tumour cells can be destroyed or inactivated, and so an explanation is required to account for the way in which the tumours which grow and develop have escaped from immunological surveillance. It has been suggested that tumour patients in general show an immunological hyporeactivity, but while a number of patients with advanced tumours have a feeble or defective immune response, this is more likely to be a result of the tumour than the cause in many patients. For example, some patients show a loss of a delayed-type hypersensitivity to agents such as tuberculin antigen and dinitrochlorobenzene (DNCB) with advanced tumour.

There are ways, though, by which immunological surveillance may be defective, both systemically and locally, which could allow a tumour to develop and grow. Patients with a primary (genetically determined) immunodeficiency are predisposed to develop leukaemias and lymphomas, but epithelial tumours are unusual in such patients. The level of immune response to a particular antigen is controlled by the immune response (Ir) genes located in the major histocompatibility complex (MHC). An individual may therefore be genetically a low responder to a particular tumour antigen and this might allow a specific tumour to develop in an individual even if the tumour carries potentially strong antigens.

Secondary immunodeficiencies are more common than primary, and can be attributed to factors such as malnutrition, drugs, infections and ageing. Dietary changes can have a profound effect on immune function, the lymphoid tissues having differing sensitivities to deficiencies or excesses of dietary components. The thymus and T lymphocytes are highly sensitive to elemental zinc with a decrease in natural killer and helper T cell function in deficiency states. Immune dysfunctions occur with iron, folic acid, and vitamin A and B deficiencies, and essential fatty acids and vitamin E excesses. Somewhat surprisingly, nutritionally deprived animals have been shown to have enhanced tumour immunity and severe protein restriction does not appear to reduce cell-mediated tumour cell killing. The immunosuppressive characteristics of drugs, especially those used in transplant recipients, are well documented and recent evidence suggests that the different subpopulations of immunocytes have different steroid susceptibilities. Tobacco and alcohol remain popular self-prescribed drugs that can cause immunosuppression with prolonged use. Viral, bacterial and protozoal infections may alter the immune system, many of the effects on the subpopulations of immunocytes being unclear. Ageing is associated with immunological hyporeactivity and recent evidence implicates an age-associated T cell defect, while monocytes do not show impaired function. These age-acquired immunological defects are possibly associated with the major histocompatibility complex although environmental factors are intimately involved.

The immune response can also be modified locally to allow tumour cells to escape from immunological surveillance. Dense fibrous tissue with its associated poor vascularity may make tissues less penetrable by immunocytes, and areas of chronic inflammation may deplete the tissues of normal immunocytes. Non-immunogenic particulate matter such as silica can non-specifically activate macrophages which may then have a local, immunosuppressive role, and ultraviolet radiation selectively depletes antigen-handling Langerhans cells from the epidermis.

Even when the immune system is intact, tumour cells may escape immunological surveillance because of the existence of humoral (blocking) factors in the serum and extracellular fluid, which are capable of interfering in some way with the effector limbs of the immune response. For example, it has been suggested that antibody, possibly without any cytotoxic activity, may coat tumour cells and protect them from effector cells associated with lethal, specific cell-mediated immune responses. The blocking factors rapidly disappear from sera when tumours are surgically removed, indicating that the agent responsible is not antibody, and it is now thought that the blocking factor is the tumour antigen itself, possibly in the form of a complex with antibody. Tumour cells, like other cells, shed their surface antigens as they grow and these soluble tumour antigens, either as free antigen or complexed with antibody, may combine with the specific receptors on cytotoxic T cells or natural killer cells and thus prevent them exerting an effect on the tumour cells themselves.

An alternative way in which tumours could escape from immunological surveillance is the suggestion that there is specific stimulation of T suppressor cells in association with a tumour due to the production of immunosuppressive substances by the tumour itself. Many cancer patients contain in their peripheral blood a population of cells, probably monocytes, which inhibit T cell proliferation, and these cells may be important in tumour escape from immunological surveillance.

Suggested mechanisms for the immunological escape of tumours which have little or no evidence in their support are that resistant tumour cells are selected out by the immune response in a similar way that antibiotic-resistant bacteria are selected out, that too little tumour antigen is present initially to promote an immune response and when an immune response develops the tumour mass is so great that it cannot be controlled, and that tumour cells replicate faster than the immune response can be adequately mounted.

It must be realized that there are many stages in the development and growth of a tumour, and that immunological factors influencing the initial stages of tumour development may have a quite different influence in the later stages of tumour growth and metastatic spread. For example, immune reactions occurring locally in the early stages of tumour growth are likely to occur in the presence of an excess of antigen which could protect some of the tumour cells from the immune response. With continued growth of the tumour, this excess antigen may spread to the regional lymph nodes where it could complex with antibody, the antibody now being in excess. The complexes formed could then pass into the general circulation with dissemination of the tumour. All antibody could in time be complexed with antigen, until eventually antibody may not be produced and so a state of immunological hyporeactivity would have developed. While much of the evidence for these ideas is lacking, they do illustrate some of the complexities involved in the relationship between tumours and related immune responses.

IMMUNOTHERAPY FOR TUMOURS

Numerous trials of different types of immunotherapy both for tumour patients and experimental animals have been carried out since the early years of this century. Many of the trials carried out have not been carefully analysed, mainly because the way that they were carried out defied adequate analysis. Apart possibly from a limited role in the management of acute leukaemia and malignant melanoma, satisfactory methods for the treatment of tumours by immunotherapy have not been established, but the strong hope remains that appropriate types of tumour immunotherapy will be available in the future. It is likely that any form of immunotherapy will only be effective if the tumour load has first been reduced to a low level by other methods of treatment, e.g. surgery, radiotherapy, chemotherapy. In theory, there are three ways in which tumour immunotherapy may be effective – amplification of the effectiveness of the immune response, sensitization of the tumour cells to the immune response, and removal of the factors inhibiting the immune response.

It is unclear at present what role is played by each of the effector mechanisms in antitumour immunity. In particular it is not known which mechanisms are important and which are unimportant. As a consequence, methods of generally enhancing immunological reactions have to be adopted. Methods of specific active immunotherapy using active immunization with whole tumour cells or extracts, and specific passive immunotherapy using antisera either prepared in animals or from patients whose tumours have undergone spontaneous regression, have failed to produce any clear pattern of therapeutic effect. Non-specific boosting of immunological reactivity has been tried using a variety of stimulants, among the most promising being tuberculin antigen (BCG) and a diphtheroid organism, *Corynebacterium parvum*. In the belief that cell-mediated immune reactions are the more important in antitumour immunity, lymphoid cells from patients immunized with tumour have been transferred to tumour patients but with equivocal results. Interferon has been reported as showing antitumour activity in experimental tumours in animals, but the results of clinical trials have been disappointing. Recombinant interleukin-2 has been prepared and initial animal experiments have shown regression of established tumours following intraperitoneal injection of this lymphokine.

No method of increasing the sensitivity of tumour cells to the immune response has been established as yet. Perhaps the most promising method would be to enhance the immunogenicity of the tumour cells by infecting them with a virus, but it is wise to remember that effective methods of treatment have rarely developed from theory.

Removal of humoral factors inhibiting the immune response is still in the experimental stage. As such factors are now thought to consist of circulating tumour antigens either in the free form or as immune complexes rather than antibody, the most likely method of removing them is immunological. This would involve active or passive immunization with tumour extracts and techniques appropriate to the individual patient and his tumour.

IMMUNODIAGNOSIS OF TUMOURS

The early detection of cancer could have a dramatic effect on clinical practice, and the main hope of immunodiagnosis is that it might be a means of accomplishing this task. Immunology may be used in tumour diagnosis by the detection of tumour products in the blood or urine, by the assay of various aspects of the host's immune response to tumour antigens, or by the immunochemical demonstration of tumour antigens in biopsy material.

Malignant cells synthesize a variety of macromolecules, mainly embryonic, which may be detected by immunological means. Such tumour marker substances which have been investigated include enzymes, hormones, fetoproteins, and carcinoembryonic antigen (see page 221). For example, the placental isoenzyme of alkaline phosphatase is found in the serum of a proportion of cancer patients (but also in some patients with ulcerative colitis or hepatic cirrhosis), chorionic gonadotrophin is produced by choriocarcinoma, and alpha-fetoprotein can be detected in the serum of many patients with hepatoma or testicular teratoma. The tumour markers identified so far have their main application in the monitoring of treatment rather than in the initial diagnosis, but it is expected that specific tumour markers will be identified in the future which will be useful in the early diagnosis of tumours.

If human tumour antigens are immunogenic it should be possible to diagnose the tumours by the demonstration of either circulating antitumour antibodies or cytotoxic lymphocytes. Details of a number of techniques describing how such host responses can be demonstrated and measured have been published, but none has been substantiated in a large series of patients for general acceptance.

As described in the section on tumour antigens, monoclonal antibodies have been raised against a variety of tumour antigens, but cross-reactivity with normal cells and capriciousness in staining of tumour cells have so far precluded their use in diagnosis.

IMMUNOLOGY AND ORAL CARCINOMA

There is no reason to believe that the immunological aspects of oral carcinoma are essentially different from the immunological aspects of tumours in general. This section therefore reviews some of the particular studies that have been reported of the relationship between immunology and oral cancer. Many studies have dealt with cancer of the head and neck rather than being confined to oral cancer, but the findings of such studies are likely to be relevant to oral cancer.

Oral carcinoma has been rarely reported in patients with a primary immunodeficiency, and those cases that have been reported could well have a viral aetiology. The increased incidence of oral carcinoma in relatively young people with the acquired immune deficiency syndrome is also likely to be related to the increased susceptibility to viral infection in such patients. The viruses thought to possibly play a causal role in oral carcinoma are the Epstein–Barr virus, herpes simplex virus type 1, and human papilloma virus.

The results of immunochemical staining of sections of oral carcinoma with monoclonal antibodies raised against squamous cell tumours are comparable with those of other squamous cell carcinomas. While occasional reports have been published of antibodies reacting with tumour tissue only, the results have not been substantiated and it still cannot be said that true tumour-specific antigens have been identified. Carcinoembryonic antigen (CEA) has been reported as present in oral cancer, when it is also detectable in serum, but it has not been described in premalignant lesions. The serum level of CEA is not, however, sufficiently specific to be of value in the diagnosis of oral cancer. Blood group antigens A and B are present on cell membranes of normal oral epithelial cells and are lost in most oral carcinomas. Benign keratotic lesions show no loss of the blood group antigens but dysplastic oral epithelium shows an increasing loss of the antigens as the degree of dysplasia increases. Interpretation of results is difficult, however, as epithelium involved in wound healing also shows a loss of the blood group antigens. Other changes in the plasma membranes of oral malignant cells which have been described include the increased release of β_2-microglobulin into the serum and a loss of receptors which bind to a plant lectin (*Ricinus communis*).

Patients with head and neck cancer show an impairment in many aspects of cell-mediated immunity. For example, they may show impaired delayed cutaneous hypersensitivity reactions particularly in advanced tumours, and the reduction appears to occur earlier in patients with carcinoma than in those with sarcoma or melanoma. The number of circulating T lymphocytes is reduced in patients with head and neck cancer, although patient survival does not correlate with the T lymphocyte count. Lymphocyte transformation *in vitro* in response to a number of antigens is reduced in patients with oral cancer. The depression in cell-mediated immunity remains depressed after surgical treatment, suggesting that there may be a primary immunological change in the patients. Consistent changes in humoral immunity are less clear but humoral responses in general appear to be relatively intact.

Both lymphocytes and plasma cells accumulate locally in oral carcinoma, T and B cells being present and many of the plasma cells staining for IgG or IgA. Histological studies have shown a correlation between the intensity of lymphocytic infiltration and the improved survival of patients. It is likely that study of the local immunocytes in oral carcinoma is more relevant to understanding the relationship between the carcinoma and the immune response than study of circulating immunocytes which may not necessarily reflect the activity of local immunocytes. Preliminary results of personal keratotic and premalignant oral mucosal lesions is unresponsive to mitogen stimulation and the addition of normal peripheral blood macrophages to the cultures of lesional immunocytes does not correct this deficiency of reactivity, indicating that functional studies of lesional immunocytes in oral cancer are needed. Studies have shown that the cervical lymph nodes are well able to mount an immune response to head and neck cancer, and are not merely passive filters of tumour emboli. The prognosis in oral cancer is improved if the regional lymph nodes show a pattern of lymphocyte predominance and an expanded paracortex and an increased number of germinal centres, indicating an active response by the nodes. The immunoreactivity in the regional cervical lymph nodes does not correlate with measures of systemic immunocompetence, once again calling into question the value of only investigating systemic immune responses in oral cancer.

CONCLUSION

The role of the immune response in the protection from or elimination of tumours remains to be defined. An attempt has been made in this chapter to review the present state of knowledge related to this complex subject. It is apparent that previous lack of progress in elucidating these problems is related less to ignorance of potential effector immune mechanisms than to our lack of understanding of the fundamental events involved in tumourigenesis. Better recognition of the features which characterize the tumour cell would allow reappraisal of the relevance of host immune mechanisms and further studies are eagerly awaited.

FURTHER READING

Binnie, W. H., Rankin, K. V. and Mackenzie, I. C. (1983). Etiology of oral squamous cell carcinoma. *J. Oral Pathol.*, **12**, 11–29

Currie, G. A. (1980). *Cancer and the Immune Response.* 2nd edn. (London: Edward Arnold)

Edwards, P. A. W. (1985). Heterogeneous expression of cell-surface antigens in normal epithelial and their tumours, revealed by monoclonal antibodies. *Br. J. Cancer*, **51**, 149–60

Eskinazi, D. P., Giuseppe, A. M., Abemayor, E., Martin, S. E. and Zighelboim, J. (1985). Monoclonal antibodies against squamous cell carcinoma. *Oral Surg., Oral Med., Oral Pathol.*, **60**, 377–81

Otter, W. D. (1985). Tumour cells do not arise frequently. *Cancer, Immunol. Immunother.*, **19**, 159–62

Perlmann, P., Troye, M. and Pape, G. R. (1977). Cell-mediated immune reactions to human tumours. *Cancer*, **40**, 448–57

Robertson, M. (1985). T-cell receptor: the present state of recognition. *Nature*, **317**, 765–71

Rosenberg, S. A., Mule, J. J., Spiess, P. J., Reichert, C. M. and Schwartz, S. L. (1985). Regression of established pulmonary metastases and subcutaneous tumour mediated by the systemic administration of high-dose recombinant interleukin 2. *J. Exp. Med.*, **161**, 1169–88

Schuller, D. E. (1984). An assessment of neck node immunoreactivity in head and neck cancer. *Laryngoscope Suppl. 35*, **94** (11), Part 2

Scully, C. (1982). The immunology of cancer of the head and neck with particular reference to oral cancer. *Oral Surg., Oral Med., Oral Pathol.*, **53**, 157–69

Scully, C. (1983). Immunology and oral cancer. *Br. J. Oral Surg.*, **21**, 136–46

Woodruff, M. F. A. (1980). *The Interaction of Cancer and Host.* (New York: Grune and Stratton)

11
Immunodeficiency

C. SCULLY and S. R. PORTER

IMMUNODEFICIENCY

Immunodeficient states have only been recognized over the past 35 years or so following the description of patients with recurrent infections by a US Army physician, Ogden Bruton, in 1952. Although immunodeficiencies seemed to be rare and of little consequence to the population at large, the appearance of the acquired immune deficiency syndrome (AIDS) has dramatically altered the picture. Primary immunodeficiencies are present from birth and are either inherited (usually in a recessive manner) or arise following chromosomal defects, or damage to the fetus *in utero* (Table 11.1). More common are secondary immunodeficiencies, caused by external agents such as drugs or infections, or by malnutrition (Table 11.2).

Table 11.1 Primary immunodeficiencies

Cell-mediated and humoral defects
Severe combined immunodeficiency (various types)
Ataxia telangiectasia
Wiskott–Aldrich syndrome

Humoral defects
X-linked agammaglobulinaemia
Common variable Immunodeficiency
Selective IgA deficiency
Selective deficiencies of other immunoglobulin isotypes

Cell-mediated defects
Di George syndrome

Complement defects
Hereditary angioedema*
Complement component deficiencies

---

*Defect of C1 esterase inhibitor

Table 11.2   Secondary (acquired) immunodeficiencies

Infections

Severe acute viral	Measles, mumps, influenza, Epstein–Barr virus
Chronic viral	HTLV III, hepatitis B
Congenital viral	Cytomegalovirus
Chronic fungal	Chronic mucocutaneous candidosis
Bacterial	Lepromatous leprosy
	Tuberculosis
	Niesserial infection
Helminthic	Schistosomal infection

Neoplasms
Hodgkin's disease
Thymoma
Chronic lymphoblastic leukaemia
Multiple myeloma
Non-lymphoid tumours

Endocrine
Insulin-dependent diabetes mellitus
Cushing's syndrome
Polyendocrinopathy syndrome(s)

Deficiency states
Malnutrition
Kwashiorkor
Iron deficiency

Autoimmune disease
Systemic lupus erythematosus
Rheumatoid arthritis
Haemolytic anaemia
Sjögren's syndrome
Chronic active hepatitis
Myasthenia gravis

Renal disease
Uraemia
Nephrotic syndrome

Miscellaneous
Severe burns
Drugs (immunosuppressants, corticosteroids)
Gastrointestinal disease (intestinal lymphangiectasia)
Sarcoidosis
High-dose irradiation (especially thoracic)
Down's syndrome

FEATURES OF IMMUNODEFICIENCY

Infection

Immunodeficiency principally manifests as an increased susceptibility to opportunistic infections (Table 11.3). The type and extent of infection depend on the type, severity and breadth of the immunodeficiency, the environment, and treatment received. Infection is more severe and involves a wider range of micro-organisms in disorders where the complete immune system is defective, such as severe combined immune deficiency syndrome, or where there is a profound defect of an immunoregulatory cell such as in AIDS.

Table 11.3 Opportunistic infections in immunodeficiency

Pneumonia, meningitis, encephalitis, sinusitis
*Pneumocystis carinii**
Aspergillosis*
Candidosis*
Cryptococcosis*
Zygomycosis*
Strongloidosis*
Toxoplasmosis*
Atypical mycobacterioses*
Neisseria spp.
Nocardia spp.
Serratia spp.
Pseudomonas
Legionella*
Klebsiella
*Pseudomonas aeruginosa**
*Staphylococcus aureus**
*Streptococcus pneumoniae**
*Haemophilus influenzae**
Echovirus
Cytomegalovirus*

Oral and oesophageal
Candidosis*
Cytomegalovirus*
Herpes simplex*
Herpes zoster*
Epstein–Barr virus*
Papilloma virus*
Histoplasmosis

Gastrointestinal
Cryptococcosis*
Giardiasis*
Isospra*

Brain
Polyoma JC virus*
*Toxoplasma gondii**
Papovavirus*

237

Table 11.3 contd.

Skin
Trichophyton spp.
Candidosis
Staphylococcus aureus
Mycosporum
Herpes simplex*
Herpes zoster*
Histoplasmosis*
Papillomavirus*

Genitourinary
Escherichia coli
Mycoplasma
Ureaplasma

Disseminated
*Mycobacterium fortuitum**
*Mycobacterium avium-intracellulare**
*Cryptococcus neoformans**
*Histoplasma capsulatum**
Cytomegalovirus*
Adenovirus*

---

*Often occur in AIDS

Neoplasms

Patients with some immunodeficiencies have an increased risk of developing various tumours, particularly of the lymphoreticular system. Possible mechanisms for this association include defective immunological surveillance, defective immunological responsiveness to oncogenic viruses or, more likely, chronic overstimulation or proliferation of lymphoid cells.

Other lesions

There tends to be a higher incidence of autoimmune disorders and atopy in immunodeficient individuals.

Acquired immune deficiency syndrome (AIDS)

This disorder, one of the most life-threatening infections to have emerged in this century, has all the hallmarks of a severe immunodeficiency disease.

AIDS is a group of disorders clinically characterized by a series of severe opportunistic infections and/or malignant neoplasms. It was first observed in a group of male homosexuals in California in 1981. The incidence of AIDS has since risen at an alarming rate so that it is now a worldwide problem. At the time of writing there have been over 15 000 reported victims in the USA and 225 in the UK.

By virtue of its principal routes of transmission (see below), AIDS has mainly been found in particular groups of patients (Table 11.4).

Table 11.4   Patient groups at risk to AIDS

Principally
Promiscuous male homosexuals/bisexuals
Intravenous drug addicts
Recipients of blood transfusions
Haemophiliacs

Also
Sexual partners of the above groups
Newborn children of the above groups
Individuals in none of the above groups, but with an ill-defined social and/or medical history

The aetiology of this disorder appears to be human T cell lymphotropic virus III (HTLV III), although other similar viruses have also been implicated (lymphadenopathy-associated viruses (LAV) and AIDS-related virus (ARV)). The virus has an RNA genome and specifically infects a subgroup of T helper cells (leu $-8+$/TQ$-1+$) important in T cell-dependent cytotoxicity, and brain cells. Infection of the lymphocyte gives rise to a profound deficiency of both cell-mediated and humoral immune systems and, interestingly, the phagocytic system also seems to be affected (Table 11.5).

Table 11.5   Immunological defects of AIDS

Principally
Lymphopenia
Reduced ratio of T helper (T4) to T suppressor (T8) cells
Reduced T cell function both *in vivo* and *in vitro*

Also
Decreased B cell activity (*in vitro*)
Hypergammaglobulinaemia
Immunoglobulin subclass abnormalities
Autoimmune phenomena
Circulating immune complexes

Reduced numbers of Langerhans cells
Reduced production and response to lymphokines
Defective monocyte chemotaxis and phagocytosis
Defective natural killer cell activity
Thymic dysplasia and altered thymic hormone levels

Raised serum levels of acid-labile interferon and B2 microglobulin

The incubation period of HTLV III is not known, but appears to range from 6 to 48 months or more. The incubation period is shortest in transfusion-associated and paediatric AIDS. Although found in most body fluids the virus is principally transmitted via blood (and blood products) and sexual intercourse (particularly anal intercourse).

Present knowledge suggests that the majority of patients infected with HTLV III remain symptom-free and thus form a large 'iceberg' of infection. About 20% of infected patients develop a prodromal illness consisting of malaise, low-grade pyrexia, weight loss, generalized lymph node enlargement, diarrhoea, and a non-productive cough. Oral candidosis is a common feature.

A minority of patients with the prodrome go on to develop one of a second type of illnesses called AIDS-related complexes (ARC). These can manifest in several forms, which include:

1.   Persistent generalized lymphadenopathy (PGL). This consists of persistent lymphadenopathy involving two or more extra-inguinal sites, in the absence of any current illness or drug likely to cause lymphadenopathy.

2.   Others develop a prolonged type of prodromal illness with a number of recurrent non-opportunistic infections, and some develop various lymphoreticular tumours.

Up to 20% of patients with ARC finally develop the features of full-blown AIDS. There is no other immunodeficiency, primary or secondary, which has such a profound clinical presentation. As can be seen from Table 11.3, AIDS victims can develop almost all of the infections and tumours that have been associated with immunodeficiency. *Pneumocystis carinii* pneumonia (PCP) and Kaposi's sarcoma are two of the most common clinical features of AIDS, though brain lymphoma and encephalopathy are becoming increasingly common. Patients usually succumb to the effects of one or more of these disorders: mortality in full-blown AIDS is almost 100%.

Up to 60% of AIDS patients have encephalopathy. This recently recognized complication of HTLV III infection has many clinical presentations such as dementia ('AIDS dementia'), depression or myelopathy. A particular worry is that many HTLV III infected patients are presenting not with the well-defined infections and tumours, but with CNS manifestations, and thus may not be diagnosed nor treated correctly.

Kaposi's sarcoma is a rare tumour of endothelial origin. Before 1981 this disorder only sporadically occurred in elderly men of Ashkenazi Jewish or Mediterranean extraction, and was also occasionally seen in immuno-suppressed patients, for example following renal transplantation (Figure 11.1). In the former group the tumours are usually of the lower extremities and rarely fatal. In AIDS (and immunocompromised patients), however, Kaposi's sarcoma produces violaceous cutaneous and/or mucosal lesions predominantly affecting the head and neck. It can be aggressive, disseminating to produce visceral lesions.

Three lines have been followed in the treatment of AIDS; namely control of opportunistic infections, eradication of tumours and restoration of the immune response.

PCP is the most common cause of death in AIDS patients and is usually treated with trimethoprim-sulphamethoxazole. If adverse drug reactions

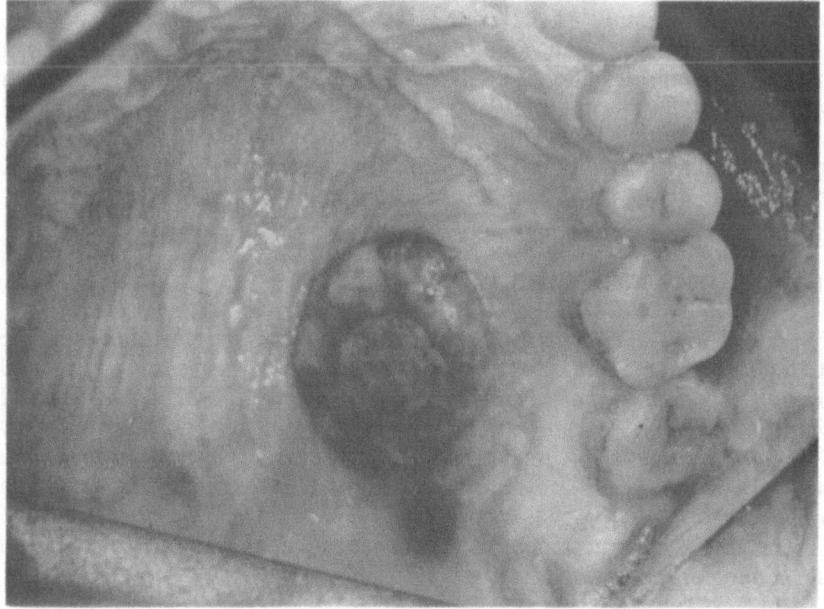

Figure 11.1   Oral Kaposi's sarcoma in an immunosuppressed patient. From, Cawson, R.A. (1986) AIDS: review. Published with the kind permission of the author and editors of the British Dental Journal

develop, or infection recurs, pentamidine isethionate or pentamidine methanesulphonate are used. Most other bacterial infections are controlled by conventional antimicrobials, but there is no effective treatment for disseminated *Mycobacterium avium-intracellulare* or cryptosporidiosis infections.

Fungal infections are treated with oral nystatin, oral ketoconazole and intravenous amphotericin. Relapses are common, and lifelong administration of ketoconazole may be the only effective treatment, although it can cause severe liver damage. Antiviral agents, in particular acyclovir, have been used both to treat opportunistic viral infections and to try and destroy HTLV III. However, although opportunistic viral infections have responded, neither AIDS nor ARC regress following this treatment.

Kaposi's sarcoma has mainly been treated with vinblastine, adriamycin or bleomycin, but none of these agents has proved uniformly successful. Radiotherapy is of some benefit in controlling severely disfiguring or painful tumours, but does not eradicate the neoplasms.

The results of immunological reconstitution have not been more favourable. Interferon, interleukin-2 and thymic hormones all produce only transient improvement in AIDS. Bone marrow transplantation is of no benefit in the treatment of AIDS, possibly because it provides HTLV III with a further group of target cells.

Attempts are now being made to reduce the viral replication with agents which inhibit RNA transcriptase, but at the date of writing the efficacy of these drugs (suramin, AL-721 and HPA-23) is unproven.

In view of the lack of any suitable treatment for AIDS, the only effective ways of reducing its incidence are likely to be by preventative measures such as testing all blood donations for HTLV III infection, heat-treating blood factors (heating to about 60 °C destroys HTLV III), and reducing sexual promiscuity and intravenous drug addiction. A vaccine against HTLV III is probably unlikely to be available until the next decade.

Head and neck manifestations of AIDS

Up to 95% of AIDS patients have head and neck manifestations (Table 11.6). The most common of these are cervical lymphadenopathy and candidal infection (Figure 11.2), both of which may present in all types of symptomatic HTLV III infection. Candidosis is severe, and often the only effective treatment is long-term ketoconazole. Herpetic infections, especially with herpes simplex and herpes zoster, are common. Aside from oral ulceration, cytomegalovirus (CMV) can cause bilateral parotitis. Adrenal gland destruction by CMV can cause hypoadrenocorticism and subsequent oral pigmentation.

Table 11.6 Head and neck manifestations of AIDS

Infections
*Candida albicans**
Herpes simplex*
Herpes zoster
Cytomegalovirus
Epstein–Barr virus
Papillomaviruses

Mycobacterioses
Histoplasmosis

Neoplasms
Kaposi's sarcoma
Squamous cell carcinoma
Lymphomata

Other
Cervical lymphadenopathy
Recurrent major oral ulceration
Parotitis
Hairy leukoplakia
Recurrent sinusitis
Addisonian pigmentation
Osteomyelitis
Rapidly progressive periodontitis
Angular cheilitis
Xerostomia

---

*These are the most common manifestations of all other secondary immunodeficiencies

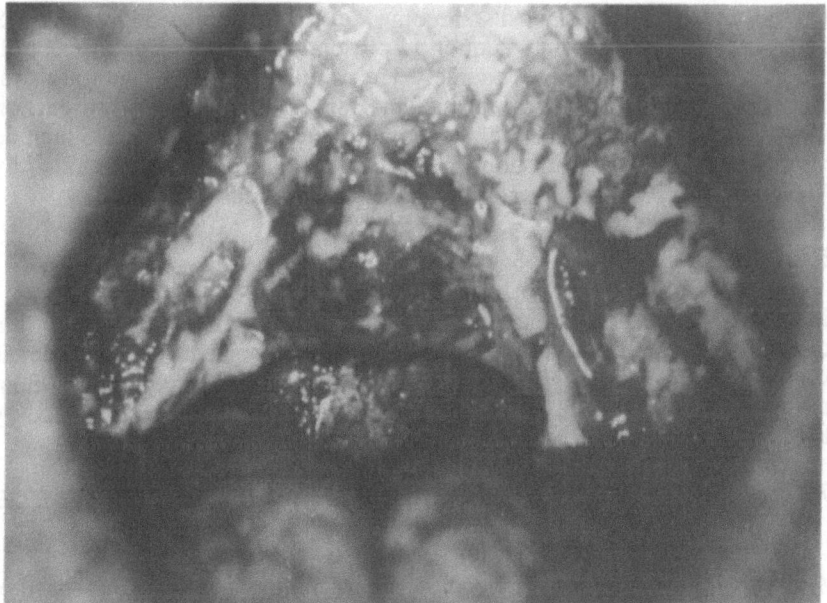

Figure 11.2 Oral candidosis in AIDS. From, Cawson, R.A. (1986) AIDS: review. Published with the kind permission of the author and editors of the British Dental Journal

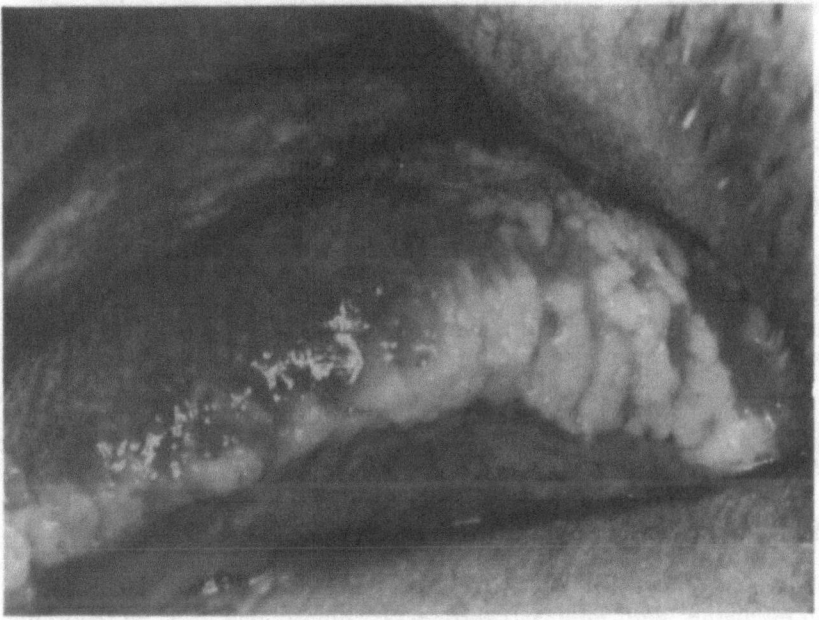

Figure 11.3 'Hairy' leukoplakia in AIDS. From, Cawson, R.A. (1986) AIDS: review. Published with the kind permission of the author and editors of the British Dental Journal

243

Oral and peri-oral Kaposi's sarcoma develop in up to 50% of AIDS patients. Kaposi's sarcoma frequently presents on the hard palate as red, blue or purple macules or nodules. Hairy leukoplakia is a unique oral feature of AIDS associated with Epstein–Barr virus and usually presents on the tongue (Figure 11.3). Other less common oral features of AIDS include rapidly progressive periodontitis, recurrent ulceration, infection by *Mycobacterium avium-intracellulare* and histoplasmosis.

Slim disease

In rural Uganda a possible variant of full-blown AIDS, known as 'Slim disease' because of marked wasting, has been reported. This disorder is similar to AIDS, although Kaposi's sarcoma occurs less frequently in Slim disease. The majority of patients with Slim disease have been infected by HTLV III.

OTHER SECONDARY (ACQUIRED) IMMUNODEFICIENCIES (TABLE 11.2)

Mild secondary immunodeficiencies are common and account for the infectious complications of many disorders; for instance oral thrush following cytotoxic therapy or the bacterial respiratory complications which may accompany severe influenza, and are much more common than primary disorders. Often the exact immunological deficiencies are not known.

PRIMARY IMMUNODEFICIENCIES

Primary immunodeficiencies are more common in males than females. The immunological defects of primary humoral immunodeficiencies, although present from birth, do not usually become clinically obvious until the levels of maternally acquired immunoglobulins have diminished. Thus the first 3 months of neonatal life may be infection-free. A classification of these disorders is shown in Table 11.1. Most of these clinical conditions are extremely rare and therefore only the more well-characterized will be discussed. Oral manifestations are summarized in Table 11.7.

PRIMARY DEFECTS OF BOTH CELL-MEDIATED AND HUMORAL IMMUNITY

Severe combined immunodeficiency (SCID)

This is a group of disorders characterized by an inability to mount normal cell-mediated and humoral responses. Inheritance can be sporadic, autosomal dominant or recessive, and consanguinity may account for up to 50% of affected cases.

There are several possible aetiologies of SCID, which include lack of

Table 11.7 Head and neck manifestations of primary immunodeficiencies

Disorder	Manifestations
Severe combined immunodeficiency	Candidosis (including CMC) Viral infections Oral ulceration Absent tonsils Recurrent sinusitis
Sex-linked agammaglobulinaemia	Cervical lymph node enlargement Oral ulceration Recurrent sinusitis Absent tonsils
Common variable immunodeficiency	Recurrent sinusitis Candidosis (including CMC)
Selective IgA deficiency	Tonsillar hyperplasia Oral ulceration Viral infections Parotitis
Di George syndrome	Abnormal facies Candidosis (including CMC) Viral infections Bifid uvula
Ataxia telangiectasia	Recurrent sinusitis Oral ulceration Facial and oral telangiectasia Cervical lymphomata Mask-like facial expression
Wiskott–Aldrich syndrome	Candidosis Viral infections Purpura
Hereditary angioedema	Swellings of face, mouth and pharynx
Chronic benign neutropenia	Oral ulceration Severe periodontitis
Cyclic neutropenia	Oral ulceration Severe periodontitis Eczematous lesions of the face
Chronic granulomatous disease	Cervical lymph node enlargement and suppuration Candidosis (including CMC) Enamel hypoplasia Acute gingivitis Oral ulceration
Myeloperoxidase deficiency	Candidosis (including CMC)
Chediak Higashi syndrome	Cervical lymph node enlargement Oral ulceration Periodontitis
Job's syndrome	Abnormal facies

adenosine deaminase or other similar enzymes, defective thymic function and absence of stem cells in the bone marrow.

The single most common feature of SCID is failure to thrive in the first 3–6 months of neonatal life. Recurrent and persistent oral candidosis, upper and lower respiratory infection, (including *Pneumocystis carinii* pneumonia), diarrhoea, malabsorption and rashes also occur. Virtually all lymphoid tissue (e.g. tonsils, Peyer's patches and thymus) is absent and lymph nodes are depleted both of T and B lymphocytes.

Bone marrow transplantation is the only effective treatment for SCID: before this treatment became available the mortality rate was 100%. Histocompatibility between donor tissue and recipient must be achieved, otherwise there is high risk of graft versus host disease occurring.

Graft versus host disease

In graft versus host disease the lymphocytes of the donor tissue mount an immunological response against the recipient of the graft. The acute disorder appears 8–20 days after transplantation and manifests as fever, haemolytic anaemia, a lichenoid rash, hepatosplenomegaly and pancytopenia leading to death. A chronic low-grade type of illness characterized by jaundice or rashes can also occur. Lichenoid lesions and a Sjögren's syndrome-like disorder are oral complications of graft versus host disease.

Wiskott–Aldrich syndrome

Wiskott–Aldrich syndrome is characterized by thrombocytopenia, susceptibility to infections and severe eczema (TIE syndrome). It is inherited as an X-linked recessive trait. Serum levels of IgA and IgE are raised while IgM is low and IgG normal. There is a progressive fall in lymphocyte numbers and function such that profound lymphopenia can become apparent by 6 years of age. Both *in vitro* and *in vivo* cell-mediated responses can be depressed. Defects of neutrophil chemotaxis have also been observed. Progressive thrombocytopenia also occurs in Wiskott–Aldrich syndrome.

Associated infections include recurrent otitis media, sinusitis and pneumonia due to *Streptococcus pneumoniae* and *Haemophilus influenzae*. Staphylococcal skin infections can be troublesome.

Both the immunodeficiency and thrombocytopenia of Wiskott–Aldrich syndrome can be corrected by bone marrow transplantation. The eczema is managed with topical corticosteroids.

PRIMARY DEFECTS OF THE HUMORAL IMMUNE SYSTEM

Sex-linked agammaglobulinaemia (Bruton's syndrome)

Bruton's syndrome is characterized by lack of all immunoglobulins, due to an intrinsic defect of B cell or plasma cell maturation. Cell-mediated immunity is normal.

Upper and lower respiratory infections, skin infections, mouth ulcers (Figure 11:4) chronic diarrhoea, meningitis, arthritis and osteomyelitis are common. Most viral infections run a benign course, but echovirus infections are not well controlled and can give rise to arthritis, hepatitis and encephalitis. Paralytic poliomyelitis following oral immunization with live vaccine is a major hazard.

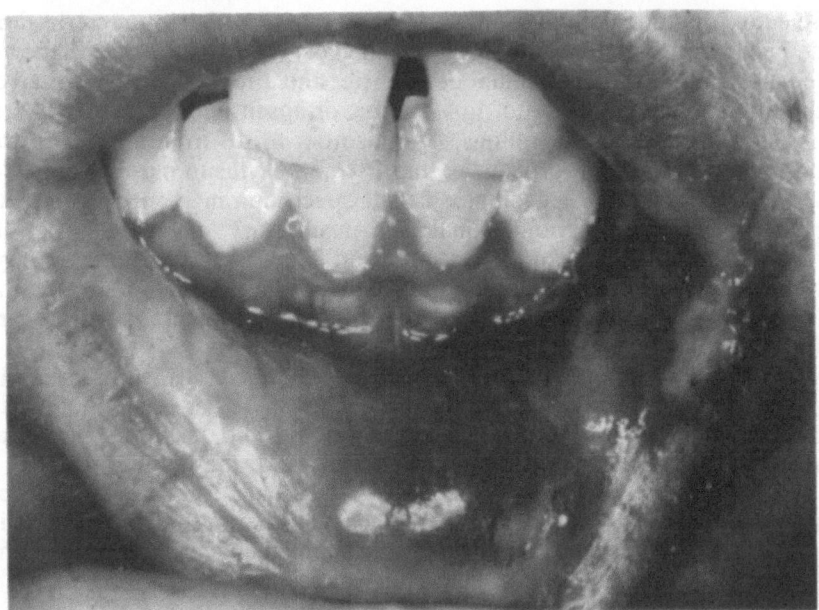

Figure 11.4 Agammaglobulinaemia (hypoimmunoglobulinaemia)

Intramuscular injections of immunoglobulins are the mainstay in the management of this disorder. These effectively replace IgG and to a lesser extent IgA and IgM. The infections in sex-linked agammaglobulinaemia can be treated by high-dose antimicrobial therapy (co-trimoxazole).

Common variable immunodeficiency (CVID)

CVID is the term given to a group of disorders in which there are reduced levels of B cells and all classes of immunoglobulins. In addition, up to a third of affected patients have low levels of T lymphocytes and reduced delayed hypersensitivity. Both sexes can be affected. Despite being a primary immunodeficiency the clinical features of CVID do not manifest until usually the third decade, when recurrent upper and lower respiratory tract infections, autoimmune disease (haemolytic anaemia, thrombocytopenia, neutropenia and pernicious anaemia), achlorhydria, malabsorption and milk allergy may occur. Patients with common variable immunodeficiencies are at particular risk of developing lymphoreticular neoplasms. This disorder is managed in the same manner as sex-linked agammaglobulin-aemia.

Selective hypogammaglobulinaemias

Selective immunoglobulinaemias are a group of disorders characterized by deficiencies of only one immunoglobulin class. Selective IgA deficiency is the most common of all immunodeficiencies and affects about one in 600 of the population. The levels of IgA are low or absent, and secretory IgA is absent from mucosal secretions. The disorder arises from a block in the normal differentiation of IgA-bearing B lymphocytes to plasma cells.

The clinical features encompass a wide spectrum ranging from complete health to severe gastrointestinal and respiratory infections. Allergic disorders, including asthma, eczema and gluten-sensitive enteropathy, frequently occur and some patients are hypersensitive to IgA in plasma infusions. Autoimmune haemolytic anaemia and rheumatoid arthritis are found with higher frequency.

Deficiencies of IgG subclasses, particularly IgG2, can also occur in patients with selective IgA deficiency: this increases susceptibility to infection, probably because most antibodies to bacteria, such as *Haemophilus influenzae* and pneumococcus are of the IgG2 subclass.

The clinical problems of selective IgA deficiency can be managed by conventional means, although IgA replacement therapy may be of value in severe cases. Hypersensitivity to the IgA supplements is a life-threatening hazard in the treatment of selective IgA deficiency.

PRIMARY IMMUNODEFICIENCY ASSOCIATED WITH CHROMOSOMAL DEFECTS

Ataxia telangiectasia

In this autosomal recessive disorder normal DNA repair mechanisms are defective such that chromosomal mutations are not corrected. Ataxia telangiectasia affects both sexes and consists of cerebellar ataxia, progressive mental defect, telangiectasia and ovarian or testicular defects. Patients with this disorder have a markedly greater risk of developing malignant tumours, particularly those of lymphoid origin.

T cell differentiation is defective, cell-mediated responses are reduced, and serum levels of IgA (and occasionally IgG and/or IgE) are reduced, while IgM levels are raised.

Patients are prone to respiratory infections including bronchiectasis. Ataxia begins when the child starts to walk, and progressively worsens. Speech is slurred and, due to muscle hypotonia and skin atrophy, the facial expression can be mask-like. Mental development ceases in about a third of affected children.

Telangiectasia appear after about 3 years of age, initially involving the bulbar conjunctivae, although later the ears, eyelids, face (butterfly rash), neck, antecubital fossae and upper thorax can be affected. Intra-oral telangiectasia can occur on the hard and soft palates. There is no effective treatment for patients with ataxia telangiectasia.

PRIMARY IMMUNODEFICIENCY ASSOCIATED WITH *IN-UTERO* DAMAGE

Di George syndrome

This rare disorder arises from the effects of either trauma or teratogenic drugs during the first trimester, such that the third and fourth branchial arches fail to differentiate correctly. This disorder is characterized by reduced cell-mediated immunity, aplasia or hypoplasia of thymic tissue, hypoparathyroidism and cardiovascular defects. Pharyngeal (and sometimes facial) deformities can also occur.

The cardiovascular deformities include Fallot's tetralogy, right-sided aorta and aortic atresia, and are the major complications of this disorder. Hypoparathyroidism results in convulsions and tetany. Oesophageal atresia and aberrant arteries about the oesophagus may cause dysphagia.

Most children succumb to the complications of the cardiovascular system or hypocalcaemia. Because of the defect in cell-mediated immunity, those who survive these problems are prone to chronic respiratory infections, viral infections and chronic candidosis. Hypertelorism, low-set notched ears, micrognathia and shortened philtrum of the lip can occur in some patients with Di George syndrome.

Fetal thymic implants can correct the immunological defect of Di George syndrome. Calcium and vitamin D supplements ensure that serum calcium levels are maintained at an adequate level.

PRIMARY IMMUNODEFICIENCIES OF THE PHAGOCYTIC SYSTEM

Phagocytosis is primarily the function of polymorphonuclear neutrophil leukocytes and macrophages. Phagocytes adhere to vascular endothelium, pass to sites of inflammation by chemotaxis and then engulf (phagocytose) and kill opsonized micro-organisms. Primary defects can arise in any of these functions (Table 11.8).

Table 11.8   Primary functional disorders of phagocytes

Defective chemotaxis
Chediak–Higashi syndrome
Job's syndrome
Schwachman syndrome
Actin dysfunction
Papillon-Lefèvre syndrome

Defective phagocytosis and/or killing
Chronic granulomatous disease
Myeloperoxidase deficiency
Glucose-6-phosphate dehydrogenase deficiency
Glutathione deficiency
Chediak–Higashi syndrome

REDUCED NUMBERS OF PHAGOCYTES

See Chapter 9.

PRIMARY DISORDERS OF PHAGOCYTIC FUNCTION

Chediak-Higashi syndrome

This rare autosomal recessive condition is often a result of consanguinity. Affected children have oculocutaneous albinism and, as a result of defective neutrophil chemotaxis and phagocytosis, recurrent bacterial infections.

The presence of unusually large lysosomal granules and a defective microtubular system prevent leukocytes from undergoing normal locomotion. Poor fusion between the lysosomal granules and phagocytic vacuoles, and a deficiency of hydrolytic enzymes, accounts for the poor bactericidal activity of the neutrophils.

Ascorbic acid may prove effective in increasing phagocyte activity.

Job's syndrome

This is an autosomal dominant condition characterized by defective neutrophil chemotaxis, raised levels of serum IgE and eosinophilia. Affected individuals suffer from recurrent bacterial infections of the skin, eyes, respiratory tract and joints. An eczematoid rash may also occur. Despite the raised levels of IgE, allergic reactions are uncommon.

Children with Job's syndrome have distinctive coarse facial features such as a broad nasal bridge, fleshy nose, macrostomia and a class III skeletal profile.

Chronic granulomatous disease

In this disorder bacterial killing by neutrophils is inadequate as there is defective production of bactericidal free oxygen radicals. Chronic granulomatous disease is mainly a disease of males, inherited in an autosomal dominant or recessive manner, each form having a different biochemical anomaly. Phagocytosis is normal, but the bacteria are not killed. Rather they are carried to the lymphoid tissue where they can give rise to suppuration and granuloma formation.

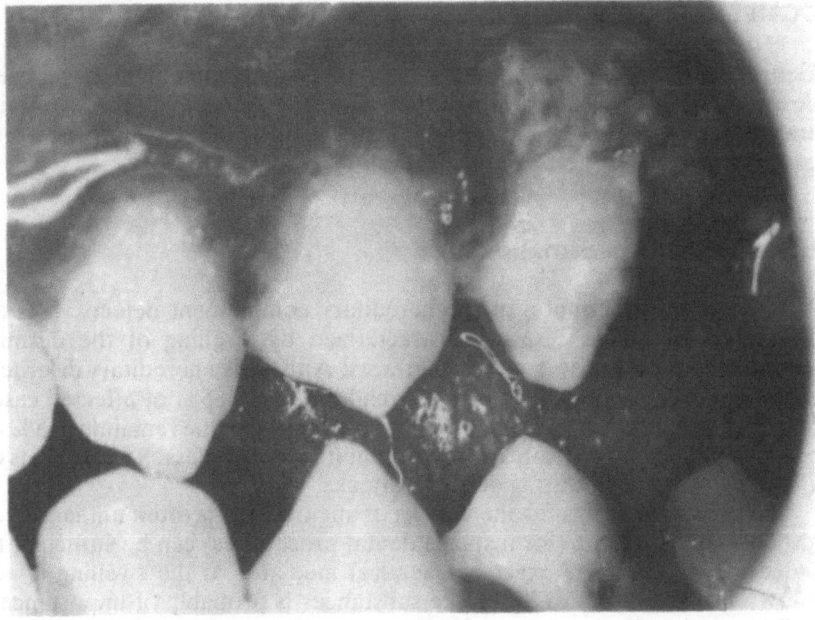

Figure 11.5 Chronic granulomatous disease

Catalase-producing micro-organisms such as *Staphylococcus aureus* are particularly troublesome in this disorder, giving rise to suppurative infections of lymph nodes, liver, bone, skin and respiratory tract.

The oral features of this disorder include enamel hypoplasia, severe acute gingivitis and recurrent candidal infections (Figure 11.5).

Prolonged treatment of infections with high doses of antibiotics is usually required. Rifampicin may be of particular benefit since it can readily penetrate cell membranes and eradicates bacteria surviving within the neutrophils. Defective killing by the neutrophils may be reversed with amantidine and chloroquine.

PERIODONTAL DISEASE AND IMMUNODEFICIENCY

While periodontal disease is not usually accentuated by defects of the cell-mediated or humoral systems, patients with neutropenias or disorders of neutrophil function (Chediak-Higashi syndrome, chronic granulomatous disease, Papillon-Lefèvre syndrome, diabetes mellitus and Down's syndrome) may suffer severe acute gingivitis and periodontal destruction. Similarly, patients with juvenile periodontitis may have defects of neutrophil chemotaxis (see Chapter 4).

COMPLEMENT DEFICIENCIES

Genetic defects of most of the components of complement have been described but are rare. These are transmitted as autosomal recessive traits and give rise to systemic lupus erythematosus-like disease and/or recurrent pyogenic bacterial (neisserial) infections.

Hereditary angioedema

This is the most common of the hereditary complement defects. It is an autosomal dominant disorder characterized by swelling of the dermis, subcutaneous tissues and mucosal surfaces. Although a hereditary disorder, it usually does not manifest until late childhood. In 85% of affected cases there is a lack of C1 esterase inhibitor (C1inh) while in the remaining 15% of patients the levels of C1inh are normal but it is functionless. Serum levels of C3 and C4 diminish during swelling attacks.

The precise stimulus for the attacks of angioedema is often unidentified, although mild trauma (for instance dental procedures) can be sufficient to induce an attack. The exact biochemical mediator of the swelling is not known but activation of kinin-like substances is probably of importance.

Commonly affected areas of swelling are the extremities, face (Figure 11.6), oesophagus and intestinal mucosa. The swelling of hereditary angioedema increases over the initial 12–18 hours, then slowly subsides over the next 48–72 hours. Abdominal pain, nausea, vomiting and a non-pruritic erythematous rash can occur. Death due to airway obstruction can be as high as 33% in some groups of untreated patients.

Attenuated androgens (such as danazol or stanozolol) or antifibrinolytic agents (aminocaproic acid or tranexamic acid) can be given as prophylaxis to control the swelling tendency. There are no regularly effective therapeutic measures for acute attacks of angioedema. Gastrointestinal and laryngeal involvement may require hospitalization, and tracheostomy or intubation may be necessary to maintain an airway.

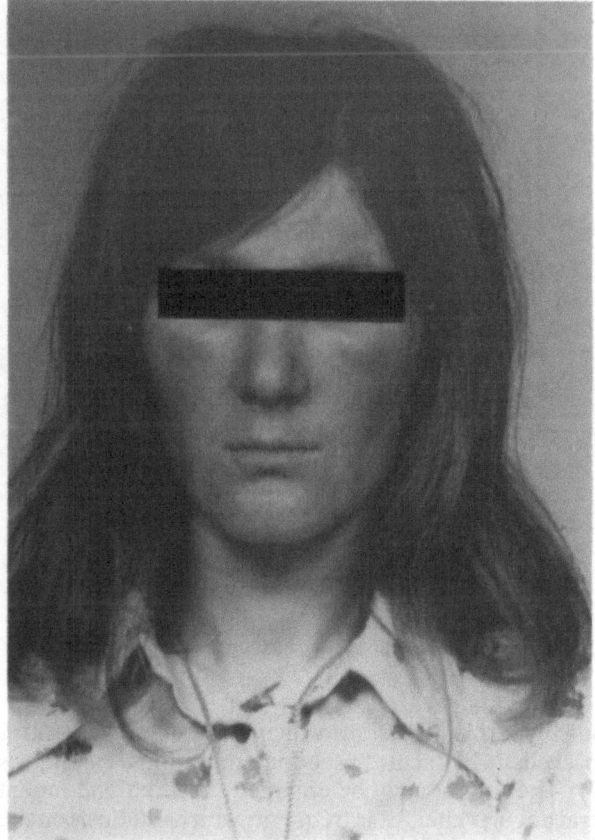

Figure 11.6 Hereditary angioedema showing infra-orbital swelling

CHRONIC MUCOCUTANEOUS CANDIDOSIS

Chronic mucocutaneous candidosis (CMC) is the term given to a group of disorders characterized by chronic candidal infection of mucosa and skin. CMC is the manifestation of a range of underlying immune defects. It is often an accompanying feature of primary immunodeficiencies, particularly defects of cell-mediated immunity, although it may also be seen in disorders of neutrophil function such as chronic granulomatous disease and myeloperoxidase deficiency. Chronic mucocutaneous candidosis is a common feature of type I multiple endocrinopathies (candidosis endocrino-pathy syndrome) and can occasionally arise in previously apparently healthy individuals (see also Chapter 5).

Patients with CMC usually have defects of cell-mediated immunity, particularly defective *in vivo* and *in vitro* responses to *Candida albicans* antigen.

The candidal infection most frequently occurs in the mouth, giving rise to

253

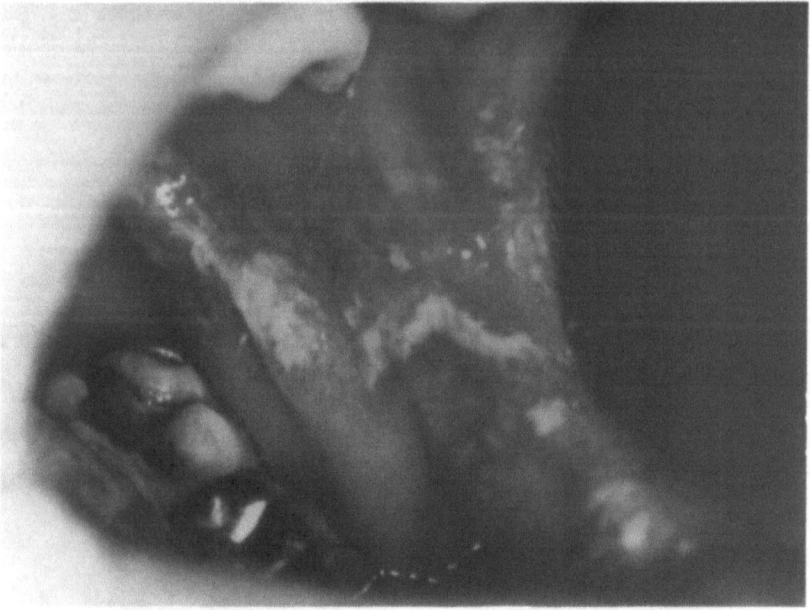

Figure 11.7   Candidal infection of chronic mucocutaneous candidosis

painful chronic hyperplastic lesions which involve any mucosal surface and are often preceded by acute pseudomembranous candidosis (thrush) (Figure 11.7). The tongue may be enlarged, fissured and indented by the teeth. Bilateral angular cheilitis is frequent; with candidosis endocrinopathy syndrome the teeth may be hypoplastic. Oesophageal involvement can cause strictures and dysphagia, while laryngeal infection may lead to hoarseness. The vulva and vagina are the other common mucosal sites of infection.

Skin lesions are usually chronic red serpiginous plaques, although granulomatous lesions may also occur. Fingernails and toenails can be affected (Figure 11.8).

The fungal infection of chronic mucocutaneous candidosis is managed by long-term antifungal agents and, not surprisingly, resistance to these drugs frequently develops. Correction of any immunological defect usually only produces a mild improvement in the clinical picture. Correction of endocrinopathies does not eradicate the severe candidal infection.

HEAD AND NECK MANIFESTATIONS
OF PRIMARY IMMUNODEFICIENCIES

These are summarized in Table 11.7. The incidence of dental caries appears in general to be no greater in patients with immunodeficiencies than the

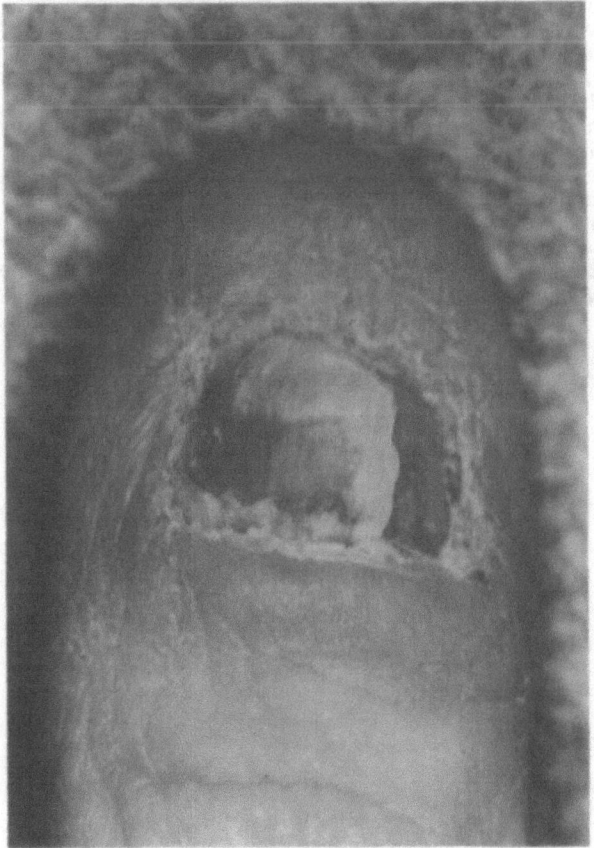

Figure 11.8 Nail involvement in chronic mucocutaneous candidosis

normal population, although some may develop rampant decay as a result of long-term use of syrup-based medicaments, while others have less oral disease as a consequence of long-term antimicrobial therapy. Tetracycline staining may occasionally be seen.

FURTHER READING

Asherson, G. L. and Webster, A. D. B. (1980). *Diagnosis and Treatment of Immunodeficiency Diseases*. (Oxford: Blackwell Scientific Publications)

Hill, H. R. (1981). Immunodeficiency diseases. *Prog. Clin. Pathol.*, **8**, 205–38

Porter, S.R. and Scully, C. (1986). Candidosis endocrinopathy syndrome. *Oral Surg.*, **61**, 573–8

Porter, S. R., Scully, C. and Cawson, R. A. (1984). Acquired immune deficiency syndrome: Update 1984. *Br. Dent. J.*, **157**, 387–91

Rosen, F. S., Cooper, M. D. and Wedgwood, J. P. (1984). The primary immunodeficiencies (Part I). *N. Engl. J. Med.*, **311**, 235–42

Rosen, F. S., Cooper, M. D. and Wedgwood, J. P. (1984). The primary immunodeficiencies (Part 2). *N. Engl. J. Med.*, **311**, 300–10

Scully, C. (1981). Orofacial manifestations in chronic granulomatous disease of childhood. *Oral Surg.*, **15**, 148–51

Scully, C. and Gilmore, G. (1986). Neutropenia and dental patients. *Br. Dent. J.*, **160**, 43–6

Scully, C., MacFadyen, E.E. and Campbell, A. (1982). Orofacial manifestations in cyclic neutropenia. *Br. J. Oral Surg.*, **20**, 96–101

Scully, C. and MacFarlane, T. W. (1983). Orofacial manifestations in childhood malignancy: clinical and microbiological findings during remission. *J. Dent. Child.*, **50**, 121–5

Scully, C. and Cawson, R. A. (1982). *Medical Problems in Dentistry.* (Bristol: Wright PSG)

Scully, C., Cawson, R. A. and Porter, S. R. (1986). AIDS – review. *Br. Dent. J.*, (In press)

Scully, C. and Lehner, T. (1980). Disorders of immunity. In Jones, J. H. and Mason, D. K. (eds.) *Oral Manifestations of Systemic Disease.* pp. 102–74. (London: Saunders)

12
Mucocutaneous Allergic Reactions

F. F. NALLY and J. J. H. GILKES

ALLERGY

General considerations

The body can protect itself against infection by certain processes collectively known as immunity. These processes occur in some form in all individuals. They may be of benefit in producing antibodies to micro-organisms or vaccines. However, immunity in its wider application also encompasses those responses to any foreign material, including foreign serum, grafts, metals, chemicals, and drugs.

During the development of immunity a harmful reaction may occur, namely allergy or hypersensitivity. Many years ago Von Pirquet introduced the term 'allergy' to describe those reactions, both immune and hypersensitive, which occurred in animals, resulting from exposure to antigens. More recently this term has been restricted to hypersensitivity states. Therefore, it can now be regarded as an altered state of reactivity of tissues to a substance, the allergen, that has been introduced to the body on a previous occasion. Occasionally, an abnormal reaction to a substance may occur in an individual who has had no previous exposure to it. No specific antibody or sensitized lymphocytes can be detected. This type of reaction is termed idiosyncrasy and is not an allergic manifestation.

Allergies could be considered as environmental diseases, although there is a marked variation in the degree of responsiveness in individuals to certain allergens, and this variation is probably genetically controlled. For example, an excess of IgE antibodies to common antigens is produced in atopic subjects. Also, there are other factors that can influence the entry of antigens into the body. These include the permeability of the skin and mucous membranes, barrier enzymes in the gastrointestinal tract, and the presence of micro-organisms which may act as adjuvants and facilitate the absorption of antigens from the site of infection.

Allergies may be either humoral (antibody) or cell-mediated. The response is highly specific for a foreign substance, the antigen, and repeated exposure usually produces an increased ability to react.

An antigen is a substance that produces humoral antibody or sensitization of certain cells. When they react in the body an observable clinical response is found. Examples of humoral reactions include anaphylaxis, angioedema, urticaria, and allergy to local anaesthetics. Contact allergy, either dermatitis or stomatitis, is a cell-mediated reaction.

Many antigenic substances can involve responses. Foreign protein, either bacterial or in food, is the classical one. However, certain substances, including drugs which are of low molecular weight, can only stimulate antibody production if they are combined with a protein. These substances are haptens and are important sensitizing agents in contact allergy. If an allergy to a drug develops, the magnitude of the reaction bears no relation to the pharmacological actions of the drug. It will also disappear after inactivation or elimination of the drug. Further exposure after a certain time interval may produce a more serious or even fatal reaction. For example, the first allergic manifestation to penicillin can be urticaria or a harmless skin rash. If this is not identified as a warning, further administration, after a period, could result in fatal anaphylaxis. A better understanding of the various mechanisms involved can be obtained by dividing them into four main types.

Types I, II, and III are subdivisions of the humoral responses in which an identifiable antibody plays a major role. In type IV, or cell-mediated reactions, it is the T lymphocyte which becomes sensitized. This classification was introduced by Gell and Coombs, who also mentioned a 'stimulatory' response, and this is sometimes included as a fifth type. It should be emphasized that a given clinical state, such as asthma or anaphylaxis, may be a manifestation of more than one type of hypersensitivity.

TYPE I – ANAPHYLACTIC REACTIONS

Type I reactions are expressions of immediate hypersensitivity which can be manifest in many organ systems in the body. The clinical features may be systemic or local and they will depend on the mode of entry of antigen into the body. It should be emphasized that the classification of type I reactions into systemic and local anaphylaxis is ill-advised, because when an individual produces a positive local response to a diagnostic skin test, he should be considered to be systemically hypersensitive. The reason for this would be evident if this same individual is given an excess of the same antigen locally or given the antigen by injection; he could develop a systemic anaphylaxis which could be fatal. Although anaphylaxis and angioedema will be described in more detail later in this chapter, they will be included here in order to compare them with the other types of hypersensitivity.

Immunological aspects of pathogenesis

If a small dose of an antigenic substance such as egg albumen is injected into an animal, there will be no obvious effect. This first injection is termed the 'sensitizing dose'. If a second injection (a 'shocking dose') is given about 2 weeks later, the animal will quickly develop the signs of generalized anaphylaxis which may be fatal. The animal has produced antibodies to the initial injection during the period between the two injections. The response is the result of an antigen–antibody reaction which releases pharmacologically active substances in many parts of the body. In the guinea pig this is particularly marked in the respiratory system, where contraction of the smooth muscles of the bronchi and bronchioles, together with capillary dilatation, will be found as the cause of respiratory distress.

The classical example of type I reaction in man is the wheal and flare on the skin, resulting from penetration of an antigenic agent. IgE immunoglobulin (reaginic antibody) in the patient's serum binds to the surface of mast cells and basophils. IgE antibody then reacts with the newly introduced antigen on the cell surface, which results in the release of pharmacological mediators. The amount and distribution of these active agents will determine the nature of the clinical response, i.e. local or general.

The Prausnitz–Kustner (PK) test in man can demonstrate this IgE-mediated mechanism. Firstly, the intracutaneous injection of the suspected allergen in the allergic patient will produce the characteristic wheal and flare. Then serum from this patient is injected intracutaneously in a normal individual to produce serum transfer of reagin antibody. Eighteen hours later a further intracutaneous injection of the suspected antigen will produce a wheal and flare, indicating a positive result. This procedure, regarded as a type of passive cutaneous anaphylaxis, is no longer routinely used because it can be potentially dangerous; among the hazards is the increasing risk of transferring serum hepatitis. Besides, total serum IgE and serum IgE antibody levels can now be estimated.

Role of pharmacological mediators

Histamine is probably one of the most important mediators of anaphylaxis. It is derived from the intracytoplasmatic granules of mast cells, basophils, platelets, and possibly other cells. Its precursor is histidine, which is in combination with heparin. The main effect of histamine is to damage vascular endothelium and cause increased capillary permeability. Clinically, erythema, urticaria, and angioedema will occur. In addition, histamine causes bronchiolar constriction and contributes to respiratory distress. There appear to be two mechanisms of histamine release. The first is the result of an antigen–antibody reaction on the surface of the mast cell, which produces dissolution and expulsion of granules from the cell. The antibody here is IgE and the reaction does not require complement. 5-hydroxytryptamine, also known as serotonin, is present as a precursor in mast cells and platelets. It is known to be a mediator of anaphylaxis in certain species and will cause increased capillary permeability and contraction of smooth muscle. It only plays a minor role in type I reactions in man.

Slow-reacting substance (SRS-A) is mainly produced in lung tissue. It does not exist as a precursor, but is generated during a type I reaction from arachidonic acid in membrane phospholipid by the lipoxygenase pathway. SRS-A has been synthesized *in vitro* and is known to cause increased capillary permeability, contraction of smooth muscle, and is not affected by antihistamines. Prostaglandins have been shown to have similar biological activities and are probably related to alteration in intracellular levels of cyclic AMP. Their precise role in type I reactions in man has yet to be determined.

Eosinophil chemostactic factor (ECF-A) exists as an acidic peptide precursor in mast cell granules. It is released in type I reactions and has a homeostatic role at the cellular biochemical level. Eosinophils are found in blood and tissues in anaphylaxis and are attracted by released histamine. They take part in detoxification in that they produce histaminase which inactivates histamine; aryl sulphatase B inhibits SRS-A, and platelet activating factor (PAF) is neutralized by phospholipase D.

The kinins have histamine-like effects on smooth muscle and capillaries. They have been demonstrated in the plasma in early anaphylaxis in many species. They are formed by the action of esterases on kallikreins. The active kinin is bradykinin, which can produce prolonged contraction of smooth muscle and is inactivated by plasma kininases. Bradykinin formation can be inhibited by C1 esterase inhibitor which is usually reduced or absent in hereditary angioedema and could account for the increased activity of the kallikrein system in this condition.

Although the release of heparin is known to contribute to anaphylaxis in dogs, its role in man is not significant.

Role of antibodies

In type I reactions, antibodies are mainly of the IgE class of immunoglobulins. They have a strong attraction for tissues and are known as reaginic or homocytotropic antibodies. They bind through their Fc region to specific receptor sites on the surface of mast cells. This Fc region of the molecule is heat-labile and therefore heating IgE antibody will destroy its ability to passively sensitize. IgE serum levels are higher than normal in patients with bronchial asthma, although the level is not directly proportional to the severity of the condition. This is probably because manufactured IgE quickly disappears from the circulation because of its autologous tissue-binding properties. IgG antibodies can also act as reagins although the extent of their contribution to the allergic state in humans is not yet resolved.

Role of antigens

There are many antigens capable of inducing type I reactions. Examples are foreign proteins such as antiserum, pollen, certain foods, insect bites, diagnostic agents and drugs. With the attached IgE antibody on its surface the exquisitely sensitive process of bridging or cross-linking adjacent IgE molecules by the specific antigen results in the release of mast cell granules. Complement is not required in this reaction. This bridging process of antibody by antigen produces a membrane signal which allows ionic calcium to enter the cell, and activates the adenyl cyclase–cyclic AMP system. It is known that expulsion of mast cell granules is enhanced by a drop in cyclic AMP or a rise in cyclic GMP. A knowledge of the effects of certain drugs on these intracellular cyclic nucleotides can help in the prevention and management of type I reactions.

TYPE II – CYTOTOXIC REACTIONS

These reactions are also 'immediate' types of hypersensitivity and many tissues in the body can be implicated. Examples of type II reactions include certain autoimmune diseases, transfusion reactions, drug-induced reactions and antibody-mediated graft rejections.

Immunological aspects of pathogenesis

This type of reaction will occur when an antigen is present on the surface of a cell, and induces the development of specific antibody. Cell death will occur either by phagocytosis by opsonic adherence, or by immune adherence through the action of C3. Cell damage may also take place through activity of the entire complement mechanism.

The antibody is usually of the IgG or IgM class. The thyroid gland is one of the most frequently involved, and leads to Hashimoto's thyroiditis. However, cell damage may not occur in hyperthyroidism where the combination of circulating antibody with fixed antigen may produce stimulation of the gland. In this case the mechanism appears to be an increase in long-acting thyroid stimulator (LATS), which is a specific IgG, and this binds to the TSH receptor in the gland, increasing its activity.

In myasthenia gravis, autoantibodies, which require complement, have been found to block neuromuscular transmission by damaging acetylcholine receptors.

In systemic lupus erythematosus, red and white cells and platelets can be destroyed by type II reactions and result in haemolytic anaemia, agranulocytosis and thrombocytopenic purpura.

Certain drugs may become attached to formed elements of blood and the resultant complex involves specific antibody productions. In this way chlorpromazine can be associated with haemolytic anaemia and quinine or amidopyrine with agranulocytosis.

TYPE III – ANTIGEN–ANTIBODY COMPLEX REACTIONS

The classical reactions of type III are serum sickness, which is the systemic form, and the Arthus reaction, the local form. Similar immunological responses occur in each.

Immunological aspects of pathogenesis

Type III reactions result from the formation of antigen–antibody complexes which are deposited in tissues and cause cell damage. A reaction may start within 3 days of introducing antigen or it can take up to 12 days to develop. The clinical result of the formation of these complexes will depend on the relative concentrations of antigen and antibody as well as their absolute amounts. Complexes will be rapidly deposited locally if there is a large amount of antibody available relative to antigen. Alternatively, if excess of antigen is present, then soluble intravascular immune complexes will be formed and will be widely distributed, causing a variety of systemic reactions.

The Arthus reaction is brought about if the antigen provokes a response at the site of introduction. The antigen will react locally with precipitating antibody and form immune complexes in the walls of blood and lymph vessels. The resultant vasculitis may last up to 24 hours. The reaction within the vessel wall activates the complement system. Anaphylatoxins will be released as split products of C3 and C5, and these will cause histamine release with vascular permeability changes. C3, C5 and C67 exert positive chemotaxis on polymorphonuclear leukocytes, attracting them to the site. They contribute to tissue damage by releasing proteolytic enzymes.

If the antigen–antibody complexes form intravascularly, they can remain in the lumen and continue to circulate. As a result, widespread distribution may gradually occur and give rise to various clinical features including fever and lymphadenopathy. Serum sickness is a good example of type III reaction. It is an adverse response after the injection of a foreign (heterologous) serum. It includes malaise, fever, skin rashes, arthralgia and lymphadenopathy. It also occurs following administration of certain drugs such as penicillin and sulphonamides. During the initial immune response there is antigen excess leading to the formation of soluble antigen–antibody complexes which diffuse into the tissues, activate complement and initiate the inflammatory response. As antibody titres rise, insoluble complexes are formed which are quickly cleared by the reticuloendothelial system. Other examples of conditions associated with immune complex deposition in tissues include some forms of disseminated malignancy, systemic lupus erythematosus, Hashimoto's thyroiditis, rheumatoid arthritis, coeliac disease and ulcerative colitis. Many cases of glomerulonephritis are due to complexes.

TYPE IV – DELAYED HYPERSENSITIVITY REACTIONS

This type is found in many hypersensitivity reactions to viruses, bacteria, and fungi; in reactions to simple chemicals; in the process of rejection of transplanted tissue; and probably include defence mechanisms against some neoplasias. Therefore defence and allergic reactions are closely associated.

Immunological aspects of pathogenesis

Type IV reactions are not uncommon; they do not depend on circulating antibody, and take up to 48 hours or more to reach a maximum response. The underlying mechanism is the combination of antigen with the T lymphocyte and therefore cell-mediated responses, or delayed hypersensitivity, are appropriate terms. The classical example of this reaction is the tuberculin test. This can be demonstrated in a sensitized individual by the intradermal injection of the tuberculin antigen. The local response, which is usually indurated and erythematous, will become gradually apparent after a latent period. The time taken to reach peak intensity will depend on (a) the degree of sensitivity, (b) the amount of antigen, (c) the nature of the antigen, and (d) the species. In man it may be as long as 72 hours. The lesion can be partially or completely prevented by corticosteroids, but not with antihistamines. The site of injection shows a gradual perivascular infiltration of lymphocytes and macrophages with the release of a number of soluble factors or cytokines with tissue destruction potential.

Delayed hypersensitivity can only be transferred passively by using specifically sensitized T lymphocytes. Serum from patients is insufficient because type IV reactions are not mediated by humoral antibodies.

Type IV delayed sensitivity reactions can be produced by a wide variety of antigens, including fungi, bacteria, some viruses and foreign proteins. Examples are the cavitation and caseation found in tuberculosis, the granulomatous skin lesion in leprosy, the skin rashes in measles, smallpox and herpes simplex infections. Drugs are also important sensitizers and this fact not only applies to patients, but is an occupational hazard in medical and dental personnel. Examples of chemicals which can induce type IV sensitivity are: preservatives such as p-aminobenzoic acid, formalin, cetrimide, methylmethacrylate, and rubber gloves. Mercury sensitivity is particularly important in dentistry. The drug or chemical, acting as a hapten, probably combines with a protein on the surface of an epithelial cell, making it antigenic.

ANAPHYLAXIS

General considerations

Anaphylaxis is usually regarded as a state of systemic hypersensitivity or type I allergy. Simultaneous and rapid involvement of many organs occurs most commonly after exposure to a drug, insect bite, or food. Some of these allergies may be fatal. Respiratory obstruction or vascular collapse are the most common cause of death.

Immunological aspects of pathogenesis

Anaphylaxis is caused by the antigen reacting mainly with IgE antibody, although occasionally reaginic antibodies can be detected in the IgG range of immunoglobulins. The reaction releases tissue-damaging chemicals including histamine, 5-hydroxytryptamine (serotonin), slow-reacting substance (SRS-A) mainly in the lungs, bradykinin, kallidin, and prostaglandin E. Vasodilatation, increased capillary permeability, and constriction of smooth muscle caused by these chemicals account for most of the clinical features.

Systemic manifestations

Systemic anaphylaxis is an allergic emergency which can occur within minutes of exposure to an allergen. It can quickly follow insect bites, injection of serum, drugs, anaesthetics, radiological contrast media, or specific skin tests.

Clinical manifestations can involve four main systems; namely the respiratory, gastrointestinal, cardiovascular, the skin and mucosa. The first sign is often seen in the skin as angioedema, urticaria, and erythema. Respiratory distress from bronchospasm or oedema of the larynx can quickly follow and prove fatal.

Intestinal cramps, vomiting, and diarrhoea often follow the skin manifestations. If untreated, a rapid fall in blood pressure can occur due to vasodilation mainly in the mesenteric vessels, and death results from circulatory collapse or shock.

It is worth remembering that even though the clinical manifestations occur within minutes, they usually subside in a few hours, provided death does not occur from shock or laryngeal obstruction. Cell damage is usually transient and most cells recover.

Orofacial manifestations

Angioedema of the lips, face, and in the mouth may occur in anaphylaxis. Also pruritis, erythema, and urticaria can occur. Itching of the nose and palate, and nasal congestion with considerable rhinorrhoea similar to acute hay fever, may occur initially. This is followed by rapid swelling of the mucosa in the soft palate, pharynx, and larynx causing respiratory obstruction.

Such conditions as vasovagal syncope, especially after local anaesthetic injections, cardiac, hypovolaemic and neurological shock and mechanical

264

obstruction in the respiratory tract should be considered in the differential diagnosis.

Immunological diagnosis

A history of previous reactions to food, drugs, chemicals or insect bites should alert the clinician. An immediate positive skin or nasal mucosal test probably confirms the diagnosis. However, a negative result to the specific allergen does not exclude hypersensitivity. If a skin patch test is negative, it should be followed by serial dilution intradermal injections. This procedure should only be done if all the facilities for dealing with an anaphylactic attack are immediately available. The total serum IgE and serum IgE antibody levels can also be estimated (see atopic eczema).

ANGIOEDEMA

General considerations

The acquired type of angioedema is one form of local anaphylaxis which is of considerable importance in dentistry. A painless swelling occurs rapidly under normal-looking skin. The lips, tongue, face, eyelids, or nasopharynx are common sites of involvement. Rarely laryngeal oedema can occur although this is more likely to be found in the hereditary form of the disease (see Chapter 11). Urticaria and angioedema may occur simultaneously.

Immunological aspects of pathogenesis

Acquired angioedema results from IgE–antigen interactions which damage deep subcutaneous and submucosal blood vessels, mainly in the head and neck. This results in degranulation of mast cells with the release of histamine. IgG or IgM antibody complexed to antigen may activate the classical complement pathway, generating anaphylatoxins which can stimulate mast cells for histamine release. Histamine release may also occur after trauma, severe physical exercise, heat, or sunlight. Aspirin and the non-steroid anti-inflammatory drugs may be associated with angioedema through the action of lipo-oxygenase-derived metabolites of arachidonic acid called leukotrienes. Hypersensitivity, physical trauma such as cold, heat, exercise, or water, underlying disease, and psychogenic factors have been implicated in angioedema.

Immunological diagnosis

As in general anaphylaxis a relevant history is essential. Elimination diets and selected challenges are useful in suspect food allergies. Skin or mucosal tests are sometimes helpful in drug-induced angioedema.

ECZEMA

Atopic eczema

General considerations

Atopy is a term given by Coca in 1923 to a genetically determined disorder in which there is an increased susceptibility to asthma, hay fever, and eczema. Although many individuals with atopic disease have transferable (IgE) reagin antibodies which can be detected by the Prausnitz–Kustner (PK) test, this is by no means a universal finding. The cause of atopic eczema still remains unknown, and there are many factors responsible for its onset. It can no longer be considered to be due to a single antibody–antigen reaction. The incidence of atopic disease in the population is over 15%.

Immunological aspects

The serum concentrations of IgE in 80% of patients with atopic eczema are higher than those of normal persons. If eczema is the only manifestation of atopy the amounts of IgE are only slightly raised, but if there is also asthma and hay fever, the levels are very much higher. The levels of IgE rise with the severity of the disease, and those with the highest levels have the worst prognosis. More eosinophils are found in the blood of patients with atopic eczema than in normal persons, and eosinophilia tends to be related to the amount of IgE. It has also been shown that about 20% of the lymphocytes have IgE bound to their membranes, instead of around 2% found in the normal population.

There is a tendency for delayed hypersensitivity responses to be decreased in incidence and magnitude. It is generally agreed that the total number of lymphocytes in the blood is slightly less than normal and that the proportion of T lymphocytes is decreased. The total number and the proportion of B lymphocytes is sometimes increased.

Systemic and oral manifestations

Atopic eczema can present at any age, and is characterized by the presence of an erythematous scaling eruption which may also exhibit vesicles and crusting. The diagnosis is usually easy from the history and clinical examination. Atopic eczema does not affect the oral mucosa, and in infancy the facial eruption characteristically spares the skin around the mouth. The importance of atopic eczema to the dentist is to appreciate that these patients are more likely to develop anaphylactic reactions to drugs. These reactions are more common in atopic persons because of their increased liability to produce reagins on exposure to antigens. Patients with atopic eczema, both active and quiescent, are liable to develop generalized infections, particularly with the virus of herpes simplex eruption.

266

Laboratory tests are rarely employed in the assessment of atopic eczema. The total serum IgE can be measured by the paper disc radioimmunoassay technique (PRIST). The method to assay IgE antibodies to a specific antigen is the radio-allergosorbent test (RAST). Strongly positive RASTs are most commonly obtained with grass pollen, dust mite, and cat hair. Egg and milk IgE antibodies are only found in about 12% of atopic subjects. The RAST test correlates well with the skin prick tests to the same allergens, but their relevance to the atopic subject is variable and not always of clinical importance.

Contact eczema

General considerations

The oral mucosa, like the skin, is subject to two types of local reaction: primary irritation and contact sensitivity. Primary irritant eczema denotes an inflammatory reaction produced by a noxious substance such as an acid or solvent. The oral mucosa is more resistant to primary irritants and caustics than the skin, because of the saliva which constantly bathes it. Chemical injuries, however, can occur from the acetyl salicylic acid (aspirin) after being held near a painful tooth; also the prolonged use of hydrogen peroxide mouthwash may also produce painful superficial erosions of the oral mucosa.

Allergic contact eczema is a reaction in response to a foreign antigen producing local inflammatory changes resulting in damage to the skin or oral mucosa. The oral mucosa is less prone to allergic eczema than the skin for the following reasons:

1. Saliva dilutes and removes potential allergens.
2. The time of contact is usually brief, with the exception of dentures.
3. Protein conjugates to which haptens bind are found predominantly in the stratum corneum; with the exception of the gums and hard palate there is no horny layer in the mouth.
4. The good blood supply and rapid absorption of water-soluble allergens again prevent prolonged contact with the mucosa.

Immunological aspects

Contact hypersensitivity reactions are the protopye of cell-mediated immune responses in clinical immunology and allergy. The local responses affecting the skin and mucous membranes are called allergic contact dermatitis and are a form of delayed-type hypersensitivity. The essence of contact sensitivity reactions is that low molecular weight environmental chemicals (haptens), such as chromate salts, come in contact with the skin or mucous membranes, and combine with cutaneous macromolecules to constitute an immunogenic hapten–carrier complex. This leads to the

267

sensitization of T cells. Upon rechallenge or continuous contact, sensitized T cells react with the complex composed of haptenic sensitizer and macromolecules. This leads to a delayed local inflammatory response that constitutes a contact eczema.

Systemic and oral manifestations

For the reasons we have already mentioned, the oral mucosa is less prone to contact hypersensitivity reactions than the skin. A contact allergic reaction in the mouth is often difficult to diagnose. There may be little in the way of erythema, and the patient may only complain of loss of taste, numbness or a soreness in the involved area. Sometimes the lingual papillae disappear. The mucous membrane reactions range from barely visible erythema, to an angry reaction with oedema. Vesicles are not common, as they quickly rupture to form erosions. In reactions to denture base materials or fixatives there is often a sharp dividing line between the affected and normal mucosa; however, irritation from an ill-fitting denture can produce a similar picture. Allergic stomatitis is often accompanied by cheilitis, and the reaction sometimes spreads to the surrounding circumoral skin, especially with reactions produced by ingredients of certain toothpastes. Occasionally a substance to which the patient is sensitized, when placed in the mouth, will produce an eczematous reaction on other parts of the body.

Mercury

Reports of sensitization to metallic mercury are rare. Amalgam dental fillings are an alloy of mercury with other metallic powders, usually silver and tin and copper. Once the amalgam fillings have been inserted there is no significant release of mercury. There are no reports of allergic stomatitis produced from amalgam fillings. However, contamination with free mercury is possible during the insertion of the filling, causing transient problems on the oral mucosa of someone who is sensitive to mercury. There have also been reports of generalized urticaria and flare-up of eczematous sites in patients who are allergic to mercury. It is more controversial as to whether trace amounts from the fitted amalgam fillings are capable of aggravating atopic eczema, or causing a wide variety of illnesses, such as weakness, headaches, and instability.

Sensitivity to mercury is usually acquired from organic or inorganic salts. The organic salts such as phenylmercuric acetate are found in herbicides, fungicides, antiseptics, in contraceptives, and as a preservative. The inorganic salts, such as mercuric chloride, were at one time used in ointments, and as an antiseptic. It is a potent sensitizer and is no longer used. There is a cross-over sensitivity between the metallic mercury and the salts. Sensitivity can be tested by patch testing. The patch tests are applied to the skin on the back (mercury trichloride 0.05%) and left in position for 48 hours. It is then removed and the site examined. A positive reaction is shown by erythema and possibly a vesicular eruption. If there is no reaction at 48 hours, the site should again be examined at 72 hours, before a negative reaction is recorded.

Nickel

Nickel is a potent sensitizer and allergic contact stomatitis and cheilitis can occur from nickel-plated instruments used in dental procedures. Many nickel-sensitive patients have acquired allergic stomatitis and cheilitis by holding nickel-plated objects, such as needles, pins, and metal lipstick holders, between the lips. Metallic chromium is not a sensitizer and in chromium nickel dentures it is the nickel which is responsible for any allergic reaction as it penetrates the micropores in the chrome-plated objects.

Essential oils

In dentistry, essential oils are chiefly used as pharmaceutical aids, as mild antiseptics, and as flavourings for toothpastes. The essential oils, particularly clove oil and cinnamon oil, may cross-react with balsam of Peru, which is used in dental cement liquids. Eugenol is the main constituent of clove oil, oil of carnation, pimento oil, and oil of bay. Eugenol is used in periodontal dressings, zinc oxide cement and impression pastes. These substances have been identified as causing allergic stomatitis and cheilitis.

Acrylic denture materials

Acrylic plastics are used in the manufacture of dental plates. The most commonly used plastic is methyl methacrylate. The acrylic monomer usually contains an inhibitor, or stabilizer, such as hydroquinine, while the polymer contains an inhibitor such as benzoyl peroxide. When the monomer and polymer are mixed in the cold, the benzoyl peroxide initiates the reaction and a hard, solid, high molecular weight polymer is formed. The mixture can also be heat-cured when no inhibitor is required. In the heat process the reaction is complete, but after cold cure small amounts of monomer will probably be left unpolymerized. This residual monomer can induce stomatitis and angular cheilitis in the sensitized individual.

Impression material – Dental impression material is more likely to cause a contact eczema to the hands of the dentist who mixed the material than to the patient who is having an impression taken. The sensitivity is usually due to the catalysts methyldichlorobenzene sulphonate and methyl-*p*-toluol-sulphonate in Impregum and Scutan.

Toothpastes

Most powder and paste toothpastes contain flavouring, colouring agents, abrasives, and soaps. In addition they contain glycerine from propylene glycol, antiseptics, preservatives, fluorides, and ammonium compounds. They are capable of causing stomatitis and cheilitis. Care should be taken when patch testing with the toothpaste as it may cause skin irritation; it is therefore preferable to ascertain the specific sensitizing ingredient.

Patch testing

The method of investigating a contact hypersensitivity reaction is by patch testing. The suspected sensitizing agents should be made up in a petroleum base at a concentration that does not cause irritation of the skin. It is then applied in a small non-sensitizing aluminium cup to the skin on the back, and left under occlusion for 48 hours. The patches are then removed and the site inspected again after a further 48 hours. A positive reaction is shown by an erythematous reaction, which can become vesicular. Attempts have been made to patch test the mucosa itself by incorporating suspected agents in orabase and applying to the inner side of the lip, but it is difficult to maintain contact with the mucosa for more than a few hours.

FIXED DRUG ERUPTIONS

Fixed drug eruptions appear as round, or oval, erythematous plaques with or without vesicles. Lesions recur in the identical area following each administration of the responsible drug, may be single or multiple and may increase in size and number with each administration of the drug, some lesions often becoming bullous. The lesions may occur anywhere on the skin and mucous membrane but are most common on the palms, soles, glans penis and lips. They are typically dark red or violet but can become pigmented. The lesions are often only slightly pruritic and there are few or no constitutional symptoms. Although the erythematous lesion may fade in a few days, those that become pigmented may last months or years. Hyperpigmentation is most common in the Negro, in whom there may well be diffuse hypermelanosis of extensive areas of trunk, face and limbs. The genital and oral lesions may be involved in association with skin lesions or alone.

The number of drugs capable of producing fixed drug eruptions is very large. Cross-sensitivity to related drugs may occur and there are occasional reports of recurrence induced by drugs which appear to be chemically unrelated. Sometimes the inducing drug can be administered without exacerbation. Well over 50 drugs and food additives have been reported to cause fixed eruptions. The drugs most commonly responsible are listed in Table 12.1.

Table 12.1 Drugs causing a fixed drug reaction

Phenazone (Antipyrine)	Quinine
Phenolphthalein	Tetracycline
Barbiturates	Phenacetin
Sulphonamides	Oxyphenbutazone
Dapsone	Chlordiazepoxide

Immunological aspects

Fixed drug eruption can be caused by drug allergy, but little is known of the mechanism. The most likely possibility is circumscribed cell-mediated hypersensitivity, and some eruptions have occurred after systemic drug administration at sites of previous contact eczema. Experiments with epidermal transplants suggest that the epidermis is not the primary site of the reaction.

A serum factor has been reported to appear during the acute phase of the eruption that has skin-reactive and/or autologous lymphocytic mitogenic activity, the latter being enhanced if the drug is added. The application of the suspected drug to the site of the healed fixed drug eruption often leads to a false positive reaction because the site may remain irritable for several weeks. If this method of proving the cause of a fixed drug eruption is used, unrelated drugs should first be applied as controls.

A challenge dose of the suspected drug, usually at the therapeutic dose, is normally given to confirm the diagnosis if the patient is on several drugs.

The appearance of the skin or mucosal lesions are usually characteristic, although a biopsy is sometimes taken to help confirm the diagnosis. Fixed drug eruptions are characterized histologically by a papillary–dermal mononuclear cell infiltrate that hugs the dermoepidermal junction. Extensive basal cell degeneration can lead to bullae formation as well as pigmentary incontinence.

ERYTHEMA MULTIFORME

General considerations

Erythema multiforme is a heterogeneous clinical syndrome due to a wide variety of provoking factors (Table 12.2). The variety of erythema multiforme (EM) which comes closest to Hebra's description in 1866 is herpes-associated erythema multiforme (HEM). This occurs largely in young healthy adults, has an acral distribution, and is characterized by mucosal lesions. The whole episode lasts about 3 weeks, and follows a herpes simplex infection. The other main subdivision which can often be distinguished by clinical presentation, histological and immunofluorescent changes is sulphonamide-associated erythema multiforme (SEM). This is not a recurrent illness and tends to be more severe, with larger and more widespread blisters and more severe mucosal involvement.

Cases of EM have also been subclassified clinically into EM minor, where there may be cutaneous lesions only or with cutaneous lesions plus involvement of a single mucosal surface, usually the mouth. If the skin together with at least two mucosal surfaces was involved a diagnosis of EM major (Stevens–Johnson syndrome) was made.

Table 12.2 Some of the causes of erythema multiforme

Viruses	**Endocrine factors**
Herpes simplex	Menstruation
Adenoviruses	Pregnancy
Infectious mononucleosis	
Coxsackie B$_5$	**Drugs**
Mycoplasma pneumoniae	Penicillin
	Sulphonamides
Bacteria	Barbiturates
Syphilis	Anticonvulsants (hydantoins)
BCG vaccination	Tetracycline
Gonorrhoea	
Staphylococcus	**Neoplasm**
Vincent's disease	Leukaemia
	Internal carcinoma
Physical factors	Lymphoma
Sunlight	Polycythaemia
Cold	
X-ray therapy	**Collagen disorders**
	Dermatomyositis
Fungi	Lupus erythematosus
Coccidiodomycosis	Polyarteritis nodosa
Dermatophytosis	Rheumatoid arthritis
Histoplasmosis	

Immunological and histological aspects

The pathogenesis of EM is unknown, but histological and immuno-fluorescent studies give some ideas. Biopsy of a target lesion shows subepidermal separation at the centre of the lesion with necrosis of the keratinocytes in the overlying epidermis. The dermal changes consist of papillary dermal oedema, vascular dilation and a perivascular mononuclear cell infiltrate.

Keratinocyte injury is more severe in SEM while spongiosis, exocytosis of inflammatory cells, liquefactive degeneration of basal zone, and leuko-cytosis is more common in HEM. Mononuclear inflammatory cells found in association with individually necrotic keratinocytes, similar to those observed in graft versus host disease, are also more common in HEM, while scattered necrotic keratinocytes, extensive epithelial necrosis or a confluent zone of basal cell necrosis prevail in SEM.

Direct immunofluorescent studies have demonstrated C3 and less commonly IgM in a granular pattern at the dermoepidermal junction. The most common location is in an area of epithelial damage but underlying a relatively intact epithelium. C3 and IgM are also found in a granular distribution around superficial dermal blood vessels. Fibrin is found in a bandlike distribution at the dermoepidermal junction in regions of necrosis or blister formation.

The mononuclear infiltrate and histological absence of vasculitis would argue against EM representing an immune complex-mediated damage. It would appear that important immunological events affect the epithelium, and it has been proposed by some authors that in EM, foreign antigens sequestered within the epithelium are an immune stimulus, and that specific cytotoxic mechanisms are involved in the epidermal cell damage.

Systemic and oral manifestations

EM is usually an acute self-limiting inflammatory disorder of the skin and mucous membranes, characterized by distinctive iris or target lesions.

These lesions are dull red, flat maculopapules which may remain small or may increase in size centrifugally to reach a diameter of 1–2 cm in 48 hours. The periphery remains red and the centre becomes cyanotic or even purpuric. The lesions appear in successive crops at intervals for a few days and fade in a few weeks. The extent is variable – classically the backs of the hands, palms, wrists, forearms, feet, elbows and knees are affected; less commonly the face, neck and trunk. Sometimes only the hands are involved. There is often blistering of the mucous membrane on the lips and buccal mucosa. In the vesiculo-bullous form many of the skin lesions will blister and the oral mucosa will be more severely involved.

The severe bullous form (Stevens–Johnson syndrome) produces a severe and characteristic illness. There may be a prodromal illness for a few days although the onset is usually sudden. The oral mucous membrane shows extensive bulla formation followed by erosions and a greyish-white membrane leading to characteristic crusting of the mouth and lips. The eye changes are often limited to severe catarrhal or purulent conjunctivitis but bulla formation can occur. The changes can regress but blindness, corneal opacities and synechiae are possible sequelae. Genital lesions are frequent. The skin lesions are variable in extent but often widespread and bullous. There are marked constitutional symptoms associated with fever. There is a pneumonitis in about 20% of patients but the radiological changes within the lungs are often greater than the symptoms. Renal involvement with haematuria or even renal tubular necrosis has been reported, and may lead to progressive renal failure.

The aetiology is unknown but many different agents and diseases have been known to precipitate an attack of EM. In over half the cases, however, no provocative factor can be found. There are also a small group of patients who present with attacks of blistering, erosions and crusting of the mucous membrane who never develop the characteristic target lesions on the skin. The diagnosis of EM in these patients is therefore difficult to confirm.

273

Laboratory tests

The diagnosis of EM is usually straightforward and can be made clinically from the characteristic skin lesions. Patients who only have lesions in the mouth should have a biopsy taken of an early lesion, but often the changes are non-specific inflammatory changes and although compatible with, are not often diagnostic of, EM. Electron microscopy shows that the damaged basement nembrane remains in the floor of the bulla.

Immunofluorescent studies on a biopsy will be negative for IgA, IgG or C3 on the basement membrane zone (BMZ) and indirect IMF will detect no circulating antibodies to the BMZ. C3 and IgM may be seen in a granular pattern around the vessels in the dermis and beneath the damaged intact epithelium.

FURTHER READING

Askenase, P. W. (1983). Contact hypersensitivity reactions. In Kerr, J. W. (ed.) *International Congress of Allergology and Clinical Immunology*. pp. 109–20. (London: Macmillan)

Champion, R. H. and Parish, W. E. (1979). Atopic dermatitis. In Rook, A., Wilkinson, D. and Ebling, F. (eds) *Textbook of Dermatology*. pp. 349–61. (Oxford: Blackwell Scientific Publications)

Eyre, J. and Nally, F. F. (1971). Nasal test for hypersensitivity. Including a positive reaction to lignocaine. *Lancet*, **1**, 264–5

Fisher, A. A. (1973). Contact reactions of mucous membranes. In Fisher, A. A. (ed.) *Contact Dermatitis*. pp. 307–35. (Philadelphia: Lea and Febiger)

Howland, W. W., Golitz, L. E., Weston, W. W. and Huff, J. C. (1984). Erythema multiforme, clinical, histopathologic and immunologic study. *J. Am. Acad. Dermatol.*, **10**, 438–46

Kauppinen, K. and Stubb, S. (1985). Fixed eruptions: causative drugs and challenge tests. *Br. J. Dermatol.*, **112**, 575–8

Nally, F. F. and Storrs, J. (1973). Hypersensitivity to a dental impression material. *Br. Dent. J.*, **134**, 244–6

Roitt, I. M. and Lehner, T. (eds) (1980). *Immunology of Oral Diseases*. (Oxford: Blackwell Scientific Publications)

Stites, D. F., Stobo, J. D., Fudenberg, H. H. and Wells, J. V. (1982). *Basic and Clinical Immunology*. 4th edn. (Los Altos, California: Lange Medical Publications)

Index